Coronavirus and Vulnerable People

Addressing the Divide in Harm and Responses and Exploring Implications for a More Peaceful World

A Volume in Peace Education

Peace Education

Laura L. Finley and Robin Cooper, Series Editors

Coronavirus and Vulnerable People: Addressing the Divide in Harm and Responses and Exploring Implications for a More Peaceful World (2022)
edited by Laura L. Finley and Pamela D. Hall

Lessons for Creating a Culture of Character and Peace in Your Classroom (2022)
by Edward F. DeRoche, CJ Moloney, and Patricia J. McGinty

The New Peace Linguistics and the Role of Language in Conflict (2022)
by Andy Curtis

Humanities Perspectives in Peace Education: Re-Engaging the Heart of Peace Studies (2021)
edited by Nicole L. Johnson

Peace is Everyone's Business (2021)
edited by Lowell Ewert and Frederick Bird

Experiential Learning in Higher Education: Issues, Ideas, and Challenges for Promoting Peace and Justice (2021)
edited by Laura L. Finley and Glenn A. Bowen

Difficult Discussions: Issues and Ideas for Engaging College Students in Peace and Justice Topics (2020)
edited by Laura L. Finley and Robin Cooper

The United Nations and Higher Education: Peacebuilding, Social Justice and Global Cooperation for the 21st Century (2020)
by Kevin Kester

Gender, Sexuality and Peace Education: Issues and Perspectives in Higher Education (2018)
by Laura L. Finley and Robin Cooper

Sustainable Peace in the Twenty-First Century: Bridging the Gap from Theory to Practice (2017)
by Dilip Vasudeo Kulkarni

Peace Jobs: A Student's Guide to Starting a Career Working for Peace (2016)
by David J. Smith

Peace Education Evaluation: Learning from Experience and Exploring Prospects (2015)
edited by Celina Del Felice, Aaron Karako, and Andria Wisler

(Book series titles continued on next page)

Teaching Peace Through Popular Culture (2015)
edited by Laura L. Finley, Joanie Connors, and Barbara Wien

Peace and Conflict Studies Research: A Qualitative Perspective (2014)
edited by Robin Cooper and Laura Finley

Understanding Peace Cultures (2014)
edited by Rebecca L. Oxford

Peace Education from the Grassroots (2013)
edited by Ian Harris

The Language of Peace: Communicating to Create Harmony (2013)
edited by Rebecca L. Oxford

More Than a Curriculum: Education for Peace and Development (2013)
edited by Johan Galtung and S. P. Udayakumar

More than a Curriculum: Education for Peace and Development (2013)
edited by Johan Galtung and S. P. Udayakumar

Think, Care, Act: Teaching for a Peaceful Future (2011)
by Susan Gelber Cannon

Building a Peaceful Society: Creative Integration of Peace Education (2011)
by Laura L. Finley

Books, Not Bombs: Teaching Peace Since the Dawn of the Republic (2010)
by Charles F. Howlett and Ian Harris

Spirituality, Religion, and Peace Education (2010)
edited by Edward J. Brantmeier, Jing Lin, and John Miller

For the People: A Documentary History of The Struggle for
Peace and Justice in the United States (2009)
by Charles F. Howlett and Robbie Lieberman

Peace Education: Exploring Ethical and Philosophical Foundations (2008)
by James Page

Transforming Education for Peace (2008)
edited by Jing Lin, Edward J. Brantmeier, and Christa Bruhn

Encyclopedia of Peace Education (2008)
edited by Monisha Bajaj

Educating Toward a Culture of Peace (2006)
by Yaacov Iram

Coronavirus and Vulnerable People

Addressing the Divide in Harm and Responses and Exploring Implications for a More Peaceful World

Editors

Laura L. Finley and Pamela D. Hall
Barry University

IAP

INFORMATION AGE PUBLISHING, INC.
Charlotte, NC • www.infoagepub.com

SECTION II

ACKNOWLEDGMENTS AND DEDICATION

Laura L. Finley and Pamela D. Hall

Laura L. Finley wishes to thank all the contributors for sharing their perspectives and for the inspiration they provide during these challenging times. Each contributor worked hard to submit his or her chapter quickly so that this book will be timely and thorough. She also wishes all her love to her amazing husband, David Bekerman, and her daughter, Anya Finley, both of whom offered love and support throughout the process. Finally, Laura Finley wishes to devote this book to her wonderful colleagues on the Board of Directors of the Peace and Justice Studies Association. She devotes her portion of any royalties to that organization.

Pamela D. Hall wishes to thank her coeditor, Laura Finley, for suggesting this project, as well as all of the contributors who understood how important it is to address the needs of the most vulnerable during this pandemic. Pamela D. Hall would also like to thank her sisters, Annette Miles, Jacquelin Crumm, Robinette Reaves, Lisa Cotman, her nieces and nephews, and her great-nieces and nephews, who are silent motivators for her at all times. A special shout out to my niece and Goddaughter Cabrillya Wallace, who reviewed my chapter on intergenerational trauma. Most importantly, I thank my ancestors, known and unknown, whose shoulders

Coronavirus and Vulnerable People: Addressing the Divide in Harm and Responses and Exploring Implications for a More Peaceful World, pp. xi–xii

www.infoagepub.com

I stand on and whose resilience is in my DNA. Pamela would like to thank these special ancestors: my paternal grandfather, Curtis Hall, who was born a slave; my father John Hall; my brother John T. Hall; and my sweet mother, Marie Quarles Hall. Lastly, she dedicates this project to her most recent ancestor, Warren Charlie Cotman, my sister Lisa's husband, who entered the Spirit's world on July 10, 2020.

The editors would also like to thanks the staff of Information Age Publishing and acknowledge responsibility for any remaining errors in this book.

INTRODUCTION

Laura L. Finley

While all of the world is and will continue to be affected by the Coronavirus and the necessary (and perhaps some unnecessary) responses to it for some time, it has become increasingly clear that already vulnerable people have been the hardest hit. Even as we write this in May 2021, while vaccinations have become available and infection rates and fatalities in the U.S. are down, people living in poverty, the elderly, people with disabilities, people of color, students, adjunct professors, medical professionals, service workers, and underpaid laborers, undocumented immigrants, LGBTQ individuals, the homeless, abused and neglected children, incarcerated individuals, and victims of domestic violence are all groups that are suffering disproportionately due to a host of preexisting social, institutional, and structural factors. These individuals suffer personally, but also in various institutions that have long been designed by and for middle and upper-class Whites, not Black, Indigenous, People of Color (BIPOC) or the poor. It is clear that these disparities are not the result of biology or personal choices but rather are the result of systemic racism, institutionalized privilege, and deliberate policies of businesses, schools, and governments (Elving, 2020).

Many poor people and people of color work in industries that were unable to quarantine when those orders were issued. They rely on public

Coronavirus and Vulnerable People: Addressing the Divide in Harm and Responses and Exploring Implications for a More Peaceful World, pp. xiii–xvii

transportation, which continues to put them at greater risk. They often reside in population-dense areas where the virus continues to be easily to spread. Other groups of the poor in America live in rural areas that did not and still do not have ample resources to help as the virus spreads to those regions. Native Americans, many of whom live on very remote reservations already lacking adequate healthcare, electricity, running water, and other necessities, contracted the virus at disproportionate rates, which threatened to wipe out many tribal elders and thereby decimate an entire culture. On tribal lands, there is a shortage of hospitals and equipment, so persons with the virus sometimes had to be flown to other places, which is very costly and takes more time, thus can be and was deadly (Morales, 2020). Deliberate policies that demonize and disadvantage the poor have become even more glaringly obvious than before the pandemic (Super, 2020).

The elderly, many of whom are confined in assisted living facilities, are at the mercy of those charged with their care. Although things are dramatically improved as of this writing, in the early phases of the pandemic the elderly were infected at high rates, as were those caring for them. Family and friends were unable to visit due to safety concerns and protocols, leaving these people alone during the most stressful time. Undocumented immigrants have been hesitant to reach out for needed services, even testing, due to their status. College students who were already struggling under tremendous student loans and recent graduates with mounds of debt had to adapt to remote teaching while, in many cases, helping support their families. Many had only limited access to computers or the Internet and relied on campus-based jobs that were not operating (Patel, 2020). Some students deferred their admission, took a semester off, or even dropped out, while others struggled to keep up their grade point averages during remote teaching. Seasonal workers, those in retail and service, and even adjunct professors have been out of work or were on strictly limited hours, so they found it difficult to provide for their families. Not only have these been financial burdens, but they have also been tremendous mental health challenges that exacerbated existing stressors.

LGBTQ individuals, particularly youth who have been ostracized from their families, found themselves couch surfing, living in unsafe environments, or trying to survive on the streets (Human Rights Campaign Foundation, 2020). Children were living in unsafe environments with adult predators, and many were dealing and continue to deal with daily trauma from sexual abuse and assault. Homeless individuals, who are often at high risk due to preexisting conditions, were even more vulnerable to living on the streets during the pandemic. Services for the homeless are often provided in congregant settings that had to be severely limited (Centers for Disease Control and Prevention, 2020). Families had to struggle to ensure that they had some income while supporting their children's education from home, often without needed resources like computers and reliable internet services. Social services have been gutted as fewer people are able to donate and workers were required to stay home, hence people had difficulties in acquiring help for health problems, abuse, unemployment, or other issues, even though these concerns all have been found to increase during crisis times (World Health Organization, 2020). Psychologists and mental health workers have experienced fatigue from addressing clients' overwhelming needs via teletherapy, yet they continued to admirably meet the needs of the most vulnerable.

Many, if not all, of the abovementioned vulnerable groups were already experiencing adverse childhood experiences, intergenerational trauma, stress, and anxiety associated with poverty, racism, food insecurity, and structural inequalities. The pandemic has overwhelmed them, and many reached out for help in support in ways that they would not have in the past. These vulnerable populations have reached their mental, spiritual, and physical threshold. Being confined to their homes or other facilities where they lacked the much-needed physical contact with friends and families created angst that will need to be addressed for a long time after this pandemic ends. Yet, while times are more challenging than ever for many, there remains much to admire in terms of people's resilience, creativity, and hopefulness.

This edited collection seeks to highlight the many ways that COVID-19 has disproportionately affected vulnerable people in the United States. In doing so, contributors shed light on the many structural and institutional barriers involved in the transmission of the disease and fatalities from it. In Chapter 1, Luigi Esposito provides a framework for understanding the flawed response to COVID-19 in the United States. He explores how neoliberalism has shaped institutions in the United States, including the for-profit healthcare model and treatment of waged workers, and has exacerbated racial disparities.

In Section I, we highlight the voices of the vulnerable. Chapters share the personal experiences of contributors and their loved ones, highlighting how BIPOC have long experienced traumas that have been worsened by the global pandemic. Alecia Deon, a queer Black woman with sickle cell anemia, discusses how what many experienced during stay-at-home orders has always been her "normal." She shares her personal experiences with broken institutions and systems that remain ill-equipped to help people like her. Johanna Thompson describes how women of color have been uniquely affected by COVID-19, as they make up most caregiving essential workers that had to remain at work and were thus more vulnerable to infection. She draws on literature to provide a framework for understanding and for hope. Jordana A. Hart, an immigration attorney, shares the stories of immigrants who already struggled in the U.S and how these struggles have been exacerbated. She calls for a rehumanizing of the approach to immigration in the United States. Fanya Jabouin-Monnay and Karine Champagne highlight the plight of Haitian Americans, noting disparities in COVID-19 transmissions and healthcare access. They point out the importance of culturally appropriate mental health services. Ruban Roberts expresses the challenges people of color had in complying with stay-at-home orders, thereby exposing existing inequalities. Mureen Shaw, a nursing professor, discusses the importance of nurses who are working on the frontlines fighting COVID-19 but who are often overlooked. Christian Schlaerth discusses the ways that adjunct faculty members, who are already vulnerable to low wages, job inconsistencies, and poor treatment, are now fearful for their future. Wim Laven focuses his work on educational disparities that have been exposed during the global pandemic and offers hope for critical evaluation and a shift in emphasis toward peace and justice. Michelle Collins-Sibley describes how she related to students studying humanities during the beginning of COVID-19, showing how literature offers a model for understanding and adaptation.

In Section II, contributors address race and trauma. Pamela Hall discusses the intergenerational transmission of the trauma of slavery. A term she coined, post-slavery syndrome, requires trauma-based therapeutic strategies, even more so during the global pandemic. Roni Bennett examines how racism is a preexisting condition that explains why people of color were and remain disproportionately affected by COVID-19. In doing so, she sheds important light on systemic racism in the United States. Laura Finley offers a review of the unique ways Native Americans have suffered historically due to colonialism and how that legacy is related to the disproportionate effects of COVID-19 on reservation lands. Jordan Pate shares the voices of vulnerable teens in Miami's teen court, showing how COVID-19 has affected them physically and socially. Conswello Davis, Pamela D. Hall, and Jordan Pate, from South Florida's Chapter of The Association of Black Psychologists, discuss ways that their organization helped meet community needs for African Americans during Mental Health Awareness Month in May 2020. Likewise, Charlene Desir, Elizabeth Louis, and Pascale Denis provide insight into how Haitian Americans can heal from generations of oppression that have been exacerbated by COVID-19. They call for the importance of Soufrans Ayisyen, or the understanding of Haitian suffering, to lead to skills, knowledge, resilience, and healing.

Similarly, Guy Jeanty and Remy Nelson provide information and tools for healing using this Haitian cultural background. LaTasha Russell shares her experience offering telehealth during COVID-19 stay-at-home orders while also making sure that she took care of herself and her family. She offers important advice for others providing therapy from home. Conswello Davis emphasizes the importance of Kemetic yoga as a healing tool.

In the end, Mark Lance and Matt Meyer describe how COVID-19 may have shed important light on disparities but also encouraged radical nonviolent organizing for social change.

We conclude this volume with recommendations for the future and words of hope.

REFERENCES

Centers for Disease Control and Prevention. (2020, April 7). *Homelessness and COVID 19-FAQs*. https://www.cdc.gov/coronavirus/2019-ncov/community/homeless-shelters/faqs.html

Elving, R. (2020, April 12). What coronavirus exposes about America's political divide. *NPR*. https://www.npr.org/2020/04/12/832455226/what-coronavirus-exposes-about-americas-political-divide

Human Rights Campaign Foundation. (2020). *The lives and livelihoods of many in the LGBTQ community are at risk amidst COVID-19 crisis*. https://assets2.hrc.org/files/assets/resources/COVID19-IssueBrief-032020-FINAL.pdf?_ga=2.197327274.405561699.1587150412-1981790490.1587052209

Morales, L. (2020, April 24). Navajo nation sees high rate of COVID-19, and contact tracing is a challenge. *NPR*. https://www.npr.org/2020/04/24/842945050/navajo-nation-sees-high-rate-of-covid-19-and-contact-tracing-is-a-challenge

Patel, V. (2020, April 14). COVID-19 is a pivotal moment for struggling students. Can colleges step up?" *Chronicle of Higher Education*. https://www.chronicle.com/article/Covid-19-Is-a-Pivotal-Moment/248501

Super, D. (2020, April 14). COVID-19 highlights—and intensifies—our mistreatment of the poor. *The Hill*. https://thehill.com/opinion/finance/492487-covid-19-highlights-and-intensifies-our-mistreatment-of-the-poor

World Health Organization. (2020, April 7). *COVID-19 and violence against women: What the health sector/system can do*. https://apps.who.int/iris/bitstream/handle/10665/331699/WHO-SRH-20.04-eng.pdf

CHAPTER 1

COVID-19 UNDER THE REIGN OF NEOLIBERALISM

Challenges and Possibilities in the United States

Luigi Esposito

INTRODUCTION

The COVID-19 pandemic has created a crisis unprecedented in our lifetime. As the novel coronavirus (SARS COV-2) spreads around the world and people get infected, lose their livelihoods, experience isolation, and struggle with providing essential needs for themselves and their families, millions are dealing with a heightened sense of fear, uncertainty, and despair. Simultaneously, the social, economic, and public health consequences of this crisis have not affected all countries and communities equally, nor have responses been the same. As discussed by various crisis management experts, how a particular country or community perceives, prepares, and responds to natural or human-made crises/disasters—at the level of policy, institutional practices, and everyday personal behaviors—is shaped by prevailing ideas, values, and priorities that are contextually contingent (e.g., Eriksson, 2017).

Coronavirus and Vulnerable People: Addressing the Divide in Harm and Responses and Exploring Implications for a More Peaceful World, pp. 3–25

Within the context of the United States, the prevailing perceptions and responses to the COVID-19 crisis and its consequences must be understood in relation to neoliberalism. Widely regarded as the dominant economic-political paradigm of our time, neoliberalism entails a series of pro-market policies, a set of values and governing rationality that minimizes the role of government as the guardian of the public interest; calls for minimizing social expenditure; seeks to privatize all public services; emphasizes flexible labor markets; rolls back worker protections and organized labor; celebrates unfettered competition, extreme individualism, and the pursuit of profit as the *sine qua non* of freedom; and emphasizes what is sometimes referred to as "the rule of the market" (e.g., Esposito, 2011l; Giroux, 2008; Harvey, 2005).

This chapter addresses how the prevalence of neoliberalism and its attending policies, logic, and values made the United States ill-equipped to prepare for, and deal with, the COVID-19 pandemic and its social, economic, and public health consequences. Despite current government efforts to bail out small businesses, save jobs, keep people from hunger and homelessness, and supply hospitals with much needed ventilators and personal protective equipment, the interventions were, for too long, not nearly enough. Indeed, despite these interventions, millions of working people in the United States—disproportionately racial and ethnic minorities—lost their jobs, struggled to pay their rents, relied on food banks for meals, and faced difficulty obtaining tests and other healthcare services. Although these outcomes were typically attributed to the pandemic, they must also be understood in relation to decades of neoliberal policies that have led to a precarious job market, extreme wealth and income inequality, enormous personal debt, inflated prices for housing and other essential needs, and an erosion of the healthcare and social safety net. In short, one central point that will be made in this chapter is that the current crisis has *amplified* inequalities and other problems that have been years in the making!

Furthermore, many of the responses to the challenges associated with COVID-19 have been framed within a neoliberal logic that values personal "freedom" over the common good and understands people as consumers/competitors responsible for their interests. This all downplays the need for broader structural reforms and blames poor and marginalized members of society—who often do not have the necessary resources to shelter in place, purchase/hoard essential supplies, adhere to social distancing, or wear protective gear—for their adversity. The point is also made that while this pandemic has had and will continue to have a devastating effect on millions of Americans, the consequences of COVID-19 might also forge a new path away from neoliberal hegemony.

OVERVIEW OF NEOLIBERALISM: INTELLECTUAL ORIGINS, HISTORIC DEVELOPMENT AND IMPACT ON U.S. SOCIETY

For more than four decades, neoliberalism has profoundly influenced virtually all aspects of economic, social, and political life, particularly in the United States. In general, neoliberal policies and principles gained popularity in reaction to progressive interventionist policies associated with Keynesianism. As is well known, in the aftermath of the Great Depression, laissez-faire capitalism came into question. Many turned to John M. Keynes's ideas to explain this economic debacle. Keynes argued that markets are rooted in human decisions and are not self-regulating (Esposito, 2011). Rather than "leaving markets alone," Keynes argued that avoiding financial meltdowns, economic instability, and mass unemployment requires state interventions in the form of constraints and regulations on businesses and financial institutions, as well as government spending to create jobs, lift consumer spending, stimulate the economy, and ensure social needs.

During the 1930s, President Franklin Roosevelt pushed for a series of Keynesian-like reforms that, collectively, came to be known as the "New Deal." These reforms included, among other measures, the implementation of a social security program and unemployment compensation system, a massive federal employment initiative that put millions of people back to work, tighter regulation of the industry, high taxes for the rich, and the promotion and strengthening of labor unions. In short, the idea was to build a new political economy in which all business activities were "surrounded by a web of social and political constraints and regulations" that eschewed the sorts of excesses promoted by laissez-faire capitalism while promoting full employment and the welfare of citizens (Harvey, 2005, pp. 11–12). These measures proved to be enormously successful. Throughout the post-World War II era, companies in the United States paid high wages, millions of American families had steady incomes, and millions of workers had lifetime pensions. In addition, profitable corporations and high taxation on the wealthy led to the expansion of the welfare state both in the U.S. and other Western societies.

These sorts of progressive policies were further expanded in the 1960s when President Lyndon Johnson spearheaded the so-called "Great Society"—a series of government programs designed to reduce poverty further and tackle racial inequalities. Even conservatives such as Nixon adopted these sorts of interventionist policies during the 1970s. Spurred by popular pressure, Nixon also followed Keynesian principles and presided over the expansion of several new federal regulatory agencies, including the Environmental Protection Agency and the Occupational Safety and Health Administration. In 1971, Nixon famously declared that "we are all

Keynesian now," showing how even a staunch opponent of the Left and supporter of free enterprise like himself accepted the idea that government had a central role to play in ensuring the general welfare (Smith, 2012).

In stark contrast to Nixon's claim, by the early to mid-1970s, Keynesianism's popularity began to decline. During this time, many of the political and corporate elites became increasingly open about their contempt for progressive interventionist policies. As discussed by Henrick Smith (2012, pp. 6–7), during this time, there was "a full-scale political rebellion by America's corporate leaders" who believed that Keynesian economic principles, along with progressive movements and policies, had supported an activist government that victimized the business sector and erected economic barriers to freedom and prosperity. Therefore, what was needed was a new set of ideas that would revitalize America's free enterprise system.

During this time, a group of radical economists, notably Friedrich August von Hayek, gained popularity. Hayek had founded the Mont Pelerin Society in the 1940s. This organization consisted of like-minded thinkers like Ludwig von Mises, George Stigler, Karl Popper, and Milton Friedman. All of them sought to promote a "free society" based on free-market principles (e.g., Hartwell, 2005). Committed to challenging the "rising tide of collectivism" associated with Keynesianism and activist governments, Hayek and his colleagues insisted that a planned economy is antithetical to a free society. According to these thinkers, human beings are naturally competitive, calculating, and self-serving, and any impediment to these natural human tendencies is an assault on freedom itself. According to Hayek, deploying the state's power to promote presumably lofty ideals such as equality and social justice leads society on a "road to serfdom" (Hayek, 1944). Therefore, rather than centralized planning, a free and open society must be organized around a free market.

Far from merely a theory, Hayek (1944) conceived the market as a "force of nature" that existed in perfect equilibrium, similar to an eco-system, if left untainted by political interventions. As discussed by Steger and Roy (2010, p. 15), Hayek and others associated with the Mont Pelerin Society were firm believers that an unfettered market would function as a "self-regulating engine of freedom and ingenuity" and would "spontaneously" create an optimal order. Similarly, Milton Friedman, who was very much influenced by Hayek, also made the case that as people freely pursue their self-serving interests, the market organizes their actions into an order that benefits all without central planning or political intervention. Therefore, competition was the key to a free, fair, and prosperous society, as a free competitive market operates based on a neutral and seemingly inherent logic unburdened by bureaucracy, politics, or ideology.

By the late 1970s and early 1980s, in the wake of a global oil crisis and increasing stagflation, efforts were made—by, among other leaders,

Margaret Thatcher in England and Ronald Reagan in the United States—to implement the ideas developed by the Mont Pelerin Society (e.g., Harvey, 2005; Klein, 2007). Drawing from Hayek (1944) and his colleagues, and convinced that all problems could be resolved by making governments smaller and unleashing the powers of the free market, Reagan spearheaded an agenda, often known as the "Reagan Revolution," that entailed, among other measures, cutting taxes, curbing government spending (particularly for social services), slashing regulations, privatizing healthcare and other public services, weakening social safety nets, and doing away with unionized labor as much as possible. Around the globe, but particularly within the context of U.S. society, these policies—which are today widely referred to as *neoliberal* policies by activists and academics—have become akin to economic and political orthodoxy and have, to varying degrees, shaped the political agendas of every administration since then, as well as that of many state/local governments. And while tax cuts, privatization, and deregulation have benefited the wealthy, critics argue this has come at the cost of less job security, stagnant wages, social disinvestment, and dramatic increases in the cost of healthcare, education, housing, and other essential needs (e.g., Harvey, 2005; Reich, 2007; Smith, 2012).

Important to emphasize at this juncture is that neoliberalism is not simply an economic model or set of policies but it also involves all-encompassing rationality that emphasizes fundamental values and practices demanded by market capitalism—for example, consumerism, hyper-competition, profit-driven behavior, and so forth—as not simply part of an ideology or belief system but rather as inviolable axioms that all responsible, competent people must adapt to (e.g., Brown, 2015). As such, only specific forms of human relations, attitudes, and behaviors that operate within the market's logic are promoted as functional, productive, or normal (Esposito & Perez, 2014). This governing rationality understands citizens as consumers and prioritizes competition over solidarity and personal liberty over social justice (Giroux, 2008). In short, under neoliberalism, the individual—understood as a competitive, self-serving, rational agent—takes ontological priority over any notion of the social. To borrow from Margaret Thatcher, "there is no such thing as society … there are only individual men and women" (Keay, 1987).

This emphasis on the individual is also predicated on an atomized and thoroughly depoliticized vision of the world in which people are assumed to be personally responsible for their situations and problems. Because the market is understood as apolitical, all outcomes in a competitive market system are understood as "deserved." Thus, poverty, illness, and other forms of adversity are not understood to be related to broader systemic/structural issues but rather the result of poor personal choices, habits, or practices. Because only individuals matter, all social problems are understood as private/personal troubles. Solutions, therefore, must also be sought within the personal/private realm. Thus, for example, avoiding poverty, illness, and other hardships requires that people be personally responsible, choose the right schools, obtain marketable skills, be able to afford healthcare insurance, choose the right doctor, and make good choices in terms of food, lifestyle, and so forth. In effect, because all human actions and decisions are either rewarded or punished by "the market," being a worthy citizen is synonymous with having a competitive edge and/or being responsible consumers. In this sense, to borrow from Henry Giroux (2008), the market becomes the "arbiter of social life."

THE COVID-19 CRISIS AS AN AMPLIFICATION OF NEOLIBERAL CONSEQUENCES

The current COVID-19 pandemic must be understood not as a "cause" but rather as an amplification of the consequences promoted by decades of the aforementioned neoliberal policies and axioms that have left millions of people, particularly those coming from marginalized communities, in a state of precarity and despair. As noted above, neoliberalism has framed how the federal government, many state/local governments, and much of the U.S.'s general public have prepared (or been ill-prepared) for and responded to the crisis. What follows is an overview of how this has affected: (1) public health; (2) the plight of millions of working people; and (3) already existing racial and ethnic inequities in the United States.

Public Health Under Neoliberalism

In a recent article, David Harvey (2020) discusses how neoliberalism across various countries, including the United States, has

> left the public totally exposed and ill-prepared to face a public health crisis of this sort, even though previous scares of SARS and Ebola provided abundant warning as well as cogent lessons as to what would be needed to be done. (Harvey, 2020)

Of course, what needed to be done is prepare for the likelihood that, in an increasingly interconnected world, a novel, highly infectious virus-like SARS COVID-2 would emerge and spread across an immunologically naïve population very rapidly. Preparing for such an event would require, among other measures, making the necessary public health investments (in the form of extra hospital beds, stockpiling personal protective equipment, and ensuring ample supplies of other vital gear) to protect frontline healthcare workers and minimize the risk of healthcare systems becoming overwhelmed. These measures are entirely in line with any notion that the government should act as the public interest guardian.

Yet consistent with neoliberal logic, for decades, what has been in place is a for-profit healthcare model that prioritizes competition and consumerism over universal access and equity. As is well known, the U.S.'s healthcare industry became increasingly privatized during the Reagan era, and this is how it remains today. What is particularly significant is that when applied to public health provisions, the neoliberal model has "eliminated the surplus coping capacities that would be required in an emergency" (Harvey, 2020). The unrelenting quest for short term profits, in other words, is antithetical to the investment and implementation of preventive measures that are needed to mitigate the effects of a public health crisis. After all, if corporations cannot profit from these measures, particularly in the short term, why bother? While profit-driven hospitals have an incentive to keep their beds full for well-paying customers needing joint-replacements or heart procedures, there is very little incentive to stockpile equipment. As aptly put by Elisabeth Rosenthal (2020), "There's no return on investment in being primed and positioned for the possibility of a once-in-a-lifetime pandemic."

What is particularly remarkable is that U.S. intelligence agencies, along with top public health officials, not only predicted a pandemic every year since at least 2013 but raised concerns about the obvious gaps in the country's defenses and ability to respond to such an event (e.g., Friedman, 2020). In fact, in 2017, an official at the Centers for Disease Control and Prevention (CDC) wrote an article in which they warned about the need to stockpile ventilators, writing that "hospitals must accept responsibility for the costs and resources needed to manage and maintain an excess of ventilators that are likely to be unused in the absence of pandemic-related surges in demand" (as cited in Rosenthal, 2020). The neoliberal model normalized the failure to purchase this potentially life-saving equipment, making hospitals akin to cruise ships without lifeboats.

In neoliberal fashion, the scarcity of ventilators and N95 masks, gloves, face shields, gowns, sanitizers, and other vital equipment was left up to "free-market competition," as state and local leaders had to rely on purchasing this life-saving equipment from the private sector. What resulted was that, throughout the country, state and local governments were forced into "bidding wars" that drove prices up. For example, New York Governor Andrew Cuomo described how New York was forced to pay about $45,000 for ventilators (twice the normal price), while N95 masks that normally would have cost .85 cents were selling for $7 each. As Cuomo described the situation, "it's like being on eBay with 50 other states" (as cited in Leigh,

2020). And this led to a situation where states and local municipalities were forced to dig deep into their tax-funded reserves while private companies around the globe cashed in.

A similar dynamic took place with testing. As much as President Trump insisted that "anyone can get a test," the lack of widescale testing for COVID-19 was something that was addressed continuously by critics. Conducting the tests involved a number of items—including kits, various chemicals, swaps, gloves, masks, and so forth. However, much like what happened with the ventilators, early in 2020, when it was not yet clear whether the coronavirus would actually produce a pandemic, medical manufacturers were reluctant to invest any significant amount of money into producing the items needed to make and conduct these tests for fear that such production would exceed demand (Rosenthal, 2020). This, combined with a lack of funding, technical flaws, bureaucratic red tape, and poor leadership undermined any chance to contain the virus's spread in the United States, as without early widescale testing, "Americans were left largely blind to the scale of a looming public health catastrophe" (Shear et al., 2020).

In response to the shortage of tests, personal protective equipment, ventilators, and other essential supplies, Trump was pressured to consider invoking the Defense Production Act. This is a provision that requires private companies to prioritize any government orders for products. Trump, however, was reluctant to take this necessary step. When pressed to explain this reluctance, President Trump gave two central reasons: (1) companies were already stepping up on their own to make these products and do the right thing, and (2) employing this provision was tantamount to socialism. One can clearly see the neoliberal logic that is operative here, as the implication is that the best solutions are always market based/business solutions. Any intrusion on private enterprise is tantamount to socialist tyranny. It was only in late March that Trump decided to invoke the Defense Production Act by executive order, but he "did so sparingly and slowly, mostly relying on backchannel arm-twisting and 'incentives' like forgiving liability to get business buy-in" (Rosenthal, 2020). Consistent with neoliberalism, saving lives was evidently not a big enough incentive (or at least it was secondary to profit).

The fact that the United States was ill-equipped to contain the virus in any significant way is also closely related to another common practice in the neoliberal agenda: cutting public expenditure. For example, on February 10, 2020, just 11 days before the World Health Organization (WHO) declared COVID-19 to be a global public health emergency, the Trump administration unveiled its proposed 2021 budget, cutting CDC funding 16% compared to 2020 spending levels. Although the budget was never enacted, it gives insight into how the neoliberal agenda to disinvest from public health has still been operative. Even more alarming, to cut costs in 2018, President Trump decided to disband the U.S. pandemic response team in the National Security Council, further weakening the U.S.'s defenses against the possibility of a global pandemic (e.g., Dozier & Bergengruen, 2020). The result of all this has been that the United States, an enormously wealthy, sophisticated country with some of the best scientists and medical experts globally, currently has the most COVID-19 infections and deaths compared to any other country. Recently, Trump has also announced terminating U.S. relations with the WHO, claiming this organization is controlled by China and, therefore, untrustworthy. The termination means the WHO will lose hundreds of millions of dollars from U.S. contributions. According to critics, U.S. withdrawal from the WHO and the resulting loss of funds will make "the global coronavirus response harder to coordinate," thereby putting people around the world at greater risk (Ward, 2020).

The Plight of Waged Workers: Intensifying Neoliberal Pain

Despite claims that infectious diseases do not discriminate and "we are all in this together," the consequences of COVID-19 have reinforced existing inequalities along the lines of class and race (not to mention gender). Over the years, neoliberal policies have gutted the welfare state, encouraged wage stagnation, increased the cost of essential needs (notably housing), and rolled back workers' rights and protections while giving the wealthy tax breaks; the U.S. capitalist economy was already structured in extreme inequality. Millions of American workers have, for years, lived under conditions of economic precarity. In fact, as much as President Trump and others continuously celebrated the U.S. economy before the rise of COVID-19 as "the strongest in U.S. history," the wealthiest 1% of households in the U.S.-owned more wealth than the bottom 90%; hundreds of thousands of Americans were already homeless (The State of Homelessness in America, 2019), and millions were already food insecure (Layne 2019), lacked health insurance, and had no paid sick leave. In addition, 40% of Americans struggled to afford basic needs (including housing and utilities) and are one paycheck away from poverty (Karpman et al., 2018).

During a pandemic involving a highly infectious virus, it is no surprise that low waged workers (comprised disproportionately of Africans Americans, Hispanics, and women) are bearing the brunt of the consequences, either because their jobs do not typically allow for meaningful social distancing or because they simply do not have the resources to weather what will likely be long-term unemployment. As stated by Isaković (2020), "the ability to isolate, work from home, homeschool your children, stockpile your shelves, access healthcare, and financially (and psychologically) put your life back together after the pandemic is class, gender, race, age, and geography dependent." Indeed, decades of inequality cannot be put aside as people of dramatically different means and socioeconomic backgrounds are confronted with the same disease. Those inequalities dramatically impact how people prepared for the pandemic, as well as who gets to shelter in place, who loses their job/livelihood, who gets sick, who gets hospitalized, who dies, and how they cope moving forward.

One clear disparity lies in the question of who can work at home and who cannot. Obviously, while a significant percentage of salaried, well-paid professionals can work online in their homes, a majority of wage workers do not have this option. As of this writing, approximately 40 million Americans had filed for unemployment (Romm, 2020). And while no industry has been untouched by the pandemic, evidence also shows that the first to suffer were low waged workers in service sector industries that require close, face-to-face encounters with customers. For example, drawing from data put out of the U.S. Department of Labor, the Economic Policy Institute finds that seven percent of all restaurants, hotels, and bar workers filed for unemployment within the first week of the closure orders (Van Dam, 2020). Other low-wage workers in retail stores and movie theaters, as well as hairdressers and laundry workers were also particularly hard hit (Van Dam 2020). One commonality among these service sector workers is not only their low wages but their lack of employment benefits—a condition that, under neoliberalism, has been in place for decades. The pandemic, therefore, disproportionately affected those who were already vulnerable.

Perhaps even more troubling is that the government assistance rolled out has not been distributed equally or quickly enough in some cases. On March 27, 2020, President Trump signed a $2.2 trillion coronavirus relief bill into law, which promised to provide a $1,200 check for most adult Americans and expand unemployment benefits. Critics, however, argue that the checks took several weeks to deliver. In fact, millions of Americans never received their checks, putting them at great risk of being unable to pay for essential needs when the economy was virtually paralyzed (e.g., Horsley, 2020). With respect to unemployment benefits, although there are some federal guidelines, each state has separate rules in terms of who qualifies. For one thing, workers have to earn a minimum amount even to qualify, which varies from state to state (Desilver, 2020). As a result, workers who derive a significant percentage of their paychecks from tips, such as waitresses and bartenders, may not make enough unemployment benefits or may get far less than what they might have hoped.

Furthermore, although the relief bill promised to help self-employed workers who are part of the so-called "gig economy," many of these workers may also not be eligible for employment benefits, particularly if they do not have the proper work and pay documentation, which also varies from state to state (Iacurci, 2020). The same dilemma applies to workers who work "under the table," who get paid in cash and therefore do not have the required documentation to get benefits. Unfortunately, these are not isolated cases. Citing research from the W. E. Upjohn Institute for Employment Research, Greg Iacurci points out that "29 states have a share of jobless workers eligible for benefits of less than 25 percent" (Iacurci, 2020). In addition, those who apply for unemployment benefits can only get them for a limited amount of time, which basically means that the benefits will not last long enough to sustain them for the duration of what will likely be a long unemployment spell. Some workers eligible for benefits have given up even before getting them, often pointing to crashed websites and overwhelmed phone systems that made submitting claims difficult (Van Dam, 2020).

Astonishingly, despite all these problems, recent commentators have complained about how the expansion of unemployment benefits has disincentivized many unemployed workers to go back to work, as their unemployment checks are, in many cases, larger than their wages (Morath, 2020). But rather than addressing how average wages are, in many parts of the country, incompatible with the cost of living and using this as a way to promote higher, more realistic wages, there is a common claim that these workers are being corrupt and trying to "milk the system" at taxpayers' expense. In some cases, as in the case of Florida Senator Rick Scott and South Carolina Senator Lindsey Graham, the claim has been made that low wage workers are getting "too much" in unemployment benefits (Wolf, 2020). And while there might be cases of laid-off workers preferring an unemployment check over a low waged job, the challenges and economic uncertainties already promoted by decades of neoliberal policies have created a scenario where unprecedented numbers of American workers find themselves at the brink of financial disaster.

Particularly hard hit are low-income single parents (mostly women) who are the sole providers for their families, cannot rely on the closed school systems for both free meals and a safe environment for their children, and have very little prospects for any sustained income (e.g., Smith, 2020). Ultimately, the struggling new working class—what some have referred to as "the precariat" (Standing, 2014)—are the people most vulnerable to not only the virus itself but also to COVID-19 related consequences such as prolonged unemployment, food insecurity, and homelessness. Furthermore, all of this is more likely to weaken their immune system (making them even more susceptible to illness), compromise their mental health, and further challenge their ability to make themselves whole once the pandemic subsides (Gurchiek, 2020)

COVID-19 and Racial/Ethnic Disparities

Far from "color blind," there are also clear racial/ethnic disparities in terms of who is most affected by the COVID-19 pandemic and its consequences. Available data suggest that African Americans in particular are disproportionately affected by COVID-19 related hospitalizations and deaths. According to a report published by *The Lancet* in early May 2020, in data compiled from hospitals in 14 states, African Americans represent 33% of COVID-19 hospitalizations, despite making up only 18% of the population studied (Kirby, 2020). In New York City, which has, for weeks, been considered the epicenter of the pandemic in the United States, the death rate is strikingly unequal, as there were 92.3 deaths per every 100,000 among African Americans, compared to 45.2 deaths per every 100,000 among non-Hispanic Whites (Kirby, 2020). New York City is not an anomaly. Drawing from data released in April by various states around the country, including race and ethnicity, *Vox* reporter Fabiola Cineas (2020) documents these disparities, particularly as it pertains to Blacks/African Americans. As reported by Cineas (2020):

> Black people made up 33 percent of Michigan cases and 40 percent of deaths, despite being 14 percent of the state's population. In Milwaukee County, Wisconsin, where black people represent 26 percent of the population, they made up almost half of the country's 945 cases and 81 percent of its 27 deaths. In Illinois, black people made up 42 percent of fatalities but make up only 14.6 percent of the state's population. In Chicago, the data is even graver: Black people represent 68 percent of the city's fatalities and more than 50 percent of cases but only 30 percent of the city's total population. In the South, the numbers are even grimmer. In Louisiana, black people accounted for more than 70 percent of deaths in the state population, which is about 33 percent black. (para. 7)

Among Hispanics, the disparities have not been so much about disproportionate COVID-19 related deaths and hospitalizations. However, that is clearly the case in some places—for example, in New York City, death rates as of April 2020 were 74.3 per 100,000 among Hispanics compared to 45.2 per 100,000 among non-Hispanic Whites (Kirby, 2020). However, what has been particularly problematic among Hispanics is that, like African Americans, they have experienced a disproportionate financial burden because of the COVID-19 pandemic. According to the Pew Research Center, for example, "Hispanics are more likely than Americans overall to say they or someone in their household has experienced a pay cut or lost their job because of the coronavirus outbreak" (Krogstad et al., 2020). In fact, 40% of Hispanics say someone in their household has had a pay cut, compared to 27% of the overall population.

Furthermore, 29% of Hispanics say they have been laid off or lost their job, compared to 20% of the overall population (Krogstad et al., 2020). Not only that, but Hispanics are more likely than other groups to express concern about getting COVID 19 and needing hospitalization. According to another report put out by the Pew Research Center, Hispanics (43%) and Blacks (31%) are far more likely than Whites (18%) to be very concerned about getting COVID-19 and needing to be hospitalized (Pew Research Center, 2020).

The reasons why African Americans, Hispanics, and other minorities are disproportionately affected by the COVID-19 pandemic are variegated, complex, and reflect a history of structural disadvantages. For one thing, generations of discrimination associated with segregation, redlining, and other policies/practices (both legal and de facto) have pushed a disproportionate number of African Americans and other minorities to live in densely populated areas and housing and work in jobs (e.g., checkout clerks, delivery drivers, fast food workers, janitors, meat-processing/packing workers, and other service-sector jobs) that are not only more precarious but do not allow them to stay at home, thereby putting them at greater risk. Not only that but a greater percentage of Blacks, Hispanics, and other minorities, particularly those living in urban areas, have to rely on public transportation to get to work, which also puts them at greater risk of infection (Cineas, 2020) According to the U.S. Bureau of Labor Statistics, fewer than 20% of Black workers and roughly 16% of Hispanic workers can telecommute (see Nania, 2020)

What is particularly noteworthy for purposes of this discussion is that this same legacy of racism and ethnic discrimination, combined with neoliberal policies and practices that, since the 1980s, have cut back on public expenditure, eroded the welfare state, weakened labor unions, and encouraged wage stagnation, have made African Americans, Hispanics, and other minority groups disproportionately poor. This also means that, in the current pandemic, many do not have the option of forgoing a paycheck and staying home without catastrophic consequences for themselves and their families. Generations of racism combined with decades of neoliberal policies have also led to poor health outcomes for a disproportionate number of racial/ethnic minorities. In fact, just in the last few years, in the name of "cutting costs" or being "fiscally responsible," various states have declined to expand Medicaid, which has reduced the number of low-income residents—disproportionately racial/ethnic minorities—with regular access to primary healthcare (Kirby, 2020). The end result is that various racial minority groups have poorer health outcomes. For example, in African Americans' case, data overwhelmingly shows higher rates of all sorts of unfavorable health conditions. According to the U.S. Department of Health and Human Services' Office of Minority Health, African Americans have a significantly higher death rate than whites for hypertension, heart disease, cancer, asthma, diabetes, and HIV/AIDS (Cineas, 2020). These underlying health conditions or "co-morbidities" make African Americans and other minorities more susceptible to getting seriously ill or dying from COVID-19. This is another example of how the current pandemic has amplified disparate health outcomes related to a history of racism and decades of neoliberal policies.

The same pattern is discernible among American Indians, particularly in the Navajo Nation. According to government figures, the known rate of COVID-19 infections in the Navajo Nation is about 1,691 per 100,000 people, second only after New York State in terms of per capita infections (Miller, 2020). Especially problematic is that an estimated 40% of homes in some parts of the Navajo Nation are without water, and most are densely packed with family members of multiple generations, partly due to tradition but also because of systemic poverty, high unemployment, and restrictive federal policies that led to housing shortages. Not only does the lack of water resources make essential hygiene practices like washing hands extremely challenging, but this condition has also had an enormously detrimental consequence on the health, economy, and welfare of the Navajo people. In fact, a lack of water, as well as a lack of transportation, has limited access to fresh food and healthcare, with only 13 grocery stores, 12 health facilities, and six hospitals available for an area roughly the size of West Virginia. Because of these and other conditions, Navajo tribal members also have high rates of diabetes, heart disease, and other underlying conditions that, much like African Americans, put them at high risk of getting seriously ill or dying from COVID-19. Notably, the lack of water infrastructure, which is at the root of many Navajo Nation problems, is at least partly due to decades of neoliberal policies that cut funding for essential social programs. Therefore, the tribal government was forced to increasingly rely on extractive industries (e.g., coal mining) to support those programs, thereby putting enormous strain on natural resources, including water (Curley & Dunbar-Ortiz, 2012). Here again, the current water shortages and lack of infrastructure that have made the Navajo Nation particularly vulnerable to the COVID-19 pandemic cannot be fully understood without context. The context is a history of federal neglect and decades of neoliberal policies.

NEOLIBERAL RESPONSES: PERSONALIZING THE CONSEQUENCES OF COVID-9 AND REINFORCING EXISTING INEQUALITIES

Not only has the COVID-19 pandemic magnified problems and inequalities that, for decades, have already been promoted by neoliberal policies, but those same problems/inequalities are often understood based on the prevailing neoliberal logic that personalizes them. As previously discussed, neoliberalism is not simply an economic model but an ideological project that atomizes social life by treating "society" as little more than a heap of individuals. In doing so, "personal responsibility" takes precedence over any notion of collective responsibility (e.g., Giroux, 2008). This ultra-individualistic type of rationality frames how all problems, responses, and solutions are understood under neoliberalism.

Consistent with this logic, some of the public health recommendations that have been most emphasized in the media and by healthcare experts to protect oneself and contain the pandemic is to "wash your hands," "shelter in place," and "maintain social distancing." While this might be sound advice personally, it does very little to promote solidarity and equality, especially because not everyone can take these measures. As already described above, some groups of people might have limited access to water, are confined to live in highly dense areas, in crowded homes, and/or are not given the option to work from home. Consistent with neoliberal rationality, these people are often perceived as flawed or irresponsible individuals who have only themselves to blame if they get sick. This logic is clearly illustrated in recent statements made by Health and Human Services Secretary Alex Azar. Addressing an outbreak of COVID-19 cases among workers in meatpacking plants, Azar suggested the outbreak had nothing to do with the workers' conditions at their workplaces but rather with their lifestyles at home, where they live in crowded housing, fail to maintain social distancing, and spread the infection (Bernal, 2020). While many argued that Azar had no ill-will in making these statements, he obviously exonerated the businesses that own and run the meatpacking plants of any responsibility and put the blame squarely on the individual workers—the majority of whom are immigrants and racial minorities—for getting sick and spreading the disease (Bernal, 2020). In much the same vein, Ibram X. Kendi (2020) addresses how media discussions about disproportionate infections, hospitalizations, and deaths among African Americans and other racial minorities emphasize poverty, co-morbidities, and unfavorable living conditions without directly addressing the racist history and larger structural conditions that lead to these outcomes. Without this information, many might begin to assume that these racially disparate health outcomes manifest from personal deficiencies among minorities—that is, the results of poor personal choices, irresponsible behavior, a lack of proper values, etc. In effect, without addressing these public health disparities' larger historical and systemic forces, the problem is personalized and depoliticized.

Personalizing the problem of disparate public health outcomes also leads to punitive responses, reinforcing the highly individualistic position encouraged under neoliberalism. In fact, similar to the punitive logic which, for decades, has dominated U.S. criminal justice policies and focus on "punishing" individual offenders, rather than addressing the underlying structural conditions that lead many individuals to offend in the first place, many cities and municipalities have taken a similar approach to deal with those who fail to maintain social distancing. Throughout the country, arresting and fining people for not wearing a mask or violating social distancing orders has become the norm (e.g., Jackson, 2020). While some might regard these measures as a rational way to discourage people from inadvertently spreading the virus, their enforcement often reinforces existing inequalities. Wealthy professionals who work at home and can minimize their time outside are not as likely to be arrested or fined for violating social distancing orders as are people who have to work outside their home, use public transit, and live in highly dense communities, and are already looked at with suspicion. Predictably, in New York City, over 80% of those who were issued a summons for violating social distancing orders were low-income Blacks and Hispanics, at least partly because they live in highly dense communities that are more heavily policed and have to work outside of their homes (Morales & Joseph, 2020). Nonetheless, the emphasis on punishment completely ignores these underlying structural inequalities and focuses exclusively on the individuals who fail to follow the rules.

Also consistent with neoliberal rationality, many people, particularly early in the pandemic, responded to the potential consequences of the COVID-19 crisis (which many feared would include food shortages and a scarcity of toilet paper) through ultra- individualistic measures associated with the neoliberal emphasis on competition and consumerism. For example, many people opted to "beat the crowds" and hoard food and toilet paper even before the spread of COVID-19 was officially declared a global pandemic. This is considered commendable behavior in a neoliberal worldview, as a competent/rational citizen is first and foremost one who is able to read market signals (i.e., anticipate market shortages), outdo others in pursuing their self-interests (e.g., get all the essential supplies you need before the shortages), and exercise responsible behaviors, which involves being a responsible consumer and purchasing enough goods to sustain oneself and one's family. Of course, the problem is that these measures entirely ignore others' needs who will be even more affected by the shortages because of a few individuals' hoarding. As a result, it became quite common throughout the country to see a few individuals leaving stores with personal stockpiles of food, toilet paper, and other essentials. In contrast, others—many of whom did not have the means to hoard vital supplies—were confronted with empty shelves (Reiley, 2020).

A similar dynamic encouraged a spike in gun sales. According to the FBI's National Instant Criminal Background Check System, there were

6,543,155 background checks for February and March of 2020, which is 1.8 million more than the previous year (FBI NICS Firearm Checks, 2020). As is well known, in the United States, gun sales tend to spike during crisis times. According to Jackey Powder from the Johns Hopkins Bloomberg School of Public Health,

> The rush to stock up on guns in tandem with the coronavirus pandemic is rooted in a gun-owning culture that promotes 'arming up' in preparation for a complete breakdown of society, while a smaller group of buyers is motivated by fear of increasing government authority in this time of national emergency. (Powder, 2020)

These concerns, of course, also align with the neoliberal emphasis on taking personal responsibility to pursue one's self-interests (in this case, to protect one's safety, family, and property) in the event of a societal breakdown or the possibility of a tyrannical "big government" that might infringe on one's rights. Here again, this is a personal/private solution to a social problem that can inadvertently lead to extremely problematic social/public health outcomes. For example, public health experts have expressed concern about the possibility that a spike in gun sales will encourage a rise in suicides and domestic homicides, particularly during a time of social isolation and heightened anxiety (Powder, 2020). An increase in gun ownership during a time of heightened fear and social anxiety might also lead to unequal outcomes, as decades of racialized criminal stereotypes make certain racial/ethnic minorities more likely to be perceived as a "threat" by armed individuals seeking to protect themselves and their property.

Even the recent protests against lifting all COVID-19 related lockdowns and "liberate" states, as President Trump recently encouraged in a series of Tweets, are clearly aligned with neoliberalism. In recent weeks, thousands of people in various states—including Michigan, Minnesota, Virginia, Texas, Arizona, Ohio, Washington, and California—have gathered to protest lockdown orders. These protests are being organized and/or attended primarily by various conservative groups, many of whom often show up with firearms. They include militia members, gun rights activists, former Tea Party activists, right-wing conspiracy theorists, and others (Mudde, 2020). While some are protesting these lockdowns as an overreaction that is hurting local economies and people's livelihoods, many others are taking to the streets because they believe there is an anti-Trump "deep state" infringing on their constitutional rights and regard these lockdowns, including orders to wear a mask, as nothing other than "big government" overreach. The guns these protesters often bring to these rallies are a clear "reminder" that citizens are prepared to take up arms against government tyranny. Many critics, however, argue that in their impassioned efforts to "liberate" the country, these mostly White, middle-class protesters are overlooking and/or devaluing segments of the population that are more vulnerable to getting seriously ill and/or dying from the pandemic (Hoskin, 2020). In short, consistent with the neoliberal worldview, the right for "personal freedom" and the need to "liberate" the free market economy is prioritized over public health.

CONCLUSION: SEIZING THE MOMENT AND THE NEED FOR A POST-NEOLIBERAL ETHOS

While the COVID-19 crisis has clearly exposed and amplified the problems and inequalities encouraged by neoliberalism, this pandemic might also challenge neoliberal hegemony by expanding current boundaries of "acceptable" social, political, and economic discourse. As discussed by Jeremy Lent (2020), amid this pandemic, ideas and policies that, for much of the country, have seemed "radical" or "unthinkable" might suddenly seem sensible and necessary. How crises might prompt social change has been previously addressed by Naomi Klein. In her groundbreaking book *The Shock Doctrine*, Klein suggests that crises such as military coups, financial meltdowns, or natural disasters often lead to public disorientation, and it is during these times of "shock" that the elite will often advance ideas and policies that benefit the wealthy, often at the expense of everyone else (Klein, 2007). Yet there is also another possibility. Much like the Great Depression resulted in a shift away from laissez-faire capitalism and the rise of a more regulated type of economy associated with the New Deal that benefited millions of middle and working-class people, the current pandemic might also lead to a revitalization of support for ideas and policies that might move the country forward to a more equitable and sustainable future, one away from the neoliberal paradigm.

Indeed, at a time when millions of Americans have faced (and in many cases continue to face) the prospect of illness, hospitalization, unemployment, hunger, debt, bankruptcy, and homelessness, ideas and policies such as universal healthcare, cancelling student debt, free college, universal basic income, government intervention to house the homeless, and instituting a federal living wage might suddenly seem reasonable to people who might have, just a few months ago, considered such policies "radical." The same is true of the "Green New Deal"—a set of policy prescriptions that, although often dismissed as too costly and hence "unrealistic," might be necessary to mitigate the current climate threat that, according to many scientists, threatens the survival of the human species. This era of a more interventionist government seems to be coming to fruition under the Biden administration, which has offered a $6 trillion spending proposal.

The Biden administration's plan includes lifting the US economy out of the Covid recession, renewing much of the country's infrastructure, generating millions of blue-collar jobs, securing affordable childcare for millions of American families, and levying higher taxes on corporations and the wealthiest Americans. What this all seems to indicate is that the neoliberal era of "small government" and deregulation is giving way to a different, "New Deal" type of era where the federal government plays an active role in ensuring the needs of the populace.

But beyond a shift in social and economic policies, what is also needed is a new ethos, one that moves away from the atomization encouraged by neoliberalism and emphasizes a strong collective purpose. While people might have very different opinions about what a "better society" might look like, there should be little doubt that this crisis has made clear that the personal and the social realms are inextricably linked. That is to say, one's decisions, actions, conditions, and circumstances both affect and are affected by others. To put this into the current context, if some people are ill with COVID-19, have no access to healthcare, cannot afford basic needs, and are at the brink of financial disaster, this impacts other people's health and financial stability as well, as others' illness increases the likelihood of infection. Their financial struggle implies they cannot contribute to the economy, compromising other people's financial well-being. When one takes this interconnectedness seriously, the neoliberal tendency to emphasize competition over solidarity, consumerism over citizenship, individual liberty over the common good or personal responsibility over social justice becomes untenable. Rather than encouraging people to be purely creatures of self-interests who must "outdo" others to get the things they want or need in life, efforts must be made—in schools, the media, the family, and other institutions—to encourage alternative values and modes of living that take altruism and reciprocity seriously. The idea is not to eliminate the pursuit of self-interest or succumb to a repressive form of collectivism. Instead, it promotes a non-dualistic type of individualism whereby people's actions and ambitions are informed by the realization that their personal well-being is fundamentally connected to others' well-being.

Also, as part of promoting a new ethos, more efforts should be made to help people realize that the prevailing order is not "neutral," as different groups of people have had different histories and experiences that affect their present and future in very distinct ways. A neoliberal vision of the world, of course, dismisses these differences by regarding all people as a constellation of generic self-serving individuals—what classical liberals called "homo economicus"—who are rewarded or punished by "neutral" market forces as they pursue their self-interests and compete freely, without any considerations for things like race, ethnicity, social class, gender, and so forth. Many people regard it as synonymous with "treating everyone equally," but this type of thinking is actually antithetical to equity. For example, an "equal" allocation of funding or public health resources will not correct those existing inequalities in an already unequal society. Suppose a history of racism and decades of neoliberal policies have made a Black or Native-American community twice as affected by COVID19 as a White, upper-middle-class community. In that case, the former requires double the funding. Rather than an "unfair handout," as many neoliberals might claim, that is what ensures equity.

Creating a more equitable society will obviously require a renewal of democratic energies to push the country forward in that direction. As history shows, this is never easy. After all, equity, solidarity, compassion, reciprocity, and similar values are not always compatible with the neoliberal status quo and those who benefit from this order. Nevertheless, the challenges generated by this pandemic have crystallized the failures of neoliberalism and the need to build a society based on precisely those values. What the country (and the world) will look like once this pandemic subsides is still in question. What is clear, however, is that this crisis does offer possibilities for meaningful social change. If citizens seize this opportunity and generate enough pressure to veer the country into a more equitable, post-neoliberal future where the common good is prioritized over markets and corporate interests, perhaps something positive might come out of this tragic historical moment.

REFERENCES

Bernal, R. (2020, May 7). HHS chief suggests workers are to blame for COVID outbreaks at meatpacking plants. *The Hill*. https://thehill.com/latino/496589-hhs-chief-suggests-workers-are-to-blame-for-covid-outbreaks-at-meatpacking-plants

Brown, W. (2015). *Undoing the demos: Neoliberalism's stealth revolution*. Zone Books.

Cineas, F. (2020, April 8). COVID-19 is disproportionately taking Black lives. *Vox*. https://www.vox.com/identities/2020/4/7/21211849/coronavirus-black-americans

Curley, A., & Dunbar-Ortiz, R. (2012, June 16). The international indigenous movement for self-determination. *Solidarity*. https://solidarity-us.org/p3618/

Desilver, D. (2020, April 24). *Not all unemployed people get unemployment benefits; In some states, very few do*. Pew Research Center. https://www.pewresearch.org/fact-tank/2020/04/24/not-all-unemployed-people-get-unemployment-benefits-in-some-states-very-few-do/

Dozier, K., & Bergengruen, D. (2020, March 19). Under fire for coronavirus response, Trump officials defend disbanding pandemic team. *Time Magazine*. https://time.com/5806558/administration-officials-fight-criticism/

Eriksson, J. (2017). *Threat politics: New perspectives on security, risks, and crisis management*. Routledge.

Esposito, L. (2011). Neoliberalism and the market society. In J. W. Murphy & K. A. Callaghan (Eds.), *Toward a post market society* (pp. 28–47). Nova Science.

Esposito, L., & Perez, F. (2014). Neoliberalism and the commodification of mental health. *Humanity and Societym 38*, 414–442.

Friedman, U. (2020, March 18). We were warned: When the inevitable inquiry into the government's response to COVID-19 happens, it will conclude that signs of a coming crisis were everywhere. *The Atlantic*. https://www.theatlantic.com/politics/archive/2020/03/pandemic-coronavirus-united-states-trump-cdc/608215/

FBI NICS Firearm Checks. (2020). *The Federal Bureau of Investigation*. Retrieved November 30, 1998–April 30, 2020, from https://www.fbi.gov/file-repository/nics_firearm_checks_-_month_year.pdf/view

Giroux, H. (2008). *Against the terror of neoliberalism*. Paradigm.

Gurchiek, K. (2020, May 11). COVID-19 takes a toll on employees' mental well-being. *Society for Human Resource Management*. https://www.shrm.org/hr-today/news/hr-news/pages/shrm-research-covid-19-takes-a-toll-on-employees-mental-well-being.aspx

Harvey, D. (2005). *A brief history of neoliberalism*. Oxford University Press.

Harvey, D. (2019, April 19). Anti- capitalist politics in the time of COVID-19." *Jacobin Magazine*. https://jacobinmag.com/2020/03/david-harvey-coronavirus-political-economy-disruptions/

Hartwell, M. (2005). *A history of the Mont Pelerine Society*. Liberty Fund.

Hayek, F. (1944). *The road to serfdom*. University of Chicago Press.

Horsley, S. (2020, May 4). Many Americans are still waiting for relief checks from the federal government. *NPR News*. https://www.npr.org/2020/05/04/850195207/americans-are-still-waiting-for relief-checks-from-the-federal-government

Hoskin, M. (2020, April 25). The Whiteness of anti-lockdown protests. *Vox*. https://www.vox.com/first-person/2020/4/25/21234774/coronavirus-covid-19-protest-anti-lockdown

Iacurci, G. (2020, March 30). These workers won't qualify for beefed-up unemployment in the Coronavirus Relief Package. *CNBC News*. https://www.cnbc.com/2020/03/30/heres-who-wont-qualify-for-beefed-up-coronavirus-unemployment-relief.html

Isaković, N. (2020, March 23). What has COVID-19 taught us about neoliberalism? *Women's International League for Peace and Freedom*. https://www.wilpf.org/covid-19-what-has-covid-19-taught usabout-neoliberalism/

Jackson, A. (2020, April 1). Police are arresting and fining people for violating social distancing orders. *ABC News*. https://www.abc57.com/news/police-are-arresting-and-fining-people-for-violating-social-distancing-orders

Karpman, M., Zuckerman, S., & Gonzalez, D. (2018, August). *Material hardships among nonelderly adults and their families in 2017*. Urban Institute. ,https://www.urban.org/sites/default/files/publication/98918/material_hardship_among_nonelderly_adults_and_their_families_in_2017.pdf

Keay, D. (1987, September 23). *No such thing as society*. Margaret Thatcher Foundation. https://www.margaretthatcher.org/document/106689

Kendi, I. (2020, April 14). Stop blaming Black people for dying of the Coronavirus. *The Atlantic*.. https://www.theatlantic.com/ideas/archive/2020/04/race-and-blame/609946/

Kirby, T. (2020, May 8). Evidence mounts on the disproportionate effect of COVID-19 on ethnic minorities. *The Lancet*. https://www.thelancet.com/journals/lanres/article/PIIS2213-2600(20)30228-9/fulltext

Klein, N. (2007). *The shock doctrine: The rise of disaster capitalism*. Henry Holt and Company.

Krogstad, J., Gonzalez-Barrera, A., & Noe-Bustamante, L. (2020, April 3). *U.S. Latinos among hardest hit by pay cuts, job losses due to coronavirus*. Pew Research Center. https://www.pewresearch.org/fact-tank/2020/04/03/u-s-latinos-among-hardest-hit-by-pay-cuts-job-losses-due-to-coronavirus/

Layne, R. (2019, May 1). 40 million Americans struggle to put food on the table. *CBS News*. https://www.cbsnews.com/news/food-insecurity-americans-still-go-hungry-after-a-decade-of-recovery/

Leigh, D. (2020, April 3). Coronavirus news: States forced into bidding wars for PPE. *ABC News*. https://abc7ny.com/ppe-personal-protective-equipment-coronavirus-new-york-ventilators/6073977/

Lent, J. (2020, April 12). Coronavirus spells the end of the neoliberal era. What's next?" *Open Democracy*. https://www.opendemocracy.net/en/transformation/coronavirus-spells-the-end-of-the-neoliberal-era-whats-next/

Miller, H. (2020, May 12). Navajo Nation now has more known COVID-19 cases per capita than any state. *The Huffington Post*. https://www.huffpost.com/entry/navajo-nation-most-coronavirus cases-per-capita_n_5eb932dac5b6f4fbe30599d5?guccounter=1

Morales, M., & Joseph, E. (2020, May 9). Blacks and Latinos are overwhelmingly ticketed by NYPD for social distancing violations. *CNN*. https://www.cnn.com/2020/05/08/us/social-distancing-stats-nyc/index.html

Morath, E. (2020, April 28). Coronavirus relief often pays workers more than work. *The Wall Street Journal*. https://www.wsj.com/articles/coronavirus-relief-often-pays-workers-more-than-work-11588066200

Mudde, C. (2020, April 21). The 'anti-lockdown' protests are about more than just quarantines. *The Guardian*. https://www.theguardian.com/us-news/commentisfree/2020/apr/21/anti-lockdown-protests-trump-right-wing

Nania, R. (2020, May 8). *Blacks, Hispanics hit harder by the coronavirus, early U.S. data show*. American Association of Retired Persons. https://www.aarp.org/health/conditions-treatments/info 2020/minority-communities-covid-19.html

Pew Research Center. (2020, April 14). Health concerns from COVID-19 much higher among Hispanics and Blacks than Whites. https://www.pewresearch.org/fact-tank/2020/05/05/financial-and-health-impacts-of-covid-19-vary-widely-by-race-and-ethnicity/

Powder, J. (2020, April 9). Surge of gun sales amid COVID-19 worries experts. *Johns Hopkins Bloomberg School of Public Safety*. https://www.jhsph.edu/covid-19/articles/gun-sales-surge-amid-coronavirus-anxiety.html

Reich, R. (2007). *Super-capitalism: The transformation of business, democracy, and everyday life*. Vintage Press.

Reiley, L. (2020, April 14). The industry says we have enough food. Here's why some store shelves are empty anyway. *The Washington Post*. https://www.washingtonpost.com/business/2020/04/14/grocery-stores-empty-shelves-shortage/

Romm, T. (2020, May 28). Americans have filed more than 40 million jobless claims in past 10 weeks, as another 2.1 million filed for benefits last week. *Washington Post*. https://www.washingtonpost.com/business/2020/05/28/unemployment-claims-coronavirus/

Rosenthal, E. (2020, May 6). We knew the coronavirus was coming, yet we failed. *The New York Times*. https://www.nytimes.com/2020/05/06/opinion/coronavirus-health-care-market.html

Shear, M., Goodnough, A., Kaplan, S., Fink, S. Thomas, K., & Weiland, N. (2020, March 28). The lost month: How a failure to test blinded the U,S to COVID-19. *The New York Times*. https://www.nytimes.com/2020/03/28/us/testing-coronavirus-pandemic.html

Smith, H. (2021). *Who stole the American Dream*? Random House.

Smith. K. (2020, March 18). Working moms among the hardest hit by coronavirus pandemic. *CBS News*. https://www.cbsnews.com/news/working-moms-among-hardest-hit-coronavirus-pandemic/

Standing, G. (2014). *The precariat: The new dangerous class*. Bloomsburg Academic.

Steger, M., & Roy, R. (2020). *Neoliberalism: A very short introduction*. Oxford University Press.

The State of Homelessness in America. (2019, September). *The Council of Economic Advisers Executive Office of the President of the United States*. https://www.whitehouse.gov/wp-content/uploads/2019/09/The-State-of-Homelessness-in-America.pdf

Van Dam, A. (2020, April 30). Crisis begins to hit professional and public-sector jobs once considered safe. *The Washington Post*. https://www.washingtonpost.com/business/2020/04/30/jobless-claims-industry/

Ward, A. (2020, May 29). Trump announced US withdrawal from the WHO. *Vox*. https://www.vox.com/2020/5/29/21274949/coronavirus-trump-world-health-organization-withdraw

Wolf, C. (2020, May 26). Rick Scott, who gutted Florida's unemployment system, says coronavirus stimulus will pay low-wage workers too much. *Orlando Weekly*. https://www.orlandoweekly.com/Blogs/archives/2020/03/26/rick-scott-who-gutted-floridas-unemployment-system-says-coronavirus-stimulus-will-pay-low-wage-workers-too-much

CHAPTER 2

CONJURE, DIGITAL LIFE, AND SURVIVAL

Alecia Deon

INTRODUCTION: ON WHERE WE STAND

"Whatever it is, coronavirus has made the mighty kneel and brought the world to a halt as nothing else could. Our minds are still racing back and forth, longing for a return to normality, trying to stitch our future to our past, and refusing to acknowledge the rupture. But the rupture exists. And amid this terrible despair, it offers us a chance to rethink the doomsday machine we have built for ourselves. Nothing could be worse than a return to normality. Historically, pandemics have forced humans to break with the past and imagine their world anew. This one is no different. It is a portal, a gateway between one world and the next. We can choose to walk through it, dragging the carcasses of our prejudice and hatred, our avarice, our data banks, and dead ideas, our dead rivers, and smoky skies behind us. Or we can walk through lightly, with little luggage, ready to imagine another world. And ready to fight for it."

—Arundhati Roy (2020)

Coronavirus and Vulnerable People: Addressing the Divide in Harm and Responses and Exploring Implications for a More Peaceful World, pp. 27–48

This chapter is, first and foremost, a narrative of my life experiences—some I have had in the digital sphere—and sociopolitical commentary situated within academic frameworks that gird my understanding of systemic oppression and global White hegemony. It is this lens that enables me to explain, dissect, and integrate my experiences into the historical and contemporary national dialogue around vulnerability—particularly disability, race, and poverty—during the COVID-19 outbreak in the United States in early 2020. This is a narrative of resistance and truth as my digital life, due to accessibility, is highly influenced by what is first and foremost millennial Black, Indigenous, and People of Color (BIPOC) praxis defined, developed, and engaged with as an antithesis of the sociohistorical triad of oppression—imperialism, colonialism, the plantocracy—its neocolonial offspring, and all forms of governmental, institutional, inter-/intrapersonal reproduction of historical and systemic violence.

In the present neocolonial era, systems of oppression are deployed against the most vulnerable populations in myriad ways. For example, the United States government has policies that institutionalize poverty for people with disabilities. Protests and acts of resistance by its citizens are met unduly by militarized police forces relying on biometrics. Genetic material freely given by consumers to companies specializing in the genetic analysis may have been collected under false pretense as police forces across the country can now access these databases. Coupled with the prison industrial complex and the school-to-prison pipeline, young Indigenous, Black, and Latin youth are targeted. In lieu of establishing social programs and offering resources to the vulnerable to mitigate their need and the possibility of crimes that directly result, money is funneled to neo-imperial and colonial efforts, which require that military spending exceed every other country in the world. The expansion of military oversight comes first through the violation of treaties and sheer disregard for Indigenous life. Policies that criminalize the LGBTQ (lesbian, gay, bisexual, transgender, and queer) population and enforce the lack of access to reproductive health resources for women add to their vulnerability. These are a few among a host of many inter-related and complex forms of oppression. For many, this pandemic is just one more vulnerability added to the already extensive list of potential harm caused by class, race, gender, sexual expression/orientation, ability, or lack thereof.

To belong to any or multiple marginalized populations means survival is a lifestyle of resistance. COVID-19 takes place amid a sort of awakening within the realm of health and wellness spurred by millennial BIPOC, creating, and disseminating information via social media. This movement is characterized by the rejection of this oppressive triad by turning to conjure, which is what happens when "critical theory and decolonized imagination converge to deploy African-based spirituality as a praxis of healing, resistance, and self-preservation" (deon, 2019, pp. 143–148). Digital conjure is public reclamation of African traditional religions from the disparaging sentiments of White hegemonic Christianity. The most radical within this movement are calling for BIPOC to make daily efforts tantamount to divesting from this triad as they attempt to counteract and reverse the impact of systematically worsening conditions—mentally, emotionally, physically, and financially—for the most vulnerable deployed through violent means with technological and scientific precision. Collectively, this movement and my participation in it functions on the premise that all facets of wellness for BIPOC and other vulnerable populations worldwide are antithetical to the perpetuation of global White hegemony.

WHEN RACISM REFUSES TO BE OUTDONE: GLOBAL HISTORIES, THE ROOTS OF A NATION AND WEALTH

The pandemic has triggered the crumbling of what remains of democratic principles not already decimated by the Trump Administration and it mirrors a nation's downfall in many ways. As a student of history—mainly African and Black histories—I am wary of the disastrous impact on these populations worldwide and those whose experiences I share currently residing in the United States. The current climate speaks to possibilities others seem unaware of or are unwilling to accept as realities in the 21st century: world war, civil war, genocide, and the rise of the police-state. Due to policies enacted that are relevant to the last civil war, each state is responsible for implementing protective measures; from what I have noted, Southern states with larger Black populations see surges in death and people contracting COVID-19. "Racism, specifically, is the state-sanctioned or extralegal production and exploitation of group-differentiated vulnerability to premature death" (Gilmore, 2007, p. 28).

The implications of this happening in the South takes us back to the era of the plantocracy. Race, slavery, and capitalism provide the necessary context for understanding what is happening to the Black population. Suppose the statistics were to only focus on Black America. In that case, I am certain the numbers would reflect that of nations in the Global South, maybe only slight improvements due to the access that residing in a "first world" nation provides. There is nothing that happens in the United States beyond this complex lens of race, poverty, and the plantocracy. COVID-19 is no exception.

Imperialism, colonialism, and the plantocracy were a combined effort towards a dystopian future now deployed as neocolonialism. It is obvious to see that the COVID-19 crisis is sure to widen this chasm between rich and poor permanently. Greed and empire have always walked side-by-side.

U.S.-American nationalist sentiments rely heavily on rugged individualism, a concept not in or even possible in most cultures across this world. This way of life leaves the most vulnerable, even more isolated, and lessens the possibility of survival. The irony is that many BIPOC have been living in this dystopia, but the widespread impact on the White population might be the only reason there was a response at all. We had seen this before with Franklin D. Roosevelt's visit to Appalachia, where most poor White residents inspired the New Deal's implementation to provide relief to all.

In contrast, Black residents of the United States have remained in dire circumstances since their enslavement and the post-reconstruction era. Again, we see this with the drug epidemic of the 1980s and the utter decimation of many Black communities, resulting in the federal criminalization of drug use and an unprecedented rise in the prison population. Not until recently, with the discovery of a silent drug epidemic sweeping through communities of young, White people, are we taking a more accurate look at drug abuse not as a criminal offense but a mental health issue. A consideration never is given to Black Americans. In many ways like world history, the telling of United States history has shown the global White hegemony will inflict unwarranted violence on populations throughout the Global South with explicit intentions toward empire-building until those outbreaks of violence are inevitably visited upon the White populous (Césaire & Kelley, 2000). It is not a matter of if, but when. "The other then, is biotechnology for the definition, construction, and perpetuation of the complex hegemony. Whereby the dystopian terra-forming enterprise of the colonizer—imperialism, colonialism, and the plantocracy—specifies life itself as landscape, with an ever-present sign that boldly reads: whites only" (deon, 2019, pp. 144–148). As we see the astronomical rise of wealth for men like Elon Musk, Jeff Bezos, Bill Gates, and others, we can expand the sign to read "rich, white men only."

To witness these realities even more pronounced than before is a wake-up call for many. These experiences can be radicalizing, and even amid a global health crisis, the United States' history of virulent racism and wealth disparity cannot be buried. Breonna Taylor's and George Floyd's deaths at police officers' hands caused Black Lives Matter protests to erupt in the middle of a pandemic. Not just in the United States but in places like Germany. The worldwide protests I witnessed throughout 2019 arrived promptly at our door. U.S.-American racism will not be outdone, not even by a pandemic. This country's history tells us that race is a short fuse, always ready to be ignited. The United States is a landscape of trauma for BIPOC buried beneath White denial, guilt, and shame.

When reports began to acknowledge the seriousness of COVID-19, I felt as if I was standing still in the eye of a hurricane. The flurry of anxiety, fear, worry, and eventually annoyance as it became more apparent that the extreme precautions and rapid life-altering changes were to impact life in the United States and the world for some time to come. In early 2020 we watched as the coronavirus tear through populations like a tornado. Then we watched the majority of the U.S.-American populous feeling confused and anxious yet watching it take an insidious turn, ever so predictably, to buying guns. They had not taken to the streets to protest the government for the same reasons the rest of the populous eventually did. No, White Americans took to the streets to demand their rights to haircuts. There is somehow an endless undertone of privilege or possibly denial. Maybe both. Indeed, unfettered privilege leads to certain protection and security from the realities of this world. The fact is that I was prepared to count 2020 and 2021 as a loss when the virus reports first came out, and only two or three months in, many people decided that the precautions and staying home were just too much.

The sheer disregard for others is the worst permutation of an uneducated and undisciplined populous. Compared to the other "world powers," the United States seriously lags in education, health, and science. The reliance on the freedom narrative and the idea of independence has almost become a form of violence in the face of the COVID-19 outbreak, which will require collaborative thinking and behavior severely lacking in the U.S.-American populous. There are too many fractures in the consciousness of this population. Racism, poverty, the belief that it is perfectly normal to have certain people die—primarily the elderly and disabled—homophobia and transphobia, and sexism continue to make their presence known. The government's lack of action has further fractured this nation, and marginalized populations are seen as a drain on resources and unworthy of life.

There are minor whisperings in the media about the reality of living in a police state where protesters are being kidnapped and murdered. Now with the deployment of surveillance technologies, the fight becomes that much harder. In the age of social media and the desire to document everything, this turns out to be an ugly clash of cultural norms and state violence. Amidst the chaos, I wonder why more people are unwilling to call the United States response to the COVID-19 pandemic genocide? When other countries closed their borders and implemented multilayered strategies to serve and protect their citizenry, this government's lack of response sent a clear message to the vulnerable about who mattered and who did not. This message is not one we are unfamiliar with, but the widespread and tangible destruction is scarring. The decision to send children back to school and reopen college campuses is truly one of the more unforgivable aspects of this government's response. In the way of economic relief, some people received one $1,200 stimulus check, which—as I scrolled through comments on Twitter, I realized—helped stymie the descent into poverty for many. There are widespread layoffs while large corporations are going through an economic boom. Money and other resources are funneled into militarizing police forces while we are in the midst of an eviction crisis. No passports are being issued. Food inspections were halted at one point. Significant efforts to dismantle the United States Postal Service before the election is one more blow to the democratic ideals this nation holds yet never bothered to create as a reality for the most vulnerable. I happened across photography credited to Thomas J. O'Halloran from the Library of Congress of a young, Black girl being educated via television because Little Rock schools were closed to avoid integration. This photograph drove everything home for me. The fractures that I am watching widen are old and intended for the poorest, sickest, and most vulnerable of us to silently fall into and never find a way out. Sending children back to school, one $1,200 stimulus check that stymied many peoples' descent into poverty, the militarization of police forces across the country, halted food inspection, no passports being issued, and the dismantling of the United States Postal Service before the election, are among a whole host of other fractures spreading in the foundation intended for the poorest, sickest, and most vulnerable of us to fall into.

TRUTH AS A FORM OF CLOSURE FOR BIPOC: DIGITAL WELLNESS MOVEMENTS AND MENTAL HEALTH

Imperialism, colonialism, and the plantocracy was—and remains in their present permutations—about destruction from the inside out. Destruction in a place that is intangible and therefore offers no clear path to retribution. What is the value of culture and self-esteem? It is in these types of questions we find the answers that we seek. As a protest sign in Chicago read, "You've taken more than we could ever loot." Global White hegemony has indebted itself to the living, breathing descendants of their atrocities and the intangible. That does not spell freedom for them either. For whose psyche is built to celebrate the death and destruction of others while it remains unscathed? Every binary operates on an axis of power and the supposed right to destroy the other—the unforeseen, unacknowledged cost: its existence. We are dealing with a people and a culture that is sick, irreparably so.

Efforts made towards a future dystopia absent of feeling, emotion, intuition, and inner wisdom are the very foundations of global White hegemony. Through the purposeful destruction of the natural world and intentional deployment of the artificial, their power converges. This is a reality engineered to empower empire and neocolonial efforts to destroy the imagination, souls, cultural expressions, and histories of BIPOC. In response, one of our only and most powerful weapons is the truth and a sense of responsibility to future generations. We each have an obligation to each other to resist this destruction and to do so, we must remember what and who enabled our survival in the first place.

In many cultural and ethnic traditions of Africa, the griot is present in some way or another as a keeper of the people's souls. The memory. The origin. The mythology. The teachings. The music. The poetry. The griot was everything. They gave people grounding in the sense of themselves. In my time and in my roles, promises, and commitments to the populations I belong to, I conceptualized myself as a conjure woman. In many ways, I believe conjurers are the keeper of our souls and our histories, just the same as griots.

What do we do in the face of an uncaring and genocidal government? We have the histories of Africa, Latin America, and the Caribbean to remind us. We have the African and Black social and political discourse of the 1950s, an era of revolution that Malcolm X called "a tidal wave of color." We have conjured, which requires us to excavate our histories and requires us to tell the truth. We have the diaspora's ancestral practices and religious systems, a testament to cultural retentions and survival in the face of White violence. No matter how bad the realities in this country get, it will be hard to rival enslavement and the destruction of the Indigenous population. Sadly, we have been here before. And against all the odds, we survived. On the journey between this world, this reality, and the next, BIPOC has each other. Amid a rapidly changing cultural, social, political, and economic system, the increasing death, radical labor shifts, and accessibility spell permanent changes that will not be undone on the other side of this portal. The role of all affected by this government and even remotely invested in disrupting this system is to take on the responsibility for showing up for their communities in these digital spaces and, otherwise, to tell the truth.

CONJURE IN THE DIGITAL LANDSCAPE: CONTEMPORARY REIMAGININGS OF HISTORICAL REALITIES

For me, the conjure woman is a historical figure. An amalgamation of Africa and the Americas. She may very well be the reason that we survived life in the Americas. The role of the griot in African societies is significant. The griot was essentially a library of a people. The griot was the storyteller—the keeper of histories. The conjurers took on this role as African peoples were enslaved and dispersed throughout the Americas. It is a title and role I claim to honor my ancestors and to honor my history. In examining the roles we embody during times of crisis, Deepa Iyer (2020) conceptualized the following roles: storytellers, guides, weavers, experimenters, frontline responders, visionaries, builders, caregivers, disrupters, and healers.

In my work, using ancient methodologies and ways of knowing to bring emotional release, healing, closure, and forgiveness to BIPOC and other vulnerable populations, I am always forced to return to the root and to examine the environments which spurred the seed and allowed it to generate into the world we see around us. Suppose we are to do the same for this country. If we are to return to the root, we are quickly reminded that prosperity was taken from some and heaped into others' overfilled plates. Indeed, we have witnessed these institutions' chameleon-like tendencies firmly rooted in a diabolical past every couple of years or so covered over in a fresh coat of paint to obscure itself from responsibility and accountability.

> Those of us who are actively working to center ourselves are undergoing a painful process of divesting our humanity from the dystopian, terra-forming enterprise of the colonizer. We are wrestling—not with the pain of our contemporary experience—but with the historical traumas visited upon on ancestors in the construction of this world. (deon, 2019, pp. 144–148)

ANCESTRAL LIBERATION THEOLOGY

> "The romance is what we do with this horror, which is inescapable"
>
> —Césaire & Kelley (2000).

Ancestral liberation theology is all permutations of Black thought formulated within the African diaspora utilizing various means and mediums to conceptualize Black life and survival based on our ancestors' ideological formulations who lived and died in the Americas having survived the plantocracy. It is the very seed of Black existence buried within the unacknowledged ruins of the past. In the example, Toni Morrison's (1987) examination in her novel *Beloved* of Margaret Garner killed her children rather than enslaved them.

In these new roles and responsibilities, we must commit to this excavation of ourselves. The lives lived and lost in the ruins of an Indigenous people and the plantocracy to reformulate a reality not based on the negation of all that came before a colonial existence. Ancestral liberation theology then requires excavating the layers below modern life in the Americans and the Western world.

For BIPOC, this process of reclamation must incorporate storytelling, research, and community. We must be prepared to undergo a personal transformation on mental, emotional, physical, spiritual, and psychological levels. The crux of ancestral liberation theology will come through the admission and acceptance of the following truths: the system has and was designed to fail you and those like you, you must undergo a process of interrogation based on your identity, after which you must do an expansive interrogation beyond your identity that may implicate you and finally you must come to a place of reconciliation with self and others due to past ignorance and possible harm caused.

Ancestral liberation theology will remind the vulnerable that life is not paradoxical to our existence, neither race, nationality, gender, gender expression or orientation, ability, or any other part of our identity. Every form of resistance undertaken by our ancestors and presently rests firmly on this understanding. Conjure and ancestral liberation theology allows us to regain and reassert this is a reclamation of wellness.

CONCLUSION: A POETICS OF HOMAGE

"Poetic knowledge is born in the great silence of scientific knowledge."

—Aimé Césaire (2000).

Our histories and contemporary realities speak to a transformation so varied from that of the past that it looks unfamiliar to those who have not survived the same journey or lived the same life. When our ancestors were put below the decks of slave ships and forced to journey through the ugly underbelly of the Atlantic, they came to regard each other as family. The journey formed for them an unbreakable kinship bond. They were no longer African and certainly not American. The children of the diaspora lived and survived in an underbelly, not unlike this portal. The memory of their home and the ways of their homeland never left them in the face of the unspeakable. They comingled in a dance of fear, uncertainty, and unceasing death. Even though the slave ships had stopped, we discovered that there is no liberation in this place. So, we draw a line between ourselves and shrill insanity. That line is magic, healing, and loving care for each other. It is orisha, candles, and conjure. It is a belief. It is a culture. It is undying but barely hanging on. It is music. It is a dance. It is poetry. It is a responsibility. It is Staceyann Chin. Toni Morrison. James Baldwin. Nikki Giovanni. Angela Davis. Audre Lorde. It is a genius. It is innovation. It is Divine. It is unshakeable. It is power. It is Spirit. Not the story they tell us but the ones we tell each other. From the underbelly, which bore the modern world and its iterations of death and mounting, violent aspirational greed, we make a simple plea to each other to rest. To resist. In our most ancient traditions. The conjurer brought forth life, laid the well-lived to rest, and narrated the story in the time between time.

The disenfranchisement taking place on a large scale has to build on policies that institute vulnerability through lack of access, denial of necessary resources, and the criminalization of those in need. I have developed many friendships in the digital sphere in the process of speaking to these socio-historical realities of race, disability, and poverty or through aiding those in need. I mostly dedicate this chapter to them because we are collectively an array of the impact of vulnerability under "normal" circumstances. In many cases, this is a reality we have known well. Even when I attempt to comfort myself by saying I am used to living under extreme circumstances, this pandemic has so exacerbated my health and finances and forces me to make some uncomfortable and potentially damning decisions. Maybe no harder than before, but the danger of this new context is frightening. Amid this crisis, my friends Se' mana and Alexis had their son taken to a youth facility where he contracted COVID-19. In the art featured here, they express the pain and sorrow of their vulnerabilities as a parent of autistic Black and Native teens boys. In so doing, they truly captured the healing intention of Ancestral Liberation Theology and the need to speak our truths (Thompson, 2020). So in remembrance of the often forgotten, I dedicate this chapter to Oluwatoyin Salau. To my friends Se' mana and Alexis surviving these extraordinary circumstances. To all the healers and conjurers finding their power in this portal. In your honor, I forced these truths unwilling from my body.

A NEW BIRTH: SUMMER 2021 UPDATE

Today, I was gifted a copy of *Mouths of Rain: An Anthology of Black Lesbian Thought* (Jones, 2021) by a stranger with whom I might share aspects of my identity. The Blackness and the queerness. Wringing out the unnecessary and owning the reality of various hells I have found myself in due to those various identities has shaped me profoundly. None like disability and none like queerness. While every relationship I have had has at some point faltered and maybe failed to regenerate, and when I frantically searched for answers, I saw my fragilities staring back at me. I revel in them, nonetheless. I carry them and they look to be secrets until someone I have loved brushes up against my vulnerabilities and mistakes them for thorns.

In the past year I have discovered that I am too tired to pretend. While I was terrified of having to go to the emergency room or live within close quarters with someone who had contracted COVID-19, I was faced with a fact that had always been reality: the relationships I had did not factor in my vulnerabilities with care, but they formed around some version of me that everyone else was comfortable with. Needless to say, once I stopped pretending, these friendships died. It was not just the fact that people lacked empathy or thoughtfulness; sometimes they were downright mean.

When people see disability as weakness it is ironically threatening. They have to face their own mortality and the reality that nothing is certain. Living through a little over a year of COVID-19 meant in some ways watching my vulnerabilities become everyone else's as well, now. The caution and care went out the window rather quickly after people got bored. I wish I could do the same without consequences. But after three decades of frequent pain episodes destroying my tissues and organs, medical abuse, racist providers, neglectful caregivers, inaccessible services, and poverty, I know better than to take the risk. I am on the list of people that it is permissible to let die. And I get that message too often for comfort, even from people who love me. These are hard pills to swallow, all around. But I am alive. A miracle in itself. This has been a wakeup call in a lot of ways. Ways I was not ready for, but it forced me to stop lying by omission, pretending I am alright being neurodivergent and disabled in this society or in my family or circle of friends.

This portal has resulted from a number of stressors on fragile fault lines. The vulnerabilities we wrestled with beforehand inched us closer and closer to death over the past year. As we crossed the half million mark of deaths, many unacknowledged, unmourned, and unremembered, I was reminded of why I stand so firmly in my spi[ritual] practice. I think about the misinformation and confusion, the triggers, the sheer chaos engineered by people who do not have to cope with surviving realities they construct. This is fixed, sewn into the very fabric of this nation and it is soul crushing and soul stealing.

Conjure is a patchwork of techniques that keep me from falling in. It requires an honest assessment and acknowledgement of the social value of my life and demands that I push past it. It is a reminded that my value is inherent and not earned through labor in the communal construction of empire, exchanged for the price of my soul. I am tasked with honoring my ancestors and remembering those passed from this life knowing that energy is not destroyed.

In the foreword of *Mouths of Rain* (Jones, 2021), Cheryl Clarke references alexis pauline gumbs, who defined survival as "living in the context of what we have overcome," I wonder if the people forced to accept life as a digital reality this COVID year would still say digital life is not real. It is the only thing that sustained many people this past year, as it has done for disabled people and many others for some time pre-pandemic. When I needed help getting to the emergency room and could not ask my own family, it was my digital family that put together $50 so I could Uber instead of having to drive medicated and in pain, as I had done many times before. It is a running joke among millennials that we would live Tweet the end of the world. In some ways, we held to that promise. Digital fundraising and other forms of mutual aid took the place of healthcare and the government's responsibility for the wellness of its people. I dare anyone to say digital life is not real life when for decades it has been my responsibility for my own survival.

I titled this chapter "Conjure, Digital Life and Survival" partially because I could not bear to tell my whole truth. So, I told the theory. I told about the framework that helped me survive in order to avoid saying what it was I survived and was still surviving. In the time between initially writing this and now, I am profoundly changed. For the better. I can no longer pretend for the benefit of the people around me and to the detriment of myself. It is odd to say that this experience brought me to life and *Mouths of Rain* filled my lungs.

REFERENCES

Césaire, A., & Kelley. K. (2000). *Discourse on colonialism: A poetics of anticolonialism* (Joan Pinkham, Trans.). New York University Press.

deon, a. (2019). Between the worlds of the colonizer and the conjure woman. *QED: Journal in GLBTQ Worldmaking, 6*(3), 143–148.

Gilmore, R. (2007). *Golden gulag: Prisons, surplus, crisis, and opposition in globalizing California.* University of California Press.

Iyer, D. (2020, March 27). Mapping our social change roles in times of crisis. *Medium.* https://medium.com/@dviyer/mapping-our-social-change-roles-in-times-of-crisis-8bbe71a8ab01

Jone, B. S. (2021). *Mouths of rain: An anthology of Black lesbian thought.* The New Press.

Morrison, T. (1987). *Beloved.* Vintage.

Roy, A. (2020, April 3). The pandemic is a portal. *Financial Times. https://www.ft.com/content/10d8f5e8-74eb-11ea-95fe-fcd274e920ca*

Thompson, S. (2020, August 1). *School-to-prison pipeline: Disabled Black Indigenous boys in the time of Covid-19.*https://www.raisingmothers.com/school-to-prison-pipeline-disabled-black-indigenous-boys-in-the-time-of-covid-19-semana-thompson/

APPENDIX

BIA School

School resource officer waiting for you, watching you.

88 cameras for 300 K through 8.

Zero tolerance for you little black boy. They don't

care you are 10 years old, 12 years old. They wait for you
outside your house gate and drive through your community
searching for little black boys in maroon collared shirts.

Locked up in jail? Doesn't matter, you still missed 10
days of school so goodbye to you. In psychiatric
care? Doesn't matter, you signed an agreement so now
you cannot come back this year. Wait until next year when
covid-19 catches you little black boy. It can
catch you again if it wants to. BIE don't care.

Do not worry, little man. Their eyes are watching you.

—Se' mana Thompson (2020), "BIE School"

Artist Statement: I wrote BIA (Bureau of Indian Affairs) School (a haiku—a form of poetry created by Julia Mallory) while my youngest son, 11 years old, and oldest son, 13 years old, were in foster care and a youth facility during COVID-19. The series "Disabled Black Indigenous Boys in the System in the Time of COVID-19" (Thompson, 2020) is about my children's experience, every image, every collage carefully made to depict their lives up to this point in time (see Figures A.1–A.17). The poem and art reflect the reality of not only Bureau of Indian Education schools, particularly within our indigenous community, but also charter and public schools outside of our community my children have attended since kindergarten. As Black Indigenous children—disabled autistic boys —they have been surveilled, threatened, and experienced violence by the carceral state: police (city and tribal), detectives, social services (on and off the reservation), tribal court, juvenile probation, school resource officers, children's psychiatric hospital, group home, juvenile detention, a youth facility, and foster care. Their disabilities, in particular autism, attention-deficit/hyperactivity disorder, and other mood disorders, and their Blackness, their Indigenousness has been criminalized; their very humanity seen as problematic, and as Frank B. Wilderson III stated (in an interview with Tiffany Lethabo King): "Incarceration and captivity for Latinos, Asians, and Muslims is a function of a historic experience; but captivity is a constituent element of Black life."

Figure A.1

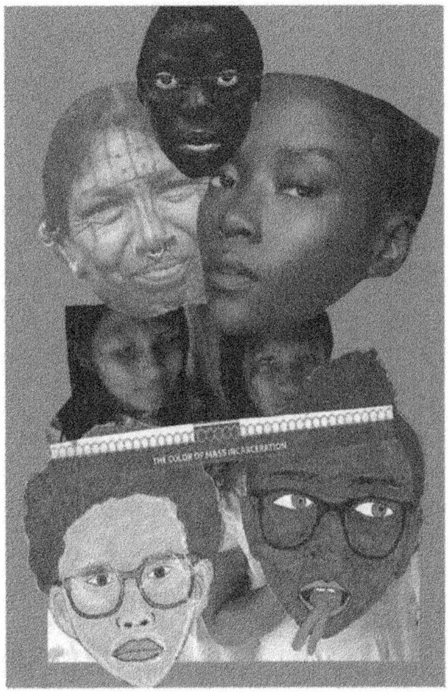
THE COLOR OF MASS INCARCERATION

Figure A.2

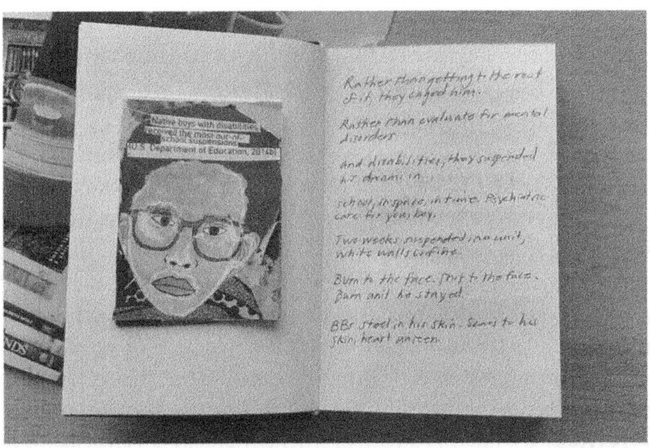
Native boys with disabilities
received the most out-of-school suspensions
U.S. Department of Education, 2014b
Rather than evaluate for mental disorders
Two weeks suspended in a unit, white walls confine.

Figure A.3

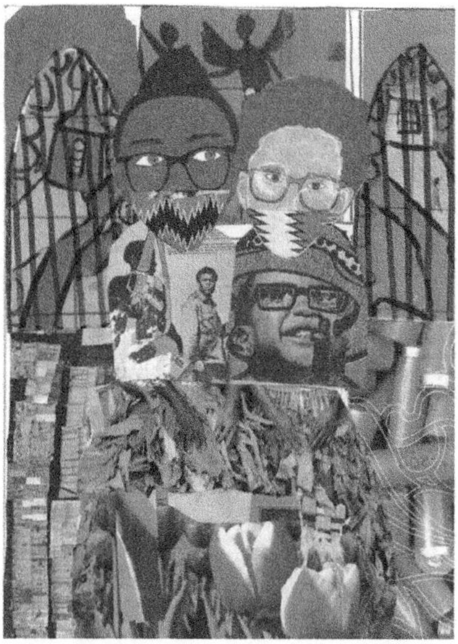

Figure A.4

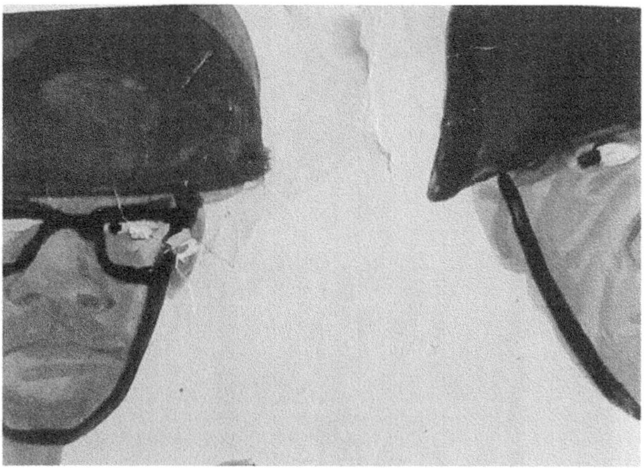

Figure A.5

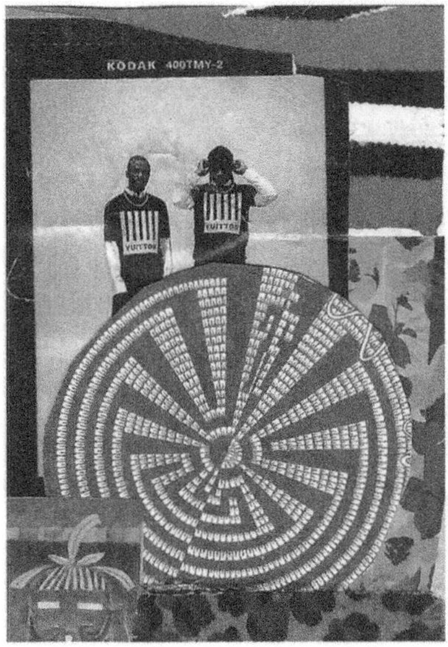
KODAK 400TMY-2

Figure A.6

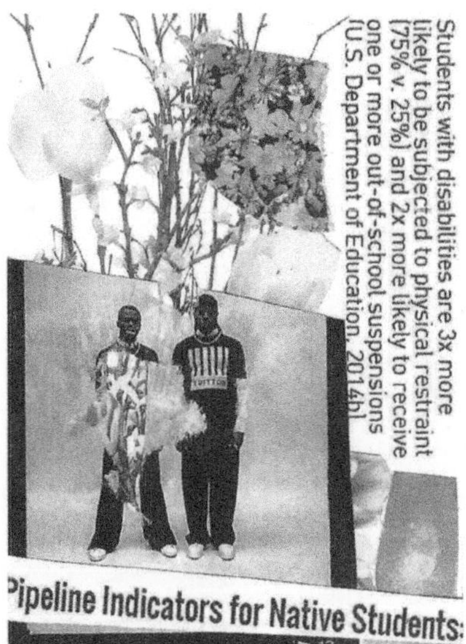
Students with disabilities are 3x more likely to be subjected to physical restraint (75% v. 25%) and 2x more likely to receive one or more out-of-school suspensions (U.S. Department of Education, 2014b)
Pipeline Indicators for Native Students:

Figure A.7

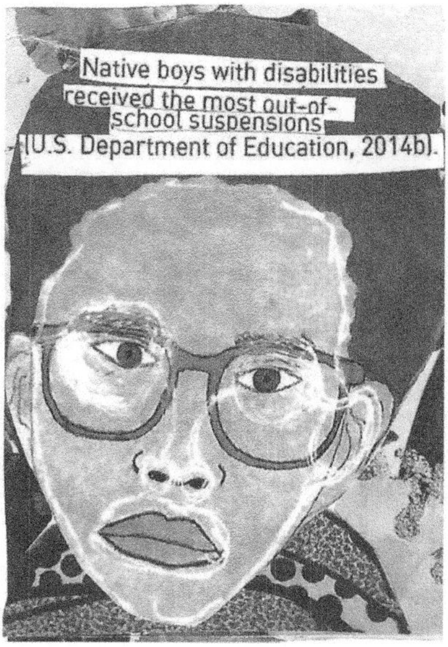
Native boys with disabilities
received the most out-of-
school suspensions
(U.S. Department of Education, 2014b).

Figure A.8

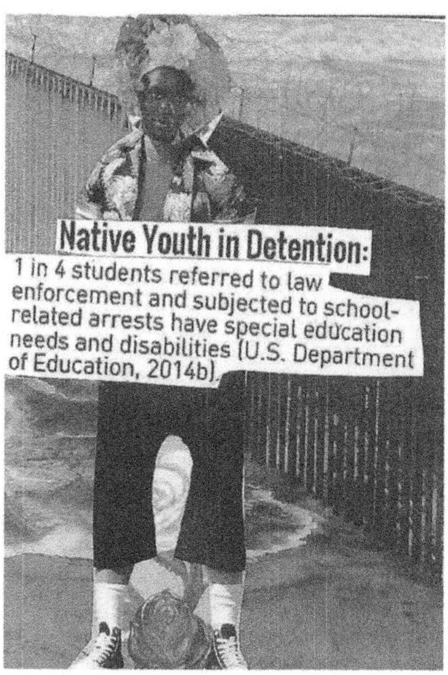
Native Youth in Detention:
1 in 4 students referred to law
enforcement and subjected to school-
related arrests have special education
needs and disabilities (U.S. Department
of Education, 2014b).

Figure A.9

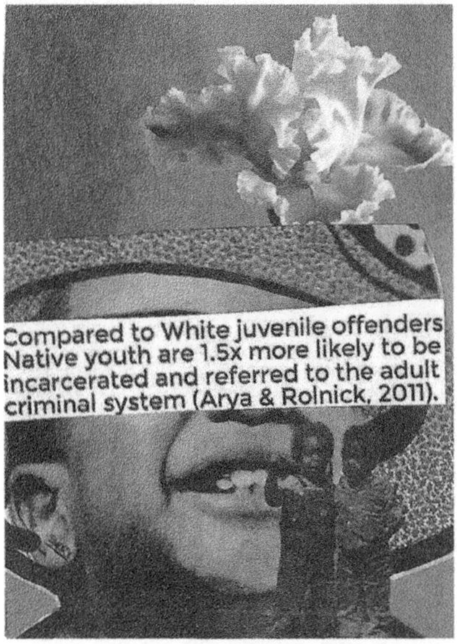

Figure A.10

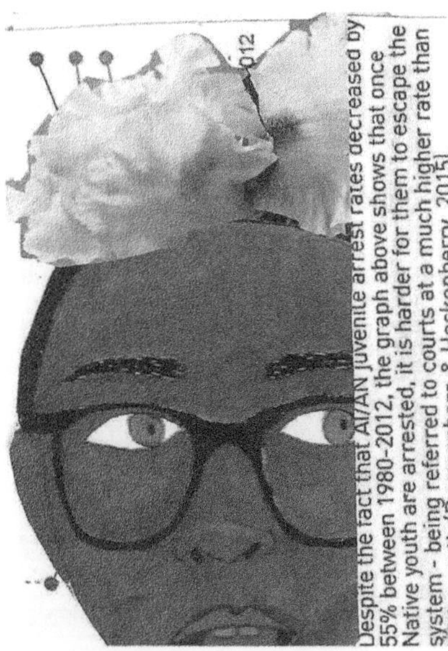
Despite the fact that AI/AN juvenile arrest rates decreased by
55% between 1980-2012, the graph above shows that once
Native youth are arrested, it is harder for them to escape the
system - being referred to courts at a much higher rate than
White youth (Puzzanchera & Hockenberry, 2015).

Figure A.11

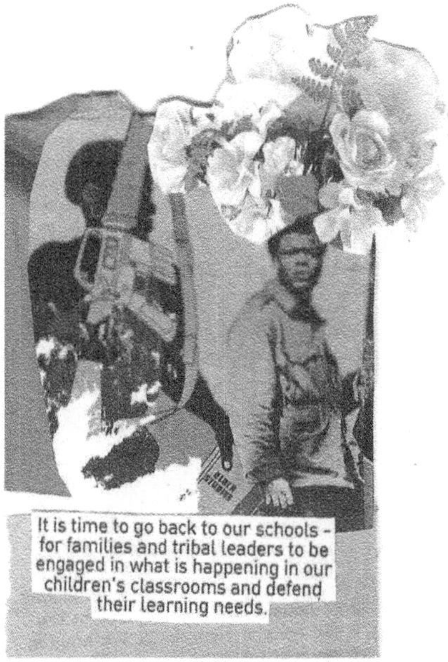
It is time to go back to our schools - for families and tribal leaders to be engaged in what is happening in our children's classrooms and defend their learning needs.

Figure A.12

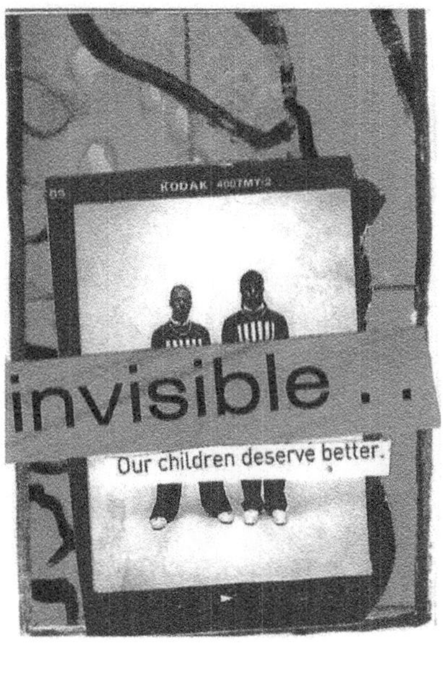
KODAK
invisible . .
Our children deserve better.

Figure A.13

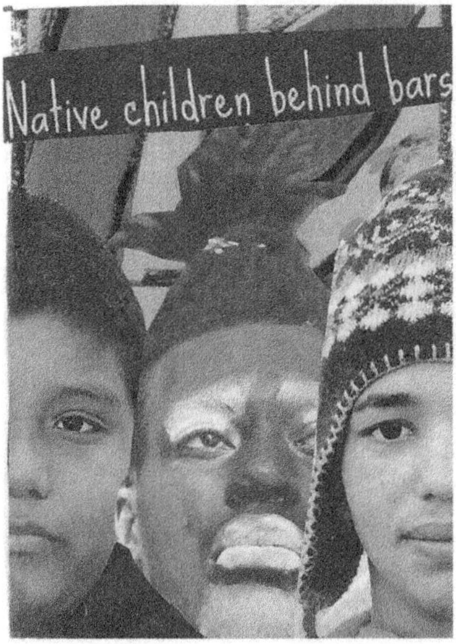

Figure A.14

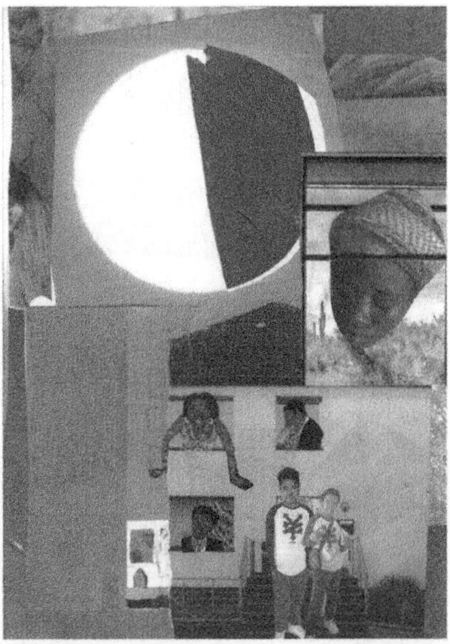

Figure A.15

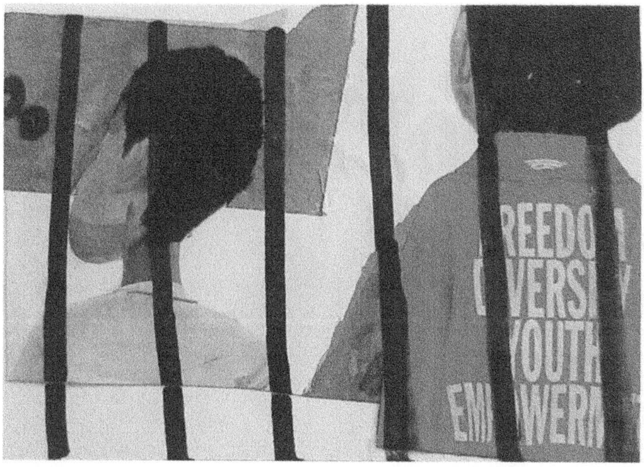

Figure A.16

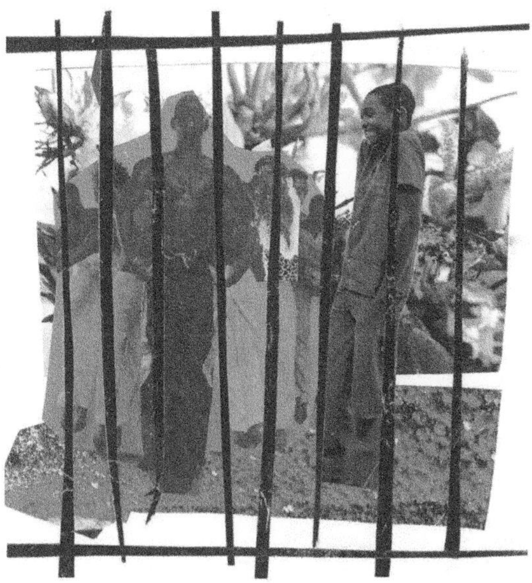

Figure A.17

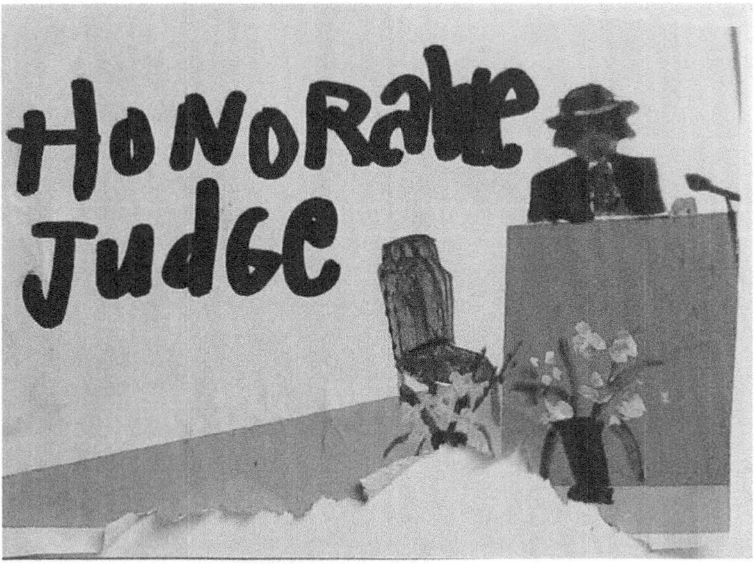

CHAPTER 3

REMEMBERING OUR POWER AND RIGHTFUL POSITION TO TRANSFORM OUR PRESENT REALITY AND ENJOY PEACE

Johanna Thompson

This chapter focuses on the intergenerational wisdom and leadership of Women of Color labeled Black through stories of resilience and resistance, mutual aid, quotes, art, activism, and organizing during this global crisis and prophesied transformation. These excerpts will provide examples of a "structural reformation" fueled by Women of Color who are labeled Black.

The coronavirus pandemic has impacted our lives in ways that we could not have imagined in our wildest dreams. In a moment, we found ourselves experiencing the greatest crisis and transformation of this lifetime. The most notable transformation is the intergenerational impacts on women and girls of color, specifically those labeled Black. The specific focus on intergenerational effects should be considered in light of the fact that COVID-19 forces the global community to face both the reality of privilege and its staunch inequities.

If we think about "privilege" as the ability not to consider or even think about something, the common societal ideology pre-coronavirus was of

Coronavirus and Vulnerable People: Addressing the Divide in Harm and Responses and Exploring Implications for a More Peaceful World, pp. 49–63

no conception that our lives would be forever altered instantaneously, it is magic, really. The reality challenges the age-old notion that *things are just the way they are and cannot change*. This pandemic demonstrates that there can be a structural reformation that shifts the inequities experienced by women and girls labeled Black and women of color daily. We recognize these inequities as hetero-patriarchal conditions, institutional racism, and capitalistic priorities that intentionally separate women of color from our humanity and history rooted in the feminine divine principles. At this moment, we have the opportunity to restore those principles with our collective power, beginning with what we believe and where we place value. Familiar rhetoric suggests that we start to reimagine the future we want; I offer an alternative thought, "*let us remember our power and rightful position to transform our present reality and enjoy peace.*"

The systems of oppression that fuel the persistent inequities previously mentioned, specifically impacting women of color, are exacerbated in this pandemic by the intentional isolation of people from one another. Women of Color labeled Black experience distinct impacts due to schools closing across the nation, as mothers struggle to find child-care while remaining in the responsibility of essential workers. Others have to relocate without planning because of financial and housing instability. Many people grapple with the loss of income and food insecurity. There are increased reports of violent shelter-in environments, relationship challenges, and shifts in familial responsibilities. Not to mention the disproportionate gaps in access to technological necessities, health disparities, greater risk, death, and the mere uncertainty of it all. Studies like that of the adverse childhood experiences (ACEs) suggest that traumatic adverse experiences have lasting effects that impact public health. Those effects span across generations. In an article published in *The Journal of Pediatrics* in July 2020, Dr. Lee Sanders asserts, "There are several ways in which the social isolation may exacerbate ACEs, job loss, school closures, and other stressors unleashed by the pandemic" (Sanders, 2020, p. 222).These adverse experiences can be defined as collective violence on our human welfare, creating a generation of *violence impacted people* (VIPs), a term I have coined to represent the interconnectedness of the ecosystem of violence to which we all have entry points. We, VIPs, will increasingly seek practices that help us heal the violence to obtain peace. Inherent in the intergenerational resilience and resistance of women of color are the keys to those practices, our ability to take pause and reflect on our lives, quickly respond, and adjust to the uncertainty of it all, immediately develop innovative systems of mutual aid, and collectively remember the vast possibilities of our future which will inevitably be different. We must practice our magic in ways that support our ability to thrive.

We are collectively experiencing the impacts of this transformation together. We must continue to share our wisdom and leadership to ensure that women of color remain visible. Women of color make up the vast majority of essential workers, providing caregiving, guidance, and protection consistent with contributions since the dawn of human existence. Women of color continue to embrace community-care techniques and cultural healing practices that lend to our resilience and resistance. We have always been an integral part of what the next iteration of human existence will look like. Our future will depend on what we remember and how we choose to lead.

At the end of 2019, I was privileged to visit Africa's continent, landing in Egypt. My travels began at The Giza Plateau and Djoser, flying down to Aswan in Upper Egypt, then leisurely journeying up the Nile visiting other sacred sites along the way. I visited nine of the Temples (Pyramids) during this first trip led by a Khemetic scholar, La Doctora, from the Khemetic School of Ancient Mysticism. The journey was transformative in my understanding of societal norms, as I witnessed ancient writings and stories etched onto the walls. Many of the people I met spoke of the transformation, the impending transition from darkness to light. We participated in many intellectual activations regarding what the age of Kheper, the winged scarab, would usher into existence. The story prophesied the transition from opposing dualities into interconnectedness, the rise of the feminine divine balancing the masculine, lifting the spell of currencia, and regeneration of a higher frequency that brings forth the peace of new beginnings. The story did not prophesy what this transition would look like or how we would experience it. However, it did prepare me to look past the pain of the losses and the unknown resulting from our pandemic to the jewels and gems that would carry us through as part of a more significant transformation. This is where the sharing begins.

Let us remember that ancient wisdom shares knowledge about a cycle of five stages of *being* represented on the Tree of Life, also referred to as the sacred Ished Tree, Persea, Lebbek, Tamarisk, Acacia, and Sycamore. The Tree of Life holds symbolic potency across many beliefs. The Egyptian story is that the Tree of Life symbolizes the Divine Plan's knowledge, which maps our destiny through a cycle of being and time. I came across this widely duplicated papyrus of the sacred tree throughout my travels, with five birds perched on branches in a circle formation. The five birds, most notably the Bennu Bird (the Phoenix), represent five stages signifying birth, childhood, youth, adulthood, and death within the cycle of life or being. Within the cycle of time, the stages represent light, the Sun's rising in the east, morning, midday, evening, and the Sun's setting in the west, darkness. Each bird grows progressively larger with each phase of being. Every soul is believed to gain significance and purpose. The Tree of Life bears the fruit of knowledge that is ready to be harvested at each stage of being. Facing east is considered the direction of life because the sun rises in the east, and facing west is regarded as the direction of death, or entering the underworld, because of the sun setting in the west. On the Tree of Life, the birds represent the first four phases of being and daylight time all face to the east; however, the bird representing death and darkness faces the west. La Doctora shared the stages as Kheper, Ra, Um/On, Atum, Amun. Kheper, the winged scarab, represents coming into being. Ra, the falcon, represents one who is rising high. Um/On represents either opening of the mouth, dividing or splitting, or full being at the sacred place of the sun. Atum represents one who is setting, and Amun is returning into the darkness. Egyptians speak of each transition period being every 500 years, and we have been in the cycle of Amun, darkness. We are currently transitioning into Kheper, coming into being, the renewal of life. The year 2020 has been full of transformations, and through it all, women of color have come into being visible and sharing our collective wisdom.

KHEPER/BIRTH/LIGHT

A Caribbean-American Fanmsaj (midwife)—birthing:

> With everything going on, the treasures of nature still exist.

When I think of the treasures of nature, I think of the birth of my two daughters. There was no experience more powerfully magical and exhaustive than growing them in my womb, birthing them forth out of my body, sustaining and protecting them as they grow and come into being. I am not the type of person who glorifies pregnancy and the birthing process as a beautiful experience. I intentionally chose diction that would capture the experience in its totality. When I describe the life-giving process as powerfully magical, I express the "treasure of nature" in its perfectly imperfect functioning. Another life formed inside of my body, taking over complete control of my being. That developing life dictated how I felt, moved, slept, ate, and functioned. People would comment that I was glowing, and I would look at them like they were crazy. All I wanted to do was sleep. Despite feeling like a human host, I felt unstoppable when it was time to deliver my firstborn. My second birth was a more tragic experience since my child was eager to come into being two months early. I spent 30 days in the hospital before the birth. On that 30th day, nature decided to exercise its power with Hurricane Katrina and my second born. I was rushed to the emergency room, where my child was cut out of me, resulting in stapling me back together while my child was whipped away to receive intensive care. I remember writing a poem to capture the story. Regardless of how they arrived, they were my creations, "my treasures of nature," my peace.

The treasures of nature also exist, playing a significant role in creating scientific and faith-based stories. As elucidated by Fayza Haikal of The American University in Cairo on the American Research Center in Egypt website:

> The origin story of how Ra spawned all that is known is both fascinating and illuminating:
>
> According to Egyptian mythology, before creation, only Darkness embraced the Primeval Ocean (Nun), out of which life would come. When the breath of life was strong and ready, the entity called Atum decided it was time for Creation to begin. An island emerged from the water to support this divinity, who manifested itself in the form of Ra, the sun god of Egypt.
>
> On a Primeval hill, Ra created out of himself the first gods, Shu (Dryness and Air), and his partner Tefnut (Humidity), who would engender other gods to complete the Cosmos: Geb the Earth god, and Nut the Sky goddess. In turn, these two birthed the Principles of life, namely Osiris, the Perfect Being, who eventually would rule over the rest of the world—which Ra was busy creating by naming the elements. And by the way, humankind happened out of the tears of his eyes.
>
> Osiris was a kind and wise ruler who taught humans agriculture and civilization. With his sister/wife Isis, who helped her husband with creativity and magic, they formed the perfect couple. Their brother Seth was strong but unruly, the opposite of his brother. In fact, Seth envied Osiris so much that he killed him to inherit his throne and rule Egypt the way he wanted. Seth's sister/ partner, Nephthys, could not stop the murder despite her love for their siblings.
>
> Killing Osiris turned out not such a bad idea. He was resurrected through his wife's magic long enough to impregnate her with son Horus, who would later avenge his father and recapture the throne of Egypt. Then Osiris departed to the Otherworld to rule over the deceased, thus ensuring resurrection and the cycle of life.

Similarly, scientific theories of abiogenesis, the natural process of the origins of life evolving from nonliving matter, explains the creation story beginning with nature. The details of abiogenesis continue to be researched. However, the prevailing scientific thought is that the transition from the nonliving to living, or *being*, arose from the waters occurring over time in an increasingly complex process. All creation stories have variation, and science is no different.

There are several primary theories for how abiogenesis occurred. In a *Nature Astronomy* article published in July of 2020, astronomers reported that carbon, an essential chemical element in the formation of *being*, is formed in the cosmos in white dwarf stars, which are the primary source of carbon in the milky way. The scientific community continues to conduct experiments to demonstrate how a volcanic gas, carbonyl sulfide (COS), may have been instrumental in the formation of peptides. It is speculated that this gas was likely present in the beginning. Since COS breaks down quickly in water, researchers propose that chains of amino acids formed on rocks near the COS source, supporting evidence for the theory that "*being*" began in underwater volcanic vents of thriving, self-contained ecosystems that still exist to this day. Like Atum in the ancient Egyptian creation story, those ecosystems regenerated to form the building blocks of living things.

Whether you identify with coming into being by experiencing the birthing process, believing the ancient Egyptian creation story, or scientific theories about the origin of life, the treasures of nature still exist and evolve. Despite "everything that's going on," this pandemic forces us to recognize how we are evolving as we live through this period of transition from *being* as we knew it to an elevated *being*. We are entering the age of the new beginning. We are coming forth, emerging out of the "primordial waters," being birthed into a rapidly advancing age of technology. Time appears to by rotating more quickly. People seem to be experiencing the powerfully magical and exhaustive birthing process. After it is complete, it will be good; there will be peace.

RA/CHILDHOOD/RISING SUN

A feminist, abolitionist revolutionary—spreading seeds of vision:

> We need to walk in the direction of Freedom.

What is the first thing that comes to mind when you hear the word freedom? As a person born in America and trained in history, I think about slavery. I know that slavery is not even a fraction of the story, but it is violence so impactful that the pain can still be felt presently. I visualize the most engaging YouTube clip (posted by Rumi, 2019) that I have ever viewed that captures the process of healing the pain of oppression and getting to peace when Nina Simone answers the question, "what's free to you?" She fidgets with her skirt and repeats the question back to the interviewer, "what's free to me? Same thing it is to you, you tell me?" She gives the interviewer the all too familiar quintessential side-eye and begins to laugh. It is one of those awkward moments when a person of privilege realizes that they have poked at the pain of oppression and the oppressed person has to search for healing grace to respond with patience.

The interviewer nervously laughs and begins to speak when Ms. Simone interrupts, saying,

> it's just a feeling, it's just a feeling, it's like how do you tell somebody how it feels to be in love? How will you tell anybody who has not been in love how it feels to be in love? You cannot do it to save your life, you can describe things, but you can't tell 'em, but you know it when it happens, that's what I mean by free.

Ms. Simone looks away and appears to be thinking about freedom, and when she is experienced freedom as a woman labeled Black raised in America. Ms. Simone recalls that she experienced freedom while performing. As if having an epiphany, Ms. Simone offers the interviewer this jewel of understanding,

> I'll tell you what freedom is to me, no fear! I mean, really, no fear. If I could have that (no fear), half of my life, (pause) no fear. Lot's children have no fear.... That's the closest way ... that's the only way I can describe it, that's not all of it, but it is really something to really, really feel.... Like a new way of seeing, like a new way of seeing something.

Nina Simone champions explaining freedom, like Isis putting back the pieces of Osiris and bringing him back to life. Ms. Simone recognizes and names aloud that children have no fear. We become seeded with societal norms that bind us in mental slavery during childhood until we unlearn and relearn how to live without fear on a path toward freedom and peace. As a person with Caribbean roots, I hear the lyrics of Bob Marley's (1979) "Redemption Song" repeating in my head, imparting knowledge to,

> Emancipate yourself from mental slavery/None, but our self can free our minds/Have no fear for atomic energy/'Cause none of them can stop the time/How long shall they kill our prophets/While we stand aside and look?/ Some say it's just a part of it/We've got to fulfill di book.

This pandemic, and the instantaneous shift away from life as we knew it, calls into question the notion that it is just a part of life that we have to fulfill. Art has always played a role in remembering and envisioning what the book should be filled with.

These legendary artists remind us of the role that art plays in directing us to "walk in the direction of freedom" towards peace. Nina Simone describes freedom as a feeling while inhaling and exhaling deeply as a heavy weight has just been lifted. During the same interview, she explains that she has felt that feeling on stage while performing her song's magical gift. Her expression of freedom resonates as deeply as the "Redemption Song" lyrics advising that we emancipate ourselves from mental slavery. Art is healing and laden with knowledge. The art of antiquity in Egypt felt like it was sharing all of the answers to achieving a harmonious balance.

Art challenges the social norms as a catalyst for change and provides an alternative way of thinking, being, imagining, and remembering to transform those social norms. Distinctly looking at historical, artistic influences, we can identify where art has been incorporated and used to create major shifts in society as pervasive and subliminal as, for example, during slavery.

There was an art to singing hymns and making patchwork quilts to send messages about actual physical freedom paths. Those songs and quilts also provided the necessary encouragement and comfort to begin the journey. During the 1960s, radio DJs played artists like Nina, Aretha, and Stevie, who incorporated revolutionary ideas into their lyrics to motivate people into action. DaVinci, Rembrandt, Warhol, and Freida Kahlo created art that sparked revolutionary shifts. Art stimulates us to think about, and challenge, how we are relating to one another. Every major cultural shift has needed to incorporate art to appeal to a mass of people. The united mass then becomes the power to disrupt, to use transformational language, to begin dialogues, to think. The pandemic is causing the need to create new language and ideas about how we will exist; the use of creativity helps us to evolve.

As demonstrated in the development of the institutions that we currently adhere to, the Temples of Egypt's artistry provides the foundation with which we derived much of our math and scientific information. We also realized the power of the pyramid's artistic attraction when using the triangular shape to create hierarchical systems and ideologies. The triangular shape did not represent a top-down, bottom-up value of social organization. The pyramid was built to be recognized from and connected to the heavens. If we use an aerial view of the pyramids rather than the limited earthly view, we can conceive an alternate social structure rooted in the foundation's strength, the four directions, the four elements, the interconnectedness. There was little mention of conflict as we know it in Egyptian sociology until Western civilization's influences began to be introduced.

Interestingly, concepts coming from the direction west, considered the direction of death and darkness, or lack of knowledge and light, are the seeds sown in childhood. Thankfully, art allows us to experience a "new way of seeing something." By incorporating art into how we are being, we are transforming and evolving our knowledge and understanding from becoming stagnant. If we did not employ art, we would risk subscribing to social norms and not transitioning to the next stages of the cycle where we return to facing east, the direction of life and light. Art has no fear. Art is a bold proclamation of vision and confidence. Art gives us concepts that expand the boundaries of generational knowledge. Art is the rising Sun on the horizon that points us in the direction to walk on a path toward freedom.

UM(ON)/YOUTH/MIDDAY

A multiethnic queer millennial—the complexities of life builds wisdom:

> Ask the Universe what is required of you and your gifts during this time and honor that and that alone. Let this incubation period birth a new world, a new normal, a new way of loving and being. Tend to the garden of self and see what blooms.

These words materialized as America received warnings that we would be entering quarantine. One of my daughters, not from my womb, made her usual distress call that she needed to keep working, secure child-care, and get a break from her two children. She knew that she could call on me to come to the rescue despite her hesitation. She would not want to hear my mouth rambling about this virus being real or they would not be quarantining us. She knew that my position would be that she should stop working so she would not be exposed. She also knew that I was not going to let her expose her children. These alarms were ringing from my lips during the period when rumors were running rampant that people labeled Black were immune to the virus and before the data revealed that we were dying at disproportionately high rates. Her children are my extended grand-children, and I am protective of all of them. I was willing to accept the labor of caring for my granddaughter, who just turned 2 years old, and my grandson, who was 2 months old. I was counting on the support of my 14-year-old daughter without really considering asking for her consent. It was late March, and we drove 30 minutes from our home, searching for the latest place they were residing. We navigated through unfamiliar streets until we arrived at the address. I spent the entire drive wondering how long it would be that they would end up being with us, especially if their mother did get infected. I chose to just put a smile on my face and crack jokes about the situation to lighten the mood. We packed their few belongings into the trunk of my car, and she informed me that I needed to get the basic necessities that she was unable to purchase, like pull-ups, diapers, and wipes.

As we pulled off, I thought of the reality of her situation, which could have been that much worse if she didn't have me to call on. I thought of the many women in her position who had no choice but to continue working despite infection warnings. I thought about the work she was doing to maintain financial stability, which was not the work of her actual gifts. I did not know about my capacity or the capacity of my 14-year-old daughter, nor did I think about how we were using, or not, our respective gifts. I did go into autopilot in the same way that I had observed so many mothers, sisters, aunties, cousins, and friends over the years during times when a need was presented. The collective gift, inherent in our magical nature, is the ability to create innovative support networks instantly. Hailing from our foremothers who made magic creating food for the soul, women in Mississippi created their own virtual health care system, and women in Miami dropped off care packages to youth participating in their programs so that they maintained a connection with the young people while beginning the practice of social distancing. Those examples are some of the collective gifts that we continue to give, which are as important as the personal gifts that we need to tend to.

Each of us was born with a gift to share with the world. Many of us have been going through the motion of life, having put those gifts aside so that we can put food on the table and take care of our loved ones, even before we can take care of ourselves. Since the beginning of our collective stories' timeline, the recurring story for women and girls labeled Black is that of caregiving as the number one priority. The more we provide for others, the more we are expected to provide, the less we can offer ourselves. The individual gifts we possess unintentionally get pushed further away from our grasp. When there is an opportunity or force of circumstance to stop, that is when we can step into our purpose. Our purpose is as ancient as Egypt's temples etched in the hieroglyphs depicting the feminine as creators and sustainers of life. We embody the essence of Ma'at each time we bring truth, balance, order, harmony, law, morality, and justice into all of the things we do. Ancient wisdom offers *heka,* the omniscient power, strength, or magic itself as the pathway. This is the untold story of our purpose and the power of the gifts of our magic. The Universe always delivers our good ... and our medicine. This coronavirus can be seen as both our good and our medicine if we are acknowledging our medicine as the lessons we need to learn to get to our good, and our good as the ability to "tend to the garden of self and see what blooms."

We can see the blossoming of women labeled Black, in real-time, with the use of technology and social media platforms allowing us to create and elevate our identities. Not only are identities elevated, but there is also the age-old trend of people looking to women of color for their wisdom and guidance. However, a woman of color makes up the second to last most disparate of demographics to be considered, as noted in Breonna Taylor's case. She was gunned down by police in her bed while sleeping, and the murderers have not been arrested. The global community continues to seek out women of color's leadership to provide solutions to address the loss of the lives of people labeled Black due to state violence manifested in health disparities and police brutality. Social media went black for a day at the request of women labeled Black. People benefitting from privilege participated in the #ShareTheMicNow campaign, which magnified "Black women and the important work they're doing to catalyze change."

As women of color and women labeled Black in particular are being magnified, I cannot help but beam at the manifesting prophecy of the rise of the feminine divine where we are seizing "this incubation period (to) birth a new world, a new normal, a new way of loving and being."

ATUM/ADULTHOOD/SETTING SUN

A 70-year-old woman living her dream and a 77-year-old female revolutionary poet—forgiving the past fosters peace:

> This virus forces us to respect the pause, be still, and give thanks in these end days.
>
> Live in tomorrow.

It is hard to consider being still amidst the pandemic, which demands we quarantine and learn the new language and social distancing rules to ensure we do not exacerbate infection rates. It is even more challenging when there is an internal struggle of whether or not to stay inside or go outside and join the revolutionary resistance of multiethnic, intergenerational bodies who flood the streets like the Nile's rising waters flooded the land to make way for a new beginning. It is a celebratory feeling to see golden sun-colored letters spelling out Black Lives Matter painted on streets, replacing the past and facing the future. How does one begin to "respect the pause" in this transformational moment? What does giving thanks look like? And how are we living through the end days?

After receiving a reminder text message from my mother, I became consumed with these questions who knows their child. The text read, "this virus forces us to respect the pause, be still, and give thanks in these end days." I understood my mother was offering advice from a faith that I was raised in, to pray and trust God. My mother intentionally reached out to share wisdom, knowledge, and support as the world seemed to be swirling into a violent reaction to our current realities. Those texts are always right on time. That advice was the catalyst to think about healing practices to engage in self-actualization. I can know myself because I know my mothers. I am the spiritual daughter of Oshun, the patron of love and sensuality. I am Geraldine's physical daughter, the daughter of Winnifred, the daughter of Isilda Deer. We are the daughters of Nu(n), Nut, Hathor, and Sekmet.

Nu represents the primordial waters, Nut the cosmos, and protector of earth. Hathor, kind and gentle, acted as the Eye of the Sun and mother of all; Sekmet, the fierce protector, was associated as Hathor's alter energy. I descend from a strong matriarchal bloodline like many women of color. The practice of pausing to honor my lineage originated from the contemporary movement to uplift women's contributions throughout our human story. The #Daughtersof campaign "examines the immediate and critical importance of self-care and healing for Black women through the lens of their matrilineal traditions," beginning with a quote from Alice Walker, "How simple a thing it seems to me that to know ourselves as we are, we must know our mothers' names" (Brainyquote, n.d.)

When we examine the feminine aspect of eschatology, the study of humanity's final events or ultimate destiny, one of the most ancient Egyptian papyruses, describes a return to the primordial waters in Chapter 175 of the *Egyptian Book of The Dead (*Faulkner & Allen, 2005). Chapter 175 provides words to ensure that we do not die a final death. Returning to Nu is where life can regenerate and be born anew. This configuration of "end days" starkly contrasts the west-facing ideology of doomsday, artistically depicted with vivid images of battles, swords, blood, angels, demons, and fear. Interestingly, there always appears to be some form of light piercing through the scene, which relates to east-facing Egyptian philosophy that we enter into the darkness and are reborn into the light. This concept eliminates the fear associated with end days and fashions, the feeling of freedom, which we can give thanks.

Sylvia Browne, who died in 2013, authored the book *End of Days: Predictions and Prophecies About the End of the World* (2008). Browne prophesied, "In around 2020, a severe pneumonia-like illness will spread throughout the globe, attacking the lungs and the bronchial tubes and resisting all known treatments." Like most prophecies, the prophecy was dismissed as society values physical evidence over individuals claiming to predict the future. Because we remember how to practice mindfulness and peace, these predictions are used to create mass panic and fear, which drives us further from recognizing our ability to control our destiny and achieve peace. Entering into the darkness is simply a phase in the cycle of existence that we emerge from renewed. If we have been in the period of Amun, this current darkness shall pass, and giving thanks in these end days is a celebratory concept for transitioning out of Amun into Kepher, where we are becoming our elevated selves.

As I think about how to become cognizant of the elevated self, self-actualization, seasoned auntie, or grandmother status in life, I am right back at the timely text from my mother. It is a much greater responsibility to tap into the elevated self. There are so many experiences and beliefs that we are healing from in our collective and individual past. That healing supports our ability to begin to "live in tomorrow." Respecting the pause is an opportunity to appreciate this period of experience and expand on an interpersonal and intrapersonal level. If you are not recognizing the concept of the elevated self, begin there. When there are obstacles outside of self, go within. Ask what you are protecting yourself from that causes movement in fear instead of faith. Moving in fear hinders our ability for growth. Pay attention to your Eye of Horus, which the ancient ones knew fit precisely in the mid-sagittal section of the human brain. It is our connection to the primal self, our five senses, and provides all the elements necessary to be able to tap into our elevated self as we focus on healing today to be able to protect our peace, enjoy a life bereft of fear, and "live in tomorrow."

AMUN/DEATH/DARKNESS

A feisty, bluest-eyed 92-year-old southern woman labeled Black still living alone in the home that she curated— the wisdom of nine decades rings loudly:

> Baby, you gots to not live in fear, these things have happened before, and we always get through; this life is not for the weak.

Her words resonated down to my core as I slipped the hot, moist mask off my face looking at this blue-eyed 92-year-old woman. She was responding to the behavior of the residents who would not come out of the house or open the door when she approached to ask if we could go around back to pick mangoes off the mango tree. The residents greeted us from behind a curtain, through a screened window, and ushered us around the back of the house with a wave of the hand. She was slightly annoyed at the disrespect. I tried to explain that people were cautious because of the lack of knowledge about the coronavirus. I explained that they would not want to come out of their homes and that she was at greater risk because of her age if they interacted with her. She sucked her teeth and motioned her hands in a way as if she was shooing away the nonsense. She then retorted, "baby, you gots to not live in fear, these things have happened before, and we always get through; this life is not for the weak." I paused for a moment, wondering if I was weak and how I should respond. I cherish every ounce of wisdom she imparts, knowing she has experienced many moons of change.

We had just pulled off from the home of one of her suitors, yes, a suitor who has a mango tree. I wanted mangos for the first time. The mangoes were particularly sweet this year, juxtaposed against the bitterness of the realities of the coronavirus. I'm wondering if the sweet is attributed to orders to quarantine and practice social distancing. On the North American continent, it has been months that we have been unable to move freely doing our normal activities that cause environmental destruction and negatively impact our ecosystem. Everything is different now. There are reports of more fish in the sea, dolphins jumping out of the water, birds in the air, locusts in Egypt, and the fruit has tasted particularly sweet. The sweetness of the fruit is a reminder that we always get through.

Women labeled Black have a tradition of finding ways to make sweet fruit of "these things that have happened before," which refers to the many trammels encountered throughout life. We descend from origin stories like that of The Distant Goddess, Hathor, also referred to as The Eye of Ra (the Sun God), who, as the story is told in *The Contendings of Horus and Seth*, was able to arouse Ra from choosing to become inert which would mean the end of the world; Hathor made the bitter, sweet (Mark, n.d.). Presently, women labeled Black embody the Hathor spirit with personalities like that of Tamika Mallory, loudly proclaiming the liberation of people labeled Black amidst continuous police violence, even through a pandemic. Like this 92-year-old, blue-eyed woman, women labeled Black reflects the balance between the feminine and masculine energies in the wake of pandemics and movements against oppression. Our elders advise that we not live in fear.

At this moment, fear takes on several different forms; the fear of not really knowing what this virus is capable of doing; the fear of how we are going to maintain our financial sustainability; the fear of keeping our children safe and educated; the fear of not being protected, physically, emotionally, and spiritually; the fear around everything we are unfamiliar with becoming a possibility.

The fears of today trigger reflection of the fears of the past. What must it have felt like to be ushered onto a boat in shackles with little care or consideration, not knowing where the destination would end? A journey that seemed endless, the loss of many lives over the vast seas, landing in an unknown place with completely different soil, air, language, culture, and interaction amongst people. Then, to be poked and prodded on this new land and have our sacred bodies handed over to foreigners to treat as less than human, coveted for our sexuality and exploited. Yet we prevailed.

Presently, it feels like we remain the bulk of essential workers being ushered to work with reckless abandon. We do not know when the new normal will begin on a voyage into a future bereft of human interaction as we've known it. This virus portends different air, language, culture, and communication. We experience the loss of human lives disproportionately high compared to people not labeled Black. Then, to be covered faceless, poked, and prodded to determine whether we are among the contagious, coveted for our resilience and resistance, while cautious not to be exploited;

the model of life is not meant for the weak. The only answer that I could muster in response to my 92-year-old blue-eyed woman labeled Black was, "yes ma'am, not choosing to live in fear, choosing to be cautious, we want to be here as long as you." I was reminded of a meme I read, "A head full of fears has no place for dreams." Our dreams are an essential part of where we remember all of the things that are possible and all of the ways in which we celebrate our gifts.

REFERENCES

Brainyquote. (n.d.). *Alice Walker.* https://www.brainyquote.com/quotes/alice_walker_146803#:~:text=Alice%20Walker%20Quotes&text=Please%20enable%20Javascript-,How%20simple%20a%20thing%20it%20seems%20to%20me%20that%20to,must%20know%20our%20mothers%20names

Browne, S. (2009). End of days; Predictions and prophecies about the end of the world. New York: Penguin Random House.

Faulkner, R., & Allen, J. (2005). *Ancient Egyptian book of the dead*. Barnes & Noble.

Mark, J. (n.d.) *Ancient history encyclopedia.* https://www.ancient.eu/Heka/

Marley, B. (1979). Redemption song. On *Uprising*. Tough Gong and Island Records.

Rumi, R. (2019, March 4). *I'll tell you what freedom is to me. No fear* [Nina Simone Video]. YouTube. https://www.youtube.com/watch?v=Y3YFrSlfZ9A

Sanders, L. (2020). Is COVID-19 an adverse childhood experience (ACE): Implications for screening for primary care. *The Journal of Pediatrics, 222,* 4–6.

CHAPTER 4

THE CORONAVIRUS AND VULNERABLE IMMIGRANTS IN THE UNITED STATES—ESSENTIAL, YET DISPOSABLE

Jordana A. Hart

> "The fear that we have as immigrants is something whose extent only we can know. We're afraid of getting sick. We're afraid of dying. We're afraid of complaining at work to our supervisors because we're not getting adequate cleaning supplies. We're ignored completely."—Maria, an undocumented Mexican worker at an apple orchard in Washington State
>
> —Villa (2020).

The United States wants to be fed during the coronavirus pandemic, yet it threatens one of the pillars of its proverbial breadbasket—undocumented migrant workers who power the agricultural industry (Corchado, 2020). It wants to be cared for during the pandemic yet fails to provide a living wage and proper protective gear to health care workers in nursing homes and hospitals, many of whom are immigrants of color.

Coronavirus and Vulnerable People: Addressing the Divide in Harm and Responses and Exploring Implications for a More Peaceful World, pp. 65–88

Contrary to the platitude of the times, we are *not* all in this together. For those who could or would not see it before, COVID-19 has provided as an x-ray of a society awash in the Contradictions that characterize White supremacist, xenophobic societies. The pandemic's health and economic effects on vulnerable immigrants in the United States—the working poor and undocumented of color—can only be viewed through this lens.

Affixing the label "essential" to millions of people that the U.S. otherwise considers low value and disposable is among the many contradictions. As we grappled with the explosive aftermath of the George Floyd murder by Minneapolis police in May 2020, the effects of the coronavirus' breath-taking assault on Black, Latinx, and certain immigrant communities of color are laid bare for all to witness: Cramped, multigenerational housing where the sick infect others; unaffordable rents and evictions; low wages for a de facto captive workforce; poorly funded public schools where the education of children without home computers is threatened; lack of medical care, health insurance, and nutritious food; and a razor-sharp anti-immigrant climate.

The flip side of this privilege coin is the "nonessential" educated middle class, working from home, forming education "pods" by communally hiring teachers so their children don't have to return to risky in-person classrooms, relying on savings to pull through, and relying on telemedicine and online grocery shopping to avoid crowds.

To be sure, COVID-19 has led to alarming and historic job losses and shuttered businesses across the board with few groups of people and few industries left unscathed. Still, we are *not* all in this together. The brutality of COVID-19 requires us to face the underprivilege of some and the overprivilege of others. This is clear when looking at unemployment maps of major U.S. cities awash in different shades of red and crimson. In New York City, it was as if parts of the Bronx were experiencing the Great Depression. At the same time, the Upper East Side faced only modest drops in employment, according to data analysts Yair Ghitza and Mark Steitz, who estimated unemployment at the fine-grained census level based on national statistics between February and August 2020 (Badger & Biu, 2020). Further, most neighborhoods in the Bronx, they found, had unemployment rates above 20%, while most south of 95th Street in Manhattan had rates half of that. The massive unemployment in Chicago's South Side, which is largely Black, and Long Beach and South Los Angeles, which are largely immigrant and Black and Latinx respectively, literally follows racial segregation patterns historically established by government "red-lining" decades ago (Badger & Biu, 2020).

As many see it, systemic racism—riddling its way through the economy, employment, health care, education, and wealth generation—is the preexisting condition for the staggering COVID-19 infection, hospitalization, and death rates in Black and brown communities in every corner of the nation. It is the underlying ingredient that has rendered these communities vulnerable while at the same time largely protecting majority white and more affluent communities. The often race-neutral, objective tones in the media and policy papers about the preexisting ill health of Black and Brown people as the basis for high infection rates "blame them for their health outcomes and not the societal conditions that created it," says Dr. Mary T. Bassett, director of the Francois-Xavier Bagnoud Center for Health and Human Rights at Harvard University and a former commissioner for New York state's Department of Health (Evelyn, 2020). The widely acknowledged disparities, which include testing shortages and delayed test results, as well as inequitable medical treatment for Black and Brown people, are not inevitable or acceptable societal norms, Bassett argues, but rather are "rooted in bias." Biases allow White and other relatively less affected communities to "other" the pandemic, viewing it at a distance. Some believe it has even shaped the careless, selfish public behavior in more conservative sectors, with some refusing to wear masks and physically distance (Evelyn, 2020).

The term "essential" typically conjures a deep positive need for something or someone precious and core to us. What does it mean, though, to be "essential" during the pandemic? Is it the worker or the work itself that is considered essential to the well-being of the rest of society during the crisis? Why are some typically low-paying, almost invisible occupations suddenly essential? According to Merriam-Webster Dictionary:

> Essential: adj. fundamental, vital, cardinal … so important as to be indispensable, implies belonging to the very nature of a thing and therefore of being incapable removal without destroying the thing itself or its character.

Among those labeled "essential" are immigrant workers given a forced choice with high stakes: Work and face illness and death—or lose your livelihood. Engaged as they are in labor that is truly fundamental to keeping the larger society going during the pandemic, these workers toil in underpaid, underprotected conditions. If they get sick and have to leave the job temporarily to isolate themselves, they risk losing pay, being fired, or even being deported. They risk infecting their families, coworkers, and neighbors.

"In America, you should always get a little suspicious when politicians suddenly start calling you a hero," writes Farhad Manjoo (2020), a *New York Times* columnist. "It's a well-worn trick; they're buttering you up before sacrificing you to the gods of unconstrained capitalism and government neglect" (Manjoo, 2020).

The public cheered appreciatively in the streets for health care workers in New York, Seattle, and other cities, even as physicians, nurses, and others urgently complained of dire shortages of personal protective equipment, furiously urged people to wear masks, and wept as their colleagues became infected and died. A nurse in Brooklyn carried a sign that said, "Please don't call me a hero. I am being martyred against my will."

The coffers of Amazon, Instacart, Uber, Whole Foods, and other mega-companies have filled as nonessential workers, who have been able to isolate and work from home, shopped for groceries and other goods online (Neate, 2020). These companies publicly thanked their legions of low-paid warehouse and store employees, drivers, and delivery people, many of them immigrants who have had to interact with the public multiple times daily, placing them and their families at risk of infection.

"We have started talking about essential workers as a category of super-heroes," said Andrew Selee, president of the nonpartisan Migration Policy Institute (MPI) and author of *Vanishing Frontiers*. Should the pandemic effects continue, we need "to think in a bold way about how we deal with essential workers who have put their life on the line for all of us but who don't have legal documents" (Corchado, 2020).

This chapter's framework about the coronavirus and vulnerable immigrants rests on the Gordian knot of U.S. immigration policy and the twin legacies of historical racism and brutal U.S. imperialism in Latin America and other global regions. We provide an overview of the health and economic impacts of the pandemic racing through immigrant communities of color; take a snapshot of some aspects of the immigrant experience during the pandemic, such as the effects on remittances immigrant workers send home despite high levels of unemployment, and the impact of the so-called "she-cession" on Latina and other immigrant women; discuss the historic, little known underpinnings of U.S. immigration law through which we can better understand the current immigration landscape; and finally, lay out a message of hope embedded in the urgent need to break barriers between people as we also find formal ways to dismantle systemic inequalities.

The Context: Anti-Immigrant Laws and Policies Before and During the Pandemic

From Chinese and Indians to Colombians, Cubans, and Nigerians to Mexicans and Hondurans, the array of U.S. immigrant communities is anything but monolithic. It forms a continuum of ethnicities, languages, economic statuses, political persuasions, education, and privilege. COVID-19 has not affected immigrant communities in the same ways. However, the Trump administration's legal and physical assault on immigrant communities, both documented or undocumented, has rocked many people's sense of belonging and their ability to weather the pandemic.

Governments globally quickly adapted their migration management tools to try to stem infected travelers from entering their countries. In the United States, the anti-immigrant spectacle, unleashed in Trumpian verbal lashes even before he took office in January 2017, was shocking even for those with low expectations of this administration. Trump cast Mexicans as "rapists and criminals" early in his presidential campaign (Ye Hee Lee, 2015), and a senior Trump senior official recently referred to immigrants of color as disease carriers (Dickerson & Shear, 2020). The administration hastily threw up legal and physical roadblocks at the southern border to hinder asylum seekers, largely from Central America and those who have made arduous journeys to the border from Africa and the Middle East (Dickerson & Shear, 2020)· Amnesty International (2018) published a report that cited U.S. Customs and Border Patrol data indicating that 6,022 families had their children taken from them at the border between April 19, 2018, and August 15, 2018.

The head of the American Academy of Pediatrics in a 2018 press releases called family separation "government-sanctioned child abuse," while the nonprofit Physicians for Human Rights called it "torture" (Habbach et al., 2020). Although the policy formally ended after a national and international outcry in the summer of 2018, the separations continued. Migrant families detained at the border are often still being given this choice: Consent to having your children released into the U.S. without you or remain together in indefinite detention. The cruelty has been compounded by the revelation of such lax government record-keeping that it is almost impossible or exceedingly complicated to reunite parents and children, among them babies. As a result, the agencies essentially lost some children by failing to keep track of them (Office of the Inspector General, 2019).

Just two weeks after his inauguration on January 20, 2017, President Trump swiftly banned Muslim travelers from several countries (ACLU, n.d.). In the name of protecting U.S. workers facing historic levels of unemployment due to the pandemic, his administration threatened to deport more than 800,000 "Dreamers," the young people brought illegally to the U.S. as children. They are currently protected from deportation and allowed to work under an Obama-era program known as Deferred Action for Childhood Arrivals or DACA. A recent U.S. Supreme Court decision, for now at least, protects the DACA beneficiaries from deportation (ACLU, n.d.). Trump also signed executive orders in April and June 2020 that suspended the issuance of family and employment visas that would allow permanent residents and certain temporary workers into the country (White House, 2020). The Trump suspensions have, in some ways, been purely symbolic due to the many exemptions built into each order and also due to U.S. embassies and consular offices in several countries remaining closed for visa processing because of the pandemic.

Trump has called the Coronavirus "foreign" and "Chinese," and there has been a commensurate increase in reported hate crimes against Asian Americans and Asian immigrants (Tien, 2020). He once stated he would prefer more immigrants from countries like Norway, not from "shithole countries" like Haiti, El Salvador, and African countries that he did not bother to name (Vitali et al., 2018). In July 2020, the government tried—and failed—to force more than a million international university students out of the country if they failed to attend in-person classes in the fall of 2020, despite the risk of contracting the virus and many universities only offering online classes to protect their students and faculty (Dicker, 2020).

As many see it, the Trump administration has used the coronavirus to justify advancing its anti-immigrant agenda in ways that have put thousands of immigrants and their home countries in jeopardy during the pandemic. The U.S. Department of Homeland Security (DHS) has continued to deport migrants, many of them infected with the virus, to their home countries. On April 10, 2020, Trump ordered visa sanctions on countries that refused to take deportees due to the pandemic and instituted penalties for eight countries so far (Hackman, 2020). For example, he imposed sanctions on Guatemala after it suspended the arrival of deportation flights starting April 6 and then indefinitely suspended such flights on April 14. Guatemalan officials reported 50 deportees, including 16 on one flight, tested positive for the virus. Despite agreeing in June 2020 not to deport infected Guatemalans, the government said the U.S. had not kept its word (Montes, 2020).

As an immigration attorney in Miami, Florida, with a majority of clients from Latin America, I listen as they describe what feels like personal stinging attacks by the government, even as they yearn to remain in this country permanently to run businesses that create jobs, go to college, and send their children to school. Like most U.S. citizens, they too are unaware of the cyclical history of racist and xenophobic laws and policies that have directly led to this Trumpian moment, causing these would-be immigrants fear, grief, and delay. Since 2017, fewer of them invoke the traditional pull factors that make the U.S. a perennially attractive destination, such as "safety" and "democracy," to explain their desire to immigrate here. They more often point to push factors such as authoritarianism, crushing poverty and violence in Venezuela, or the economic and political fragmentation and devalued currency of Argentina, or the devastation of extreme climate change on farmlands and food supply in Guatemala and Mexico.

At this writing, the U.S. has more than 5 million confirmed infections and 161,000 dead, buckling under the highest rates in the world (Fortin & Andreoni, 2020). The country struggles with massive infection outbreaks under a leaderless, corrupt federal government with a hodgepodge of contradictory national messages and no policy at all, even about the basics like face coverings and social distancing. A patchwork of often highly politicized but largely unenforced state and local efforts are all those residents can go by. Meanwhile, some in politically conservative southern states have vociferously protested mask wearing as a violation of their freedom under the Constitution. Videos have gone viral, showing a few patrons attacking store employees and destroying property when they have been ordered to mask up or leave (Aratani, 2020).

The explosive mix of unabated COVID-19 infections, economic forces of profit over humans, and anti-migrant and racist policy platforms is indeed crushing for many workers labeled "essential."

CORONAVIRUS AND HEALTH

> "When you are subjected to racism and internalized racism, it can lead to poor health outcomes ... we live in a very racist society, so it's not surprising that this is something we need to be aware of and think about as we talk about COVID-19."
>
> —Dr. Fatima Cody Stanford, obesity medicine physician Massachusetts General Hospital and Harvard Medical School (as cited in Graham, 2020).

As the COVID-19 pandemic began to emerge in the U.S. in February 2020, the virus's effects became rapidly unambiguous: Black and Brown people in hardest-hit states like New York were being infected and dying at astronomically higher rates than U.S. born Whites and more privileged immigrant groups. The high infection and death rates continued unabated for Black and Brown communities, even as a tiny percentage of the population in the Whitest states and counties.

Presuming racism is a preexisting condition for the effects of COVID-19, the data tell a story of the pandemic's racial and ethnic devastation, the depths of which experts say will not be fully understood for years.

African Americans are 13.4% of the U.S. population of almost 350 million, while Latinx makes up 18.5%, Asians 5.9%, and Native Americans and Alaska Native people 1.3%. According to the U.S. Centers for Disease Control (CDC, 2019), COVID-related hospitalizations were highest among African Americans, Native Indians, and Alaska Native people, regardless of age, followed by Latinx, which includes a significant immigrant population. According to the CDC data:

- African Americans, American Indians, and Alaska Native people are five times more likely than non-Latinx Whites to be hospitalized;
- Latinx were four times more likely to be hospitalized than non-Latinx Whites;
- Latinx between the ages of 40 and 59 have been infected at five times the rate of whites in the same age group;
- Of Latinos who have died of COVID-19, more than 25% were younger than age 60 compared to 6% of Whites.

In the context of Latinx immigrant communities, the health effects of COVID-19 have been tightly wound up with spiraling economic havoc, lack of health insurance, and insufficient access to fully funded and equipped health clinics. In 42 states plus Washington D.C., an analysis by *National Public Radio* (NPR) in May 2020 found that Latinx routinely made up a greater share of confirmed COVID-19 cases than their share of the population. In eight states, it was more than four times greater. White deaths from COVID-19 were lower than their share of the population in 37 states and the District of Columbia. For example, in Virginia, more than 12,000 cases—49% of all cases with known ethnicity—came from the Latinx community, which makes up only 10% of the population.

Some other sobering results: About 65% of positive tests in the county that is home to Chattanooga, Tennessee, are Latinos, even though they make up *just 6%* of the population. With many infected family members living in the same intergenerational homes with no other place to isolate or quarantine, Chattanooga officials assessed how to provide alternative sites like hotels where people could safely quarantine (Cano et al., 2020). According to the state's Department of Health and Human Services, Latinos account for 45% of coronavirus cases in North Carolina, where they make up only 10% of the population. In the Latino and Native American town of Guadalupe, Arizona, residents are testing positive at more than four times the entire county's rate. The zip code with the most COVID-19 cases in Maryland borders the nation's capital and is majority Hispanic (MPI, 2021). There were a record 44.7 million immigrants living in the U.S. in 2018, making up 13.6% of the nation's population that year. South and East Asians made up 27.4% of all immigrants in 2017; Mexicans were 25.3%; and other Latin Americans were 25.1%, followed by 9.0% born in another regions. European and Canadian immigrants made up a relatively small share of the foreign-born population—13.2%—in 2017 (MPI, 2021).

In New York, which was the global COVID-19 epicenter in spring 2020, data published by *The New York Times* (which has the largest and most complete database by any media organization) confirmed that all but one of the top 20 neighborhoods with the lowest infection rates were in largely white, wealthy zip codes. "We are watching, in real-time, racial disparities and the pandemic of poverty," said Bronx Assemblyman Michael Blake, whose district overlaps with one of the poorest congressional districts in the United States (Mays & Newman, 2020).

In the Rio Grande Valley along the Texas border with Mexico, 90% of residents are Latinx, many of them recent immigrants with U.S.-born children. More than a third of the families live in poverty. At the same time, half have no health insurance, including about 100,000 undocumented residents who rely on under-resourced hospital emergency rooms and local clinics for care (Dickerson, 2020). Some 60% of residents are diabetic or prediabetic and suffer some of the nation's highest obesity and heart disease rates. To avoid a medical bill that could cripple them, many only arrive at the hospital when they are extremely ill. "They don't seek health care until they are much sicker," said Sherri Abendroth, Safety and Emergency Management Coordinator at DHR in Edinburg, Texas. "So when we get them, it is longer hospital stays, more intensive treatments" (Dickerson, 2020).

Although they are disproportionately affected by the virus, Black and Brown communities appear to be short-changed even when it comes to testing and treatment, leaving a gaping hole in the available data. Hospital and death records show that Black people, Latinx, and Native Americans are disproportionately suffering and dying from severe COVID-19 disease; nationwide, Black people are dying at 2.5 times the Whites' rate, according to *Science Magazine* (Servick, 2020). Without knowing the race of everyone tested, epidemiologists say they can't uncover whether high death rates among Black people and other people of color are driven primarily by more exposure to infection, diagnosis at a later stage of the disease, a higher risk of severe illness once infected, or insufficient medical care. Understanding these drivers might inform solutions, whether that means boosting accessibility to testing, improving public health messaging in hard-hit communities, or aiming for earlier diagnosis and more supportive care. "The lack of data speaks a lot to whose lives we value and whose lives we don't," says Richard Besser, president, and CEO of the Robert Wood Johnson Foundation, who addressed a meeting on COVID-19 and Black communities organized in June 2020 by the National Academies of Science, Engineering, and Medicine (NASEM) (Servick, 2020). In summer 2020, *The New York Times* sued the CDC for access to COVID data by race and ethnicity, and the CDC finally issued it (Oppel & Gebeloff, 2020). It remains unclear why the CDC failed to issue the data on its own.

Immigrants Excluded From Federal Coronavirus Medical Care Relief

Congress passed the Families First Coronavirus Relief Act in March 2020, which authorized COVID-19 testing to be covered by publicly funded Medicaid. In April 2020, they enhanced it to add funds for Medicaid coverage of coronavirus testing for the uninsured. Still, not all immigrants are eligible for Medicaid; only "qualified" immigrants—green-card holders with more than five years in status, as well as asylees. At least 3.7 million low-income uninsured non-citizens are not covered for virus testing and treatment under Medicaid. Some 27% of the total U.S. uninsured population are noncitizens, according to the MPI (Chisti & Bolter, 2020).

There was some positive news in the act, however. Despite the omission of millions of essential workers from the two most comprehensive relief efforts enacted to date, community health centers—which provide medical care regardless of a patient's immigration status—received $2 billion in additional funding under the act. Federal health centers, including community health centers, were allocated $825 million under the Paycheck Protection Program and Health Care Enhancement Act.

CORONAVIRUS AND EMPLOYMENT

> "Our real enemy is not the virus, but our response to the virus – a response that has been degraded and deformed by the structural inequalities of our society.... The biological virus afflicting individuals is also a social virus. Its symptoms—inequality, callousness, selfishness and a profit motive that undervalues human life and overvalues commodities—were too long masked by the hearty good cheer of American exceptionalism, the ruddiness of someone a few steps away from a heart attack."
>
> —Viet Than Nguyen (2020), opinion writer and author of *The Refugees* (Nguyen, 2020).

The pandemic has raised fundamental questions about the country's history, values, and national identity. It has reframed in some quarters that ubiquitous theory of "American exceptionalism," which generally refers to the fact that the United States, alone among wealthier nations, never developed a working-class (labor) party or the type of welfare state and safety net that exist in Canada and most European nations. The pandemic has laid bare the consequences of prioritizing "rugged individualism" and the proverbial bootstraps over the role of government intervention—upending what many Americans have long considered the superiority of their brand of free-market democracy and its manifestations in the world.

"As an American, I think there is a lot of good to be said about our libertarian traditions. But this is the consequence—we don't succeed as well as a collective," said Dr. Jared Baeten, an epidemiologist and vice dean at the University of Washington School of Public Health (Leonhardt, 2020). Data show the United States, alone among wealthier nations (and even among some developing nations), has some of the highest maternal and infant mortality rates, surprisingly low testing achievement in math and science, burgeoning rates of homelessness, and other markers of an unequal society. (Leonhardt, 2020).

As the pandemic hit and the U.S. economy shut down in the spring of 2020, unemployment shot up 31% for foreign-born works (including some U.S. citizens) between February and March compared to a 16% increase among native-born Whites. The federal government did take one step early on to ensure as much as possible an unimpeded food supply chain and ongoing medical care: It bestowed the title "essential" on an estimated 55 million workers, among them many immigrants, at least six million of whom are undocumented.

Being "essential" means being exempt, whether you like it or not, from state or municipal stay-at-home orders and quarantine. According to the MPI (2020), the U.S. has an estimated 12 million undocumented immigrants. MPI says about 6 million immigrants (not necessarily undocumented) are "essential" frontline workers in the food industry, transportation, and health care and are overrepresented in certain critical occupations like doctors and home health aides, where they face heightened risk of exposure. Another estimated 6 million are within food services and domestic households, making up 20% of those sectors' total workers

Up to 75% of the country's one million farmworkers—who work the initial stepping-stone in the U.S food chain—are undocumented Mexican and Central American migrants. Many are seasonally employed and live in packed farm camps or dormitories on employer property. The virus has ravaged farmworkers as they travel up the Atlantic coast from Florida to Maine to harvest berries and other crops in summer and fall 2020. Many farms, although they are concerned about their bottom line and the threat of anything slowing down harvesting, do not allow workers to physically distance, or provide regular opportunities to wash or sanitize their hands, or wear proper masks, all of which the CDC says are required to try to limit virus outbreaks (Tully, 2020).

Meanwhile, somewhere between 30% and 50% of the U.S. meat-packing industry is comprised of undocumented workers from Mexico, Guatemala, and El Salvador and immigrants from various East African nations, according to the American Enterprise Institute (Orrell, 2020). Some of the largest plants were slammed with the virus and had to close to disinfect and add some protective dividers. In April 2020, Nebraska Governor Pete Ricketts said that workers at these facilities would face a loss of unemployment benefits unless they returned to work. However, such benefits do not apply to undocumented workers anyway. His threat followed Trump's announcement that he would invoke the Defense Production Act to reopen closed meat regardless of safety. To explain the outbreaks, Smithfield Foods' statement about their Sioux Falls, Nebraska outbreak offensively stated that the living conditions of these immigrants are "different than they are with your traditional American family." Since many of these workers lack legal status, they cannot defend themselves against exploitative or coercive labor practices. In August 2019, ICE agents rounded up and arrested hundreds at these plants (Orrell, 2020).

Many Immigrants Excluded From the Federal CARES Act

Hit not only with the race-based economic and social disparities affecting other essential workers, undocumented workers, who make up 4.8% of the entire U.S. workforce, cannot collect unemployment and so are more likely to be coerced to work even while sick, which means spreading the infection among their coworkers and families.

The U.S. Congress starting in April 2020 passed four bipartisan federal pandemic-relief packages. Many immigrants, particularly the undocumented and their U.S. citizen and legal permanent resident (green card) family members, were excluded from the most critical relief effort, the $2 trillion measure known as Coronavirus Aid, Relief, and Economic Security Act, or CARES Act. The CARES Act Pandemic Unemployment Assistance, or PUA. provided relief to unemployed workers, included gig workers for the first time, and those who were ineligible for state unemployment insurance or had exhausted state benefits.

The Act excised unauthorized workers, 4.8% of the entire U.S. workforce, although they contribute millions in tax dollars annually. Further, the CARES Act provided a one-time cash payment of $1,200 to earners making less than $75,000 and filed a tax return in 2018 or 2019 using a valid social security number (SSN). The vast majority of undocumented workers file taxes using only an IRS-issued Individual Tax Identification Number (ITIN). In so-called mixed-status families (families with documented and undocumented members), the CARES Act excluded U.S. citizens and lawful permanent residents ("green card" holders) with SSN who jointly filed with an ITIN user, making entire families ineligible. MPI has estimated that as many as 15.4 million people in mixed-status families were excluded from the $1,200 stimulus payments, including 9.9 undocumented immigrants, 3.7 million children, and 1.7 million spouses who are U.S. citizens and green-card holders (MPI, 2020). At this writing, Republicans and Democrats continue to negotiate for workers' ongoing economic protections after the protections expired July 31, 2020.

At least four states (California, Michigan, New Jersey, and Washington) and eight localities (Austin, Boston, Chicago, Minneapolis, Seattle [with King County, Washington], St. Paul, and Washington, DC, along with Montgomery County, Maryland) had stepped in, as of May–June 2020, to partially fill the gap for those left out of federal aid. For example, California has created a disaster relief fund to provide residents with one-time stimulus payments if they were ineligible for federal payments because of their immigration status (MPI, 2020).

COVID-19 IMPACT ON REMITTANCES

The migrant story of remittances does not loom large in the public imagination like deportation or family separation. Still, the outsized influence of remittances—money or goods migrants send home to their families and friends—offers insights into the immense sacrifice of many low-wage workers and the life-altering consequences to their families and communities of origin. COVID-19 was expected to create a pause in this lifeline, but a few surprising trends have emerged that have turned experts' theories upside down.

The need for remittances by the national economies of poorer countries is at once the legacy of U.S. colonialism, corporate greed, and the disastrous effects of climate change in countries like Haiti, Mexico, and Guatemala that, circularly, force more people into poverty and push family members to leave and seek work abroad in more prosperous nations. With 270 million migrants globally, remittances are lifelines between rich and developing nations, sending more money to middle-income and low-income families worldwide than foreign direct investment and official development funds combined (Cocco, 2019).

Mirian Lopez Acevedo, a graphic designer in Chiapas, Mexico, said her mother lost her full-time cleaning job in the U.S and has been unable to send for the first time in 10 years money which Ms. Lopez uses to support both her 5-year-old daughter and her grandmother. "I don't have a lot of work right now," she told *CNN*. "The truth is the salary I make is not enough." She said she used her mother's monthly funds to buy goods, pay her daughter's tuition, and grow her savings (Gallon, 2020).

Remittances make up a significant percentage of some countries' national economy—28% for Haiti, 18% for Honduras, and higher for many other countries (IMF and World Bank, 2017). Remittances to Mexico along were worth $39 billion in 2019, according to the World Bank (World Bank Group, 2020). Mexicans and Central and Latin Americans make up more than 50% of all immigrants in the U.S.· with the U.S. being the source of most remittances to these regions. The Inter-American Dialogue provides a succinct snapshot of the pandemic and Latin American and Caribbean migration:

> Thirty-six countries had 94% of all Covid-19 cases as of May 15, 2020. Migrants in these countries represent 90% of all remittances to Latin America and the Caribbean. Over 200 million migrants are living in host countries with an elevated number of Covid-19 cases. Hot spots of the global pandemic are home to the majority of migrants from Latin America and the Caribbean. (Malloy Jewers & Orozco, 2020)

Last year saw record remittances equal to $554 billion (Malloy Jewers & Orozco, 2020). In April 2020, reviewing the rapid catastrophic effects of the virus on global economies, the World Bank released data showing its expected remittances to drop globally, including by as much as 20% to Latin America and the Caribbean. The expected drop in remittances came as direct foreign investment in what the World Bank calls "low and middle-income countries," or LMICs, was expected to drop by 35%.

Remittances have built homes, classrooms, and community centers (Wainer, 2012). Households receiving remittances eat better, send their children to school rather than pushing them into the workforce, start businesses, and access better health care. According to the Inter-American Dialogue, some 94% of all remittances to Mexico and Central America come from migrant workers in the United States.

It was logical to expect that, with unemployment and lower salaries surging in the United States, especially among those in highly affected industries, migrant workers' ability to send cash home would falter. While remittances to El Salvador did fall by 40% in April 2020 compared to the same month last year, the cash flow surged back in El Salvador, Guatemala, Nicaragua, Honduras, and Mexico by June, up year-over-year in five of the first months of 2020 (Sieff, 2020). In March 2020, remittances to Mexico topped a record $4 billion. "I remember thinking, 'Oh my God, what happened here?'" said Jonathan Heath, the deputy governor of Mexico's central bank. "It's the exact opposite of what we were expecting" (Sieff, 2020). Indeed, in June 2020, Mexico recorded $3.53 billion in remittances, an 11% jump over 2019.

Experts are unclear as to the reason for the pandemic remittance phenomenon; so far at least, none of them were able to forecast it with regard to migrants in the United States. There are two theories: One is that Mexican, Central, and Latin American migrants tend to work in industries deemed essential—agriculture, construction, and food retail—and were able to remain employed, even if they took a cut in hours or pay. In 2017, more than 34% of Mexicans and Central Americans worked in construction;

14% of Caribbean migrants worked in health care; and a total of 36% of Mexicans, Caribbean citizens, Central Americans, and Latin Americans worked in food preparation and retail. The second theory is that some who lost their jobs could take advantage of federal and state unemployment packages. However, many immigrants and all undocumented workers were prohibited from such aid.

THE PANDEMIC'S "SECESSION": WHY THE COVID ECONOMIC CRISIS IS MOST AFFECTING IMMIGRANT WOMEN

Denise Frederick, a single mother from St. Lucia, worked two jobs in New York City—as a nanny and a home care provider. The family she worked for as a nanny left the city and continued to pay her full salary until July 2020, when they cut her pay to hire a nanny where they are currently residing. Frederick's home care job also cut her pay, even as she paid to commute by bus and subway during the pandemic and where she paid for her own personal protective equipment (Holpuch, 2020). She said she worries she will lose both jobs.

Betty, an undocumented housekeeper from Colombia, has worked for the same employer in Miami, Florida, caring for the three children for more than two decades. She figured out multiple new routes after the couple divorced, moved to separate homes, and shared custody. She earns $600 a week. When the pandemic struck, her employer told her to come in just twice a week when no one would be home. He continued her full pay, telling her he worried about her exposure to the virus on public transportation. Betty said:

> I have worked for this family for many years and adore the children like they are my own, but I wasn't sure what to expect with Covid. For now, I am luckier than most of the housekeepers I know who was just kicked out by their employers with no notice and no pay. These families could afford to help them.

She refused to identify herself due to her undocumented status fully.

COVID-related job losses or pay cuts for women have been nothing short of catastrophic. From February through May 2020, 11.5 million women in the U.S. lost their jobs compared to 9 million men (Holpuch, 20201) In fact, Latina immigrants had the highest jobless rate—22%, or double the rate for white men (Capps et al., 2020). As during the Great Recession of 2008–2009, immigrants are most vulnerable to job loss because they are relatively young, have lower levels of education, and are concentrated in certain "non-essential" face-to-face industries like the retail trade, leisure, and hospitality (hotels, restaurants, bars, and amusement parks).

The data between January and April 2020 on job losses for Latina immigrants who tend to be concentrated in certain occupations was breathtaking: Unemployment went from 2.8% to almost 34% in personal services, which includes domestic employees and office cleaners; from 5.5% to 38% in hotels, restaurants and other leisure and hospitality services; and from 1.3% to 9.5% in health services (Capps et al., 2020). According to a survey of the National Domestic Workers Alliance and the Institute for Policy Studies, at least 70% of immigrant nannies, housekeepers, and home care aides like Frederick lost their jobs or had a cut in pay or hours (Bayard & Freeman Brown, 2020).

Black immigrant domestic workers are at the epicenter of three converging catastrophes—the pandemic, the resulting economic depression, and structural racism (Bayard & Freeman Brown, 2020). Intersectional identities such as Black, undocumented immigrant, woman, and low-wage worker make these workers some of the most invisible and vulnerable workers in the country. Surveys conducted in March and April 2020 by the Institute for Policy Studies found up to 93% of respondents in Miami-Dade County had either lost their jobs or had a pay cut, and 65% feared being evicted or having their utilities shut off. With 66% of nannies in New York, Massachusetts, and Miami-Dade and 72% of Miami-Dade housekeepers saying they are undocumented, many workers were ineligible for the one-time federal $1,200 payment and the $600 weekly unemployment insurance under the Cares Act, which ended July 31, 2020.

"Many of the challenges that are facing women of color workers, issues around childcare, issues around lower wages, issues of lack of flexibility and lack of job security, have all been made worse by the pandemic," says C Nicole Mason, chief executive of the Institute for Women's Policy Research. "So, the situation for women who were struggling before the pandemic has only gotten worse."

Some say they the pandemic's surprising silver lining may be the emergency of a more equitable economy: Employers may have a new awareness of the importance of their workers and their humanity and realize that the ravages of the pandemic are showing that what was long considered individual problems are broken structures and systems that are failing everyone to different degrees.

U.S. Immigration History and Legacy in the Time of COVID-19

"The past is never dead. It's not even past," one of William Faulkner's oft-quoted lines aptly applies to the origin story of vulnerable U.S. immigrant communities of color as well as to why COVID-19 has ravaged certain immigrant families and workplaces (as cited in Leopold, 2012). There is a clear line from overt anti-immigrant, white supremacist policies and sentiments that gave birth to U.S. immigration law to the subpar status of many immigrant communities of color and their U.S. born children.

Until 1952, race was the stated epicenter of U.S. immigration law and policy. As the country constructed its nascent immigration laws in the 1800s, the fundamental question of who could immigrate to the U.S. turned on who was White, a definition that shifted with the waves of new immigrants. Italians, Jews, and the Irish—who early on were referred to as "white negroes" because they worked in the Northeast as unskilled laborers, maids, cooks, and waiters—shifted tacitly from non-White to White as the country moved to exclude others based on skin color and other perceived racialized traits. "From this country's inception, the laws regulating who was or could be a citizen were tainted by racial prejudice," wrote Ian F. Haney Lopez in a 1996 article titled *White by Law: The Legal Construction of Race*. "More than this, it reflects the conscious design of the U.S. immigration and naturalization laws."

Between 1790 and 1870, only white immigrants could become U.S. citizens. Congress in 1790 declared that a "free white alien" who had resided in the U.S. for two years and had good moral character could become a U.S. citizen through the legal process of naturalization. In 1857, meanwhile, the U.S Supreme Court in *Dred Scott* found, among other things, that blacks, free or slave, were not—and could not become—U.S. citizens. Congress gutted the *Dred Scott* decision in 1866 when it found "all persons born in the United States and not subject to any foreign power, excluding Indians not taxed, are hereby declared to be citizens of the United States" (Library of Congress, n.d.). Two years later, it wrote the definition into the Fourteenth Amendment.

After 1870, only Whites and U.S. born people of African ancestry could become citizens. The Chinese Exclusion Act of 1882, the first U.S. law targeting a single specific ethnic group, prohibited the Chinese—painted at the time as criminals unable to assimilate—from naturalizing. Congress virtually banned all immigration from Asia in 1917.

For U.S. immigration purposes, the fundamental legal question until 1952 was how to determine who was White. The Supreme Court took various approaches to what proved a slippery assessment, basing its legal definition on "scientific studies" and the "instinctive" opinion of the so-called everyman. In 1922, for example, it held in *Takao Ozawa* that the Japanese were not White because, "as sustained by numerous scientific authorities, they are not members of the Caucasian race," and, in 1924, Congress banned Japanese immigration (U.S. House of Representatives History, Art & Archives, 2018). White society, the Court would later conclude, was the ultimate arbiter of Whiteness.

The Supreme Court in 1923 continued in its effort to define Whiteness in the context of immigration law. In *Bhagat Singh Thind* in 1923, it was found that "a high-caste Hindu of full Indian blood" was not eligible to naturalize even though Thind argued that biologically, he was, in fact, Caucasian. The *Thind* Court said the word "white" was to be interpreted "in accordance with the understanding of the common man." Straining credulity, as some scholars see it, the Court concluded:

> It is very far from our thought to suggest the slightest question of racial superiority or inferiority. What we suggest is merely racial difference, and it is of such character and extent that the great body of our people instinctively recognize[s] it and reject[s] it through assimilation. (Justia, n.d.)

It was World War II that coaxed the U.S. away from its racial bans as it fought another racist, Hitler. Germany, in 1935, with its citizenship limited to "Aryans," was said to be the only country other than the U.S. with such racial restrictions. Indeed, the Nazis repurposed much of the Jim Crow laws from the U.S. to develop their anti-Jewish platform (Little, 2019). In 1943, the Chinese were allowed to naturalize, followed in 1946 with restrictions lifted for Indians (i.e., from India) and Filipinos. Congress in 1952 entirely reformed immigration law, officially ending all legal racial bars.

Race is no longer a legal barrier, but caste-like racism, impacting as it does all fundamental aspects of U.S. society, cycles through immigration policy, as we see today in the Trump administration and through the influential white nationalist nativists paralyzing Congress's effort to modernize and restructure immigration law.

Those who would benefit the most from U.S. immigration reform are poor, indigenous Mexicans and Central Americans who are undocumented yet central to supporting the U.S. food supply and other industries. U.S. legal and political historian Mae M. Ngai says undocumented immigrants "are at once welcome and unwelcome; they are woven into the economic fabric of the nation, but as labor that is cheap and disposable" (Ngai, 2004, p. 2).

Approaches to a More Collective and Equitable Society

To even begin to ponder actions that could bring peace and equity to U.S society means understanding the history that has brought us the social and economic depravity that COVID-19 has put on full display. We must reckon with the depths of the flawed Trump administration's response to the pandemic, one that has particularly injured Black, Latinx, and immigrant communities of color. That the Trump administration is closely allied to White supremacist movements and individuals is telling.

Coupled with the country's tendency to avoid authentically addressing White supremacy and generational racial inequities, remedies to excise these longstanding cancers do not easily come to mind. Time will tell, but the public torture-murder of Mr. Floyd, a Black man, under the knee of a Minneapolis police officer, may have uniquely jolted the nation, and indeed the world, into rethinking the bankrupt racialized social order under which we all live and which the pandemic has forced White and other privileged people to confront.

"The two struggles—Black liberation and immigrant rights—are intertwined and must be confronted together," writes the public scholar Dr. Lorgia Garcia-Pena (2020):

> We must recognize the same colonial logic, which convinced the world that it was somehow acceptable to profit from capturing and enslaving Africans and Indigenous people, continues to sustain the 'immigrant' as a racialized sub-human category of unbelonging, and racialized immigrant subjects as disposable, consumable bodies without history, aliens to the nation-state at the service of the global capita machinery.

Even the most jaded anti-racists and social justice scholars have been carefully watching the astonishing impact of the Black Lives Matter (BLM) movement on municipalities, police, and private corporations. Latinx and other BLM allies, including many immigrants, understand that uprooting white supremacy and alleviating the distressing inequalities that afflict African American people will surely right the ship for immigrants of color. COVID-19 and racism have in fact, more than ever, underscored the need for dialogue within intergenerational immigrant communities and reckoning in Latinx communities with their anti-Blackness.

A wholesale retooling of the U.S. economy and society may seem unrealistic, yet steps are being taken to reshape laws, policies, and public institutions at the local and state levels. Immigration advocates have laid out a host of proposed immigration reforms, including a return to respecting international human rights norms and laws for refugees and asylum-seekers; providing a path to legalized status for Dreamers; raising the per-country caps on family-based and employment-based visa categories; raising the seasonal visa cap for migrant farmworkers (some steps have recently been taken to ease restrictions on this important visa category for essential workers); and an end to travel bans from Muslim countries. These may come sooner than we anticipate if we get to celebrate a new administration on January 20, 2021.

The path out of racism and xenophobia is persistently blocked because both strands underpin every facet of society—medicine, banking, employment, education, criminal justice, and housing. They have a stranglehold on the White American psyche and, due to internalized oppression and colorism, on the psyche of some Latinx and other immigrants of color.

We must shift our thinking from laws and policies to our hearts and emotions, which means rehumanizing our perceptions of Black immigrants and other immigrants of color. It means trying to eliminate the notions of rugged individualism for a caring collective at the local and state levels in particular. It is what the MIT Presencing Institute calls a "shift from an ego-system awareness that cares about the well-being of oneself to the eco-system awareness that cares about the well-being of all, including oneself" (Presencing Institute, n.d.).

Breaking these person-to-person barriers must start with face-to-face grassroots meetings and dialogues to reach an understanding that we all have similar fears, expectations, and hopes, no matter who we are. People largely do not even know the genesis of the de facto barriers that keep them apart at a personal, human level. But facilitated community dialogues and small gatherings among people of different backgrounds who usually do not get a chance to meet each other have proven to move the needle. "I hope after this pandemic, the people get the point that we are in your communities, we are your neighbors, we are your friends," says Maria, the undocumented worker in Washington state (Villa, 2020).

In its own way, the coronavirus pandemic of 2020 may push us down the path toward economic equity and, for the first time, liberate all of us from the smallness and meanness that haunt so much of American life and move us toward Dr. Martin Luther King Jr's "Beloved Community."

REFERENCES

American Academy of Pediatrics. (2018, June 15). President of American Academy of Pediatricians on family separation: "Nothing less than government-sanctioned child abuse." *America's Voice*. https://americasvoice.org/press_releases/president-of-american-academy-of-pediatricians-on-family-separation-nothing-less-than-government-sanctioned-child-abuse/

American Civil Liberties Union. (n.d.). *Timeline of the Muslim Ban*. ACLU. https://www.aclu-wa.org/pages/timeline-muslim-ban

Amnesty International. (2018, October 11). *Catastrophic immigration policies resulted in more family separations than previously disclosed*. https://www.amnestyusa.org/reports/usa-catastrophic-immigration-policies-resulted-in-more-family-separations-than-previously-disclosed/

Aratani, L. (2020, June 29). How did masks become a political issue in America? *The Guardian*. https://www.theguardian.com/world/2020/jun/29/face-masks-us-politics-coronavirus

Badger, E., & Biu, Q. (2020, August 7). The beleaguered neighborhoods where workers have no work. *The New York Times*. https://www.nytimes.com/interactive/2020/08/05/upshot/us-unemployment-maps-coronavirus.html?searchResultPosition=4

Bayard, M., & Freeman Brown, K. (2020, June). Notes from the storm: Black immigrant domestic workers in the time of Covid-19. *Institute for Policy Studies*. https://ips-dc.org/black-immigrant-domestic-workers-covid-19/

Cano, R., Snow, S., & Anderson, B. (2020, June 21). *Covid-19 is ravaging America's vulnerable Latino communities*. WGBH.org. https://www.wgbh.org/news/national-news/2020/06/21/covid-19-is-ravaging-americas-vulnerable-latino-communities

Capps, R., Batalova, J., & Gelatt J. (2020, June). *Covid-19 and employment: Assessing the early fallout for immigrants and other US workers*. Migration Policy Institute. https://www.migrationpolicy.org/research/covid-19-unemployment-immigrants-other-us-workers

Centers for Disease Control and Prevention. (2020, December 10). *Introduction to COVID-19 racial and ethnic health disparities*. https://www.cdc.gov/coronavirus/2019-ncov/community/health-equity/racial-ethnic-disparities/index.html

Chisti, M., & Bolter, J. (2020, April 24). *Vulnerable to COVID-19 and in frontline jobs, immigrants are mostly shut out of U.S. relief*. Migration Policy Institute. https://www.migrationpolicy.org/article/covid19-immigrants-shut-out-federal-relief

Cocco, F. (2019, August 28). Remittances: The hidden engine of globalisation. *The Financial Times*. https://ig.ft.com/remittances-capital-flow-emerging-markets/

Corchado, A. (2020, May 10). Legalize all essential workers. *The New York Times*. https://www.nytimes.com/2020/05/06/opinion/sunday/coronavirus-essential-workers.html

Dicker, J. (2020, July 14). *Trump administration reverses course on foreign student ban*. CNBC. https://www.cnbc.com/2020/07/14/fight-heats-up-over-foreign-student-ban-as-more-than-200-schools-join-in.html

Dickerson, C. (2020, July 19). "A straight up trajectory" hits already stressed border region. *The New York Times*. https://www.nytimes.com/2020/07/19/us/coronavirus-texas-rio-grande-valley.html

Dickerson, C., & Shear, M. (2020, May 3). Before COVID-19, Trump aide sought to use disease to close border. *The New York Times*. https://www.nytimes.com/2020/05/03/us/coronavirus-immigration-stephen-miller-public-health.html

Dred Scott v. Sandford, U.S. Supreme Court. (1857). https://www.oyez.org/cases/1850-1900/60us393

Evelyn, K. (2020, July 14). A slap in the face: How racial bias dogs U.S. coronavirus response at every level. *The Guardian*. https://www.theguardian.com/world/2020/jul/14/coronavirus-us-racial-bias-black-latino

Fortin, J., & Andreoni, M. (2020, August 9). U.S caseload surpasses 5 million, leading world. *The New York Times*. https://www.nytimes.com/interactive/2021/us/covid-cases.html

Gallon, N. (2020, July 14). The world runs on remittances. Covid-19 could end that for many. *CNN*. https://www.cnn.com/2020/07/14/americas/mexico-remittances-covid-19-intl/index.html

Garcia-Pena, l. (2020, June 8). *Dismantling anti-Blackness altogether.* North American Congress on Latin America. https://nacla.org/news/2020/06/09/dismantling-anti-blackness-together

Graham, R. (2020, April 10). Being a person of color isn't a risk factor for coronavirus: Living in racist country is. *The Boston Globe*. https://www.bostonglobe.com/2020/04/10/opinion/being-person-color-isnt-risk-factor-coronavirus-living-racist-country-is/

Habbach, H., Hampton, K., & Mishori, R. (2020, February 25). *"You will never see your child again:" The persistent psychological effects of family separation.* Physicians for Human Rights. https://phr.org/our-work/resources/you-will-never-see-your-child-again-the-persistent-psychological-effects-of-family-separation/

Hackman, M. (2020, April 10). Trump threatens to deny visas to countries refusing deportees. *The Wall Street Journal*. https://www.wsj.com/articles/trump-threatens-to-deny-visas-to-countries-refusing-deported-citizens-11586577586

Holpuch, A. (2020, August 4). The 'shecession': Why economic crisis is affecting women more than men. *The Guardian*. https://www.theguardian.com/business/2020/aug/04/shecession-coronavirus-pandemic-economic-fallout-women

Justia. (n.d.). *U.S. v Bhagat Singh Thind* 261. U.S. 204 (1923). https://supreme.justia.com/cases/federal/us/261/204/

Leonhardt, D. (2020, August 7). The unique U.S. failure to control the virus. *The New York Times*. https://www.nytimes.com/2020/08/06/us/coronavirus-us.html

Leopold, T. (2012, November 11). *Famed quotation isn't dead—and could even prove costly.* CNN. https://www.cnn.com/2012/11/06/showbiz/movies/faulkner-midnight-paris-allen-lawsuit/index.html

Library of Congress. (n.d.). *Citizenship and the 14th Amendment* https://www.loc.gov/law/help/citizenship/fourteenth_amendment_citizenship.php

Little, B. (2019, May 20). How the Nazis were inspired by Jim Crow. *History.* https://www.history.com/news/how-the-nazis-were-inspired-by-jim-crow

Malloy Jewers, M., & Orozco, M. (2020, August). Immigrants, remittances and Covid-19. *Inter-American Dialogue*. https://www.thedialogue.org/wp-content/uploads/2020/08/FINAL-Migrants-Remittances-and-Covid-19_08.05.20.pdf

Manjoo, F. (2020, July 15). Please don't call them heroes. *The New York Times*. https://www.nytimes.com/2020/07/15/opinion/schools-reopening.html

Mays, J., & Newman, A. (2020, April 9). Virus is twice as deadly for Black and Latino people in New York City. *The New York Times*. https://www.nytimes.com/2020/04/08/nyregion/coronavirus-race-deaths.html

Migration Policy Institute. (2021, February 11). *Frequently requested statistics on immigrants and immigration in the United States.* https://www.migrationpolicy.org/article/frequently-requested-statistics-immigrants-and-immigration-united-states

Montes, J. (2020, June 24). US fails to prevent deportation of migrants infected with COVID-19, Guatemalan officials say. *The Washington Post.* https://www.wsj.com/articles/u-s-fails-to-prevent-deportation-of-migrants-infected-with-covid-19-guatemalan-officials-say-11593023095

National Public Radio. (2020, May 30). *What do coronavirus racial disparities look like state by state?* https://www.npr.org/sections/health-shots/2020/05/30/865413079/what-do-coronavirus-racial-disparities-look-like-state-by-state

Neate, R. (2020, July 16). Family fortunes of wealthy increase as super-rich ride coronavirus storm. *The Guardian.* https://www.theguardian.com/news/2020/jul/16/family-fortunes-of-wealthy-increase-as-super-rich-ride-coronavirus-storm

Ngai, M. (2004). *Impossible subjects: Illegal aliens and the making of modern America.* Princeton University Press.

Nguyen, V. (2020, April 19). The ideas that won't survive the coronavirus. *The New York Times.* https://www.nytimes.com/2020/04/10/opinion/sunday/coronavirus-america.html

Office of the Inspector General, U.S. Department of Homeland Security. (2019, November 25). *DHS lacked technology needed to successfully account for separated migrant families.* https://www.oig.dhs.gov/sites/default/files/assets/2019-11/OIG-20-06-Nov19.pdf

Presencing Institute. (n.d.). *About.* https://www.presencing.org/aboutus

Oppel, R., & Gebeloff, R. (2020, July 5). Fullest look yet at racial inequality of coronavirus. *The New York Times.* https://www.nytimes.com/interactive/2020/07/05/us/coronavirus-latinos-African Americans-cdc-data.html

Orrell, B. (2020, April 29). *Hypocrisy strikes: "Essential" workers and the meatpacking industry.* American Enterprise Institute. https://www.aei.org/poverty-studies/hypocrisy-strikes-essential-workers-and-the-meat-packing-industry/

Physicians for Human Rights. (2020, February 25). "You will never see your child again:" The persistent psychological effects of family separation. *Physicians for Human Rights.* https://phr.org/our-work/resources/you-will-never-see-your-child-again-the-persistent-psychological-effects-of-family-separation/

Servick, K. (2020, July 10). *"Huge hole" in COVID-19 testing data makes is harder to study racial disparities.* The American Association for the Advancement of Science. https://www.sciencemag.org/news/2020/07/huge-hole-covid-19-testing-data-makes-it-harder-study-racial-disparities

Sieff, K. (2020, August 6). Coronavirus surprise: Remittances to Mexico rise during pandemic. *The Washington Post.* https://www.washingtonpost.com/world/the_americas/coronavirus-remittance-mexico-guatemala-salvador-honduras/2020/08/05/5a1bcdbe-d5be-11ea-930e-d88518c57dcc_story.html

Tien, C. (2020, April 21). I'm Chinese. That doesn't mean I have coronavirus. *The New York Times.* https://www.nytimes.com/2020/03/07/opinion/coronavirus-asian-racism.html

Tully, T. (2020, July 5). How you get your berries: Migrant workers who fear virus but toil on. *The New York Times.* https://www.nytimes.com/2020/07/05/nyregion/nj-migrant-workers-covid-19.html

U.S. House of Representatives History, Art & Archives. (2018). *First arrivals, first reactions*. https://history.house.gov/Exhibitions-and-Publications/APA/Historical-Essays/Exclusion-and-Empire/First-Arrivals/

Villa, L. (2020, April 17). "We're completely ignored." Amid the pandemic, undocumented immigrants are essential but exposed. *Time*. https://time.com/5823491/undocumented-immigrants-essential-coronavirus/

Vitali, A., Huny, K., & Thorpe, F. (2018, January 11*)*. *Trump referred to Haiti and African Nations as 'shithole' countries*. NBC News. https://www.nbcnews.com/politics/white-house/trump-referred-haiti-african-countries-shithole-nations-n836946

Wainer, A. (2012, June). *Exchanging people for money: Remittances and repatriation* (Briefing Paper #18). Bread for the World Institute. https://www.bread.org/sites/default/files/downloads/briefing-paper-18.pdf

White House. (2020, June 22). *Proclamation suspending entry of aliens who present a risk to the U.S. labor market following the coronavirus outbreak*. Whitehouse.gov. https://www.whitehouse.gov/presidential-actions/proclamation-suspending-entry-immigrants-present-risk-u-s-labor-market-economic-recovery-following-covid-19-outbreak/

World Bank Group. (2020, April). Covid-19 crisis through a migration lens. World Bank. https://documents.worldbank.org/en/publication/documents-reports/documentdetail/989721587512418006/covid-19-crisis-through-a-migration-lens

Ye Hee Lee, M. (2015, July 8). Donald Trumps: False comments connecting Mexican immigrants and crime. *The Washington Post*. https://www.washingtonpost.com/news/fact-checker/wp/2015/07/08/donald-trumps-false-comments-connecting-mexican-immigrants-and-crime/

CHAPTER 5

A COVID-19 MOMENT

Haitian Mental Health Clinicians Reflecting on Grief and Loss

Fanya Jabouin Monnay and Karine Champagne

Corona Virus Speaks 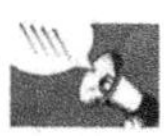

Why do you call me the invisible enemy?
Have I not Boldly revealed myself to You?
Oh, I see, you were busy
Too busy to notice my entrance!
What's that you said? You thought...
You thought I would only deal with those "Others"
Why by now you know I don't discriminate

*

Why do you insist on calling me the invisible enemy?
Is that your way of saying that I sucker-punched you?
So, you believe yourself so powerful
So untouchable, So carefree!
You failed to see my Might even as I got closer to you.

*

Coronavirus and Vulnerable People: Addressing the Divide in Harm and Responses and Exploring Implications for a More Peaceful World, pp. 89–109

Why do you insist on calling me the invisible enemy?
You don't see me yet? I know you do!
Every life extinguished, it's me
Every tear shed, it's me
Every moment of fear felt, it's me
Every traumatic breath of defeat, it's me
And yet you insist on calling me the invisible enemy
I wonder when will you really see me?
Oh, now I see, you do see me,
The World sees me!

I am Corona Virus, Global Queen indeed!! 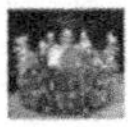

—**Dr. Fanya Jabouin Monnay**

The above poem "Corona Virus Speaks" is a self-reflection by coauthor Fanya Jabouin Monnay, penned while in lockdown. Her words emerged as she was curious about how her fellow Haitian colleagues were dealing with this pandemic. In particular, she wondered how they were dealing with the overwhelming grief and loss which dominated discussions among the members of the Haitian Mental Health Think Tank (HMHTT) in South Florida; this curiosity fueled the authors' desire to engage in the research study described in this chapter. The authors wanted to gain insight into how other Haitian mental health clinicians and practitioners reflected on grief and loss during the COVID-19 pandemic. The authors also sought to use this study as a tool to gauge the impact of this pandemic on the personal and professional lives of their fellow Haitian American mental health clinicians. This study's findings demonstrated how these clinicians, although directly affected by this pandemic, were still able to overcome their shock, reach back to their cultural roots, embrace the uncertainty found in the pandemic's chaos, and acknowledge the change and adapt to a new life rhythm. This process is what these clinicians recognize as their cultural resilience.

INTRODUCTION

The COVID-19 pandemic has brought a halt to the daily lives of most everyone globally due to the onslaught of death and grief it has unleashed. In the United States, COVID-19 became a magnifier of societal inequities for the African diaspora. The death rates are disproportionally higher in communities largely populated by people of African descent (Fortuna et al., 2020; Laster Pirtle, 2020; Millett et al., 2020). This insurmountable level of grief and loss is compounded by the social and physical distance that is required to maintain one's health and safety. Traditional African diasporic grief customs embrace a village concept to people deal with grief and loss. However, social distance protocols nullify the healing ability found within the construct of the village. As an example, for Haitians, cultural burial rituals such as the family gathering and spiritual sendoff of a loved one are now nonexistent (Denis et al., 2020). Haitian mental health clinicians have been sidelined and have had to find unique ways to connect to and support families who are in crises of unbelievable grief and loss. To this end, a group of Haitian professionals in South Florida came together during the lockdown period to support and dialogue about the immense issues and the work that lay ahead. This gathering organically grew to formally become the HMHTT, with the primary mission to support professional members in their work to heal their communities.

This chapter will provide an important snapshot of how Haitian mental health clinicians reflected on the grief and loss that they have experienced during the COVID-19 pandemic lockdown in South Florida from March to April 2020. The two authors of this study are both Haitian mental health clinicians who have worked with Haitian/Haitian American families to support their adjustment, acculturation, and overall quality of life in the United States. Some of these families are legally considered as immigrants who migrated for the chance of a better life, some as refugees and others have temporary protected status (TPS) as displaced individuals escaping tremendous strife and tribulations (Guensburg, 2017). Although in desperate pursuit of a better life, these Haitian immigrants are now faced with incredible grief and loss during COVID 19. Their lives are complicated by the day-to-day realities of life as part of the African diaspora living in the United States. As a result, psychological services from linguistically and culturally competent clinicians have enabled more adaptive coping strategies that supported the immigrant enclave to thrive and pursue the American dream. Unfortunately, this pandemic has offered a lens for scrutiny into the quality of life of the African diaspora living in the United States, revealing that many immigrants have been marginalized and silenced (Lindskoog, 2018).

AUTHORS' PERSONAL REFLECTIONS

Fanya Jabouin-Monnay, DMFT

I work in a school setting as a mental health provider, which is rewarding and stressful. Therefore, I was counting down the days to spring break and had one week left to work. I was filled with anticipation looking forward to visiting with my daughter, who was in Washington, DC, for a school internship. I was eager to be "the" tourist, and she my ever-dutiful guide. It seemed that she, too, was equally filled with eagerness. She kept reminding me to pack my allergy pills because the cherry blossoms would be blooming this time of year, and, of course, we would be in the thick of it. Boy, was I ready! However, on March 13, before leaving work for the weekend, my school administrators announced that we would need to take our school break sooner, and by the end of the next week, more information will be revealed. The verdict was that we would be working remotely probably until the end of spring break. Our school support team stayed in touch as we got busy planning and exploring best practices to connect with our students and their families. We were all caught in this web of anxiety and uncertainty, but as always, our team stayed focused, and humor was our coping tool of choice.

I knew of COVID-19 as it was on the Washington State horizon, but now it seemed more present. This point was clear as the phone calls started coming from friends and family in New York City. Moreover, my daughter was now leaving DC for home, and instead of talking about my DC excursions, my husband and I were discussing plans for her to self-isolate when she got home and her worries about us. That was the first wave of disruption and grief as COVID-19 started to pierce through and infringe upon my reality.

The second wave came rushing in like a town's crier sounding the alarm of doom. Initially, it was the pronouncement of my uncle's sudden death. I was told it was a "heart attack": appallingly, I felt relieved. But what saddened me most was that my cousin and her young son had to deal with this bereavement and loss alone. Due to mitigating efforts for COVID-19, only five people could partake in the funeral process, and no other remembrance rituals would be performed. We all took comfort in the possibility of a memorial service and family reunion next year. That was good enough for a while, and then a friend called sharing that he had lost close to a dozen friends from COVD-19. I did not know any of his friends, but he called because he wanted to connect with someone, and perhaps because I am a family therapist, I might have been a safer contact. This started me thinking how odd this was because some in our community were skeptical about this virus and felt shame for contracting it. I read about the burning of COVID-19 clinics in Haiti and the menacing threats of violence against people who may have contracted this virus.

Later that week, another cousin called to let me know that she lost her mom from COVID-19. During our conversations that followed, I heard so much pain, regret, and shame from her. She was struggling because her mom was in a nursing home at the time, a conflict I, too, am familiar with, as I had to place my dad in one years before. I kept thinking that it is such a mark of shame for a Haitian daughter not to care for her aging parents as expected. In her case, because of social distancing, she had no time for goodbyes or to see the body before the burial. That night I cried for her, her beautiful mom, my uncle, my friend, and the memories of my parents I so desperately missed. I also cried out of guilt because I felt grateful that I would be spared their loss from COVID-19.

It became a bit too much, and so for a few days, my bed and sleep were all that I knew. My husband made sure that he brought me all kinds of traditional herbal remedies to keep me hydrated and energized, but he allowed me to sleep as much as my body would bear. My body has always been the crucible for my emotions, and being immuno-compromised, it is not unusual for hibernation to show up. My body does not differentiate whether celebratory or grieving but simply is a vehicle of expression, the way I take time to process significant changes in my life. I reconnect through my body and vocalize it through my poetry. So, I hibernated, and I wrote, which yielded "Corona Virus Speaks." This also stirred up a curiosity for me. I wondered how other clinicians were fairing during this lockdown period. What issues or concerns had COVID-19 unleashed for them? Who are they sharing their impressions with, and how has this affected their work with clients? These questions became more earnest for me as I began sharing with others in the HHTT, where we held a sacred space for these unique conversations. We were giving voice to the idea of Haitian wellness and exploring our roles as clinicians providing psychological care during a period of incredible grief and loss in our community. With encouragement and this contribution's opportunity, I channeled my attention and embarked on this incredible journey of discovery.

Karine Champagne, LCSW

I excitedly moved to the Miami area to connect with culture, be closer to family, and build relationships. Little did I know that on the horizon was a pending pandemic that would shake me to my core and cement my beliefs about mental health. Before I could acclimate to this unique environment, build a solid support system, and establish a wellness routine to sustain my mental health, the COVID-19 crisis occurred. In March, my job informed us that we would be working from home "for a little while." Upon entering this quarantine, I had high hopes of finally having time to take care of my house and finally move. What occurred is a deeper appreciation of what my clients struggle with daily. I was suddenly faced with managing a chronic illness, polycystic ovarian syndrome, which includes irregular lengthy periods that left me feeling drained emotionally and physically. Due to my recent geographical move, I had limited support, limited financial resources, and the anxiety of COVID-19 but I was still required to be there for my clients.

My nickname in Creole literary translates to "laughter," Yet, laughter or joy seemed like a faraway dream many days.

I entered the mental health field in my late teens because Haitian Americans deserved the resources necessary to support their mental wellness just like everyone else. I saw this as a calling, my life's purpose, as I wanted to bear witness and help clients speak their truths. They needed to heal from their trauma, but most of all, I wanted to help them uncover that they had unique coping skills that allowed them to thrive. It is fitting that I had to put into practice and apply these beliefs to deal with my own traumatic experience during this pandemic.

I struggled to get up in the mornings and had difficulty focusing and following through with paperwork. The news, social media, and my obligations became heavy burdens that seemed too much. Staying connected was a chore, going out was anxiety-producing, and I was saddened that this was my new normal. I felt caged in and trapped. I was hypervigilant and binge-watching Netflix. This attempt to "deal" encouraged me to participate in a project where we, as clinicians of Haitian descent, could discuss how we grieve and how it has encouraged our resilience. I went through denial and then established "why this was happening." The ability to be around other clinicians to speak my truth about the way we (I) grieve was key. I showed up for my clients on those video calls, but the more I connected, the better I showed up for myself.

THE COVID-19 PANDEMIC

The COVID-19 pandemic is the megaphone that shouted out to the world Black people's pain and neglect in American society (Shadmi et al., 2020; Raifman & Raifman, 2020). This public health crisis has illuminated the consequences of marginalization and offered a masterclass for all to see and bear witness (Dorn et al., 2020; Wright & Merritt, 2020). Public health crises bring forth an exponential level of chaos, fear, incredible suffering, grief, and loss. This novel pandemic is no exception, as it presents as an enigma that is quickly spreading while its etiology and treatment protocols remain elusive to public health officials (Zhou et al., 2020; Lai, Liu, et al., 2020; Lai, Shih, et al., 2020). Moreover, the COVID-19 pandemic has significantly curtailed community responses to grieving and bereavement rituals and highlighted an emerging political narrative that does not engender a collective mourning process (Hutton, 2020). It has evoked a heightened level of panic and fear that Ho et al. (2020, p. 155) remind us "can afflict anyone irrespective of gender and sociodemographic status." They warn of a need to prepare for not only the medical impact but also the psychological impact of the pandemic. Another curious aspect of this virus is its degree of lethality to the geriatric population, immune suppressant individuals, and those with underlying chronic health issues such as diabetes, hypertension, and asthma (Tai et al., 2020). For the African diaspora within the United States, this pandemic is akin to them playing Russian roulette with their lives because of years of race-based discrepancies in healthcare systems and treatment outcomes (Samuels-Staple, 2020; Wilder, 2020).

According to the Center for Disease Control (CDC), *Life Course Report of 2011* (as cited by Goosby & Heidbrink, 2013), African Americans had a higher morbidity and mortality rate than any other ethnic or racial group. Goosby and Heidbrink (2013) attributed this discrepancy directly to systemic disparities in healthcare delivery for the overall African diaspora. These scholars contend that these race-based inequities cause undue stress, thereby resulting in further physiological and psychological harm to an already marginalized population. This marginalization of the African diaspora also results in political and economic losses (Task Force on Inequality and American Democracy, 2004), higher death rates, disproportionate levels of grief, and a diminished overall quality of life (Moore et al., 2020). This insurmountable level of grief and loss is further compounded by the social distancing and lockdown protocols required to maintain one's safety during the pandemic. However, for vulnerable and marginalized individuals, this measure appears more punitive than preventive and emphasizes the impact of structural inequities within our healthcare system (Goosby & Heidbrink, 2013). Other scholars suggest that any approach to rectifying our healthcare system's structural inequities must include active collaboration between public health stakeholders, including our governmental entities. Smith and Judd (2020, p. 158) offer that positive treatment outcomes during this pandemic require a concerted effort beyond the "biomedical viewpoint … clinical realm."

Nonetheless, our government's disjointed responses continue to amplify the risks of COVID-19 for the very people it needs to protect. One such group is the Haitian community in South Florida. In recent years, Haitian immigrants have established roots within the sociopolitical fabric in South Florida, which has resulted in an increase in political involvement, giving them more prominence in the region (Man, 2017). The Haitian population in South Florida is estimated at "more than 300,000 where "Haitian ancestry has increased much more than the growth of the overall population in Broward, Palm Beach and Miami-Dade counties in the past decade" (Man, 2017, p. 1). The Haitian diaspora lives throughout the tri-counties with the following estimation: 127,189 residing in Miami Dade, 116,818 in Broward, and 77,785 in Palm Beach counties (Man, 2017, p. 2). Besides culture, "equity gaps due to language, income, and immigration status have come into greater focus and are at risk of widening in the months ahead" (Lazarin, 2020). This means that Haitian immigrants, like many minority groups in this country, experience disenfranchisement and are disproportionately represented with poor healthcare outcomes (Williams, 2012), economic insufficiency and unemployment (Capps et al., 2020).

The State of Florida has seen an increase in the number Haitian immigrants since the 2010 earthquake that decimated the island nation (Esnard & Sapat, 2011; Sapat & Esnard, 2013). Due to Haiti's proximity to the state of Florida, this immigrant enclave has maintained close kinship connections and a clear sense of cultural identity (Kobetz et al., 2012). However, Hollenbaugh (2015) reminds us of the importance of recognizing Haitians from an all-encompassing ethnic lens. She refers to Haitian immigrants as "'triple minority' as they are immigrants, an ethnic minority, and likely underprivileged" (p. 6). Denis et al. (2020) indicated that these testing centers for COVID-19 have not been located in areas with large numbers of Haitian residents. In the early phases of the pandemic, the restrictive criteria for testing require that the individual be symptomatic. However, if the individual waited to be symptomatic, more likely than not, it was too late to find adequate treatment.

COVID-19 also poses a major financial burden on Haitian families. The Migration Policy Institute (MPI) fact sheet indicated that the effects of COVID-19 on immigrant unemployment status were directly correlated with specific industry groups during the lockdown period. Many immigrants are prominently employed within the service industry, where face-to-face interaction is paramount. To mitigate the virus's spread, these industries were compulsory furloughed or closed, causing an explosive surge in unemployment (Lyons, 2020; Sonmez et al., 2020). The effects of this global pandemic have intensified the degree of empathic stress for this group for Haitians in Florida and their kin in Haiti (Nicolas et al., 2006).

METHODOLOGY

The research utilized a case study methodology. A case study is a descriptive and exploratory analysis of a person, group, or event (Rowley, 2002). The authors conducted an in-depth investigation with a group of Haitian mental health clinicians to explore how these clinicians processed grief and loss pandemic related to their own personal and professional coping during the lockdown during the COVID-19. To follow social distancing measures, we created an online focus group to collect data. Focus groups allowed us to collect qualitative data that provide insight and meaning into Haitian clinicians' "combined local perspectives" (Grudens-Schuck et al., 2004, p. 3). The following questions guided the qualitative study:

1. How do Haitian/Haitian American mental health clinicians in South Florida understand and reflect on how COVID-19 has impacted them personally and professionally?
2. How do Haitian/Haitian American mental health clinicians in South Florida recognize and report on Haitian culture influences in their reflective practice during COVID-19 lockdown?
3. In what way do Haitian mental health clinicians in South Florida apply lessons learned of Haitian culture and their professional knowledge as they integrate new pathways for their toolkits with Haitian clients?

Participants

A total of seven participants were recruited purposefully (Tongco, 2007) and through snowball techniques from the HMHTT to take part in focus groups. The participants were diverse and represented a variety of disciplines within the mental health field. Inclusion criteria consisted of Haitian ancestry, specifically self-identification as first or second-generation Haitian and self-identification as a Haitian-Creole speaking clinician. Exclusion criteria were not actively providing clinical services currently or doing so for less than three years with Haitian clients. Six participants were first-generation Haitians, born in Haiti, and one a second-generation Haitian American. Five of the clinicians were raised in the United States, and two were raised and completed their undergraduate education in Haiti. All participants completed their graduate studies in the United States. As a group, their clinical experiences range from five to 20 years, and they work within diverse settings: private practice, higher education, medical and school settings, and community-based agencies. The name of each participant has been changed to protect their anonymity.

Meet the Participants

Terese is a family therapist who is motivated to work with her ethnic community. She joined her parents from Haiti in the United States as a prepubescent juvenile. She indicated how family separation and unification had a significant impact on her identity as a Haitian woman. Her life's work is fueled by her desire to honor and give back to her birth community and positively destigmatize mental health issues. She has over 20 years in the mental health field and works from a cultural, ecological stance that embraces individuals' experiences as sacred.

Nannie is a clinical social worker, and she is passionate about the intersection of trauma and spirituality in adolescents and their families. She is a dedicated and a strong leader in her church community and collaborates with various professionals, church leadership to raise awareness about Haitian mental health and culturally competent services. Nannie came to this country as a young adolescent and has experienced personal losses in her life. She draws on that when working with families that are experiencing grief and loss.

Alphonse is a psychotherapist, and he is in the middle phase of completing his doctoral degree. He considers himself more as an advocate and has taken leadership roles to support the Haitian community in Haiti and the United States. He emigrated to the States after completing his education in Haiti. He specializes in infant mental health and child sexual abuse issues. He has spearheaded programs focusing on the impact and cultural perception of child sexual abuse and HIV as public health issues.

Seranie is a family therapist who came to this country as a 10-year-old. She is a wife and mother of five children. She is motivated to work with families dealing with diverse issues, but her focus is to work with families dealing with abuse.

Ginette is a social worker, and she has been working with families for over 10 years. However, she indicated that "I feel like when you are Haitian, you have been working with Haitian your entire life." She takes pride in her work with Haitian families. She provides acculturation support to parents to bridge the cultural divide that may impact their roles as effective and nurturing caretakers. She is motivated to work with teens experiencing difficulties with mental illness disorders.

Edine is a mental health therapist and a doctoral candidate. She came to this country at age 6 and is proud to maintain her cultural identity. She has worked in the medical setting and especially in perinatal care. Her motivation to work with her clients is what she reported as "you really want to bring the best to your people; you want them to do better."

Jeanne is a social worker with 12 years of experience. She came to the U.S. with her family as an adolescent. She is a wife and mother of two minor children and has a close relationship with her elderly parents. She has been working in the community with children and families. In her work, she provides psychosocial and therapeutic support for children and their families. She expresses that her clients are not resonating well with "Covid-19 and telehealth."

Ethical Considerations

This study received approval from the Institutional Review Board (IRB) at Nova Southeastern University. The authors reviewed the purpose of the study, and its risks and benefits were discussed with all participants. Confidentiality, anonymity expectations, and consent for their active participation were reviewed and obtained prior to the start of each focus group. Pseudonyms were used for all participants. Participants were advised that they were free to withdraw from the study at any time. However, none withdrew their consent.

Data Collection and Analysis

A total of seven mental health professionals participated in one three-hour focus group discussion to elaborate on their personal and professional perceptions during the lockdown period of the COVID-19 pandemic from March to April 2020. The three-hour focus group was conducted and facilitated on the Zoom Meeting platform, where clinicians could reflect on their practice and that of others. Following a case study approach, the authors used an "interview guide to direct group discussion and stimulate conversation" (Dilotorio et al., 1994, as cited in McLafferty 2004, p. 189) and to "produce good conversations" (Grudens-Schuck et al., 2004, p. 4). The questions were divided into two distinct sections, which promoted conversations regarding the clinicians' personal and professional awareness about their lived experiences during the COVID-19 lockdown. The conversations were video recorded, transcribed, and analyzed to learn about participants' awareness, understanding, and their grief and loss during the pandemic lockdown, as well as about working with Haitian/Haitian American clients on grief and loss issues during these times.

SIGNIFICANT FINDINGS/DISCUSSION

Data analysis of this case study generated four themes:

1. Defining Grief and Loss During COVID-19

All seven participants acknowledged experiencing grief and loss during the lockdown. However, they differentiated their losses in concrete ways. For some, the grief and loss were conveyed as a sense of disequilibrium and purpose. For others, it was grounded in a profound spiritual loss.

Jeanne, a social worker, is one clinician who spoke about grief and loss in this way. She indicates that she had not experienced any family death so far from COVID but indicated that she and her family lost the barometer of what normal is in their lives. She expressed it in this way:

> So, I started to realize grief is not just you losing someone. Grief is everything around you; just not being connected ... something you're used to, something you're attached to every day and just all of a sudden, is taken away from you, your everyday routine. Everything that you know to, to be true to be real to be normal, is suddenly not normal. So, I think that's how in my personal life, I've learned to describe grief or the new definition of grief.

Although Jeanne expressed gratitude for not experiencing any family deaths, she still acknowledged struggling with being present in her own space and a longing to get back to her life before the pandemic. One can deduce that from her next point regarding her awareness about how COVID-19 has disrupted her family life and has robbed her family (children) of this sense of normalcy, there's a loss for them too. She explained:

> Just being in a home with my children and my husband being stuck in here. Um, I kind of started to realize we were all grieving.... They (children) are grieving their school. They grieved their classmates, um, my son would sit in front of a zoom class and start to cry while his teacher is giving a math lesson.... And I would just walk him away. So, I started to realize grief is not just you losing someone; grief is everything around you just not being ... something you're used to, something you're attached to every day and just all of a sudden is ... taken away from you, your everyday routine.... Everything, everything that you know, to be true to be real to be normal is all of a sudden, not normal.

2. Loss of Spiritual Connection

All participants acknowledged this idea of spiritual connection and how it has been impacted by the pandemic. This included not being able to go to church and struggling with the reasons for this pain. It seemed that some participants struggled with the idea that as a community, so much has been taken from them and now even the ability to collectively worship has been denied.

Here is a type of loss of spiritual connection, as indicated by one of the participants. Edine, a mental health practitioner, acknowledged experiencing losses from the death of loved ones. She shared:

> This whole pandemic has opened a lot of that for me (grief), our family has lost five people ... and I have family in New York and in Boston, and we lost a total of five ... right now we have people ill, and so it's just it's.... As a child, I wasn't really much of a funeral attendee. You know-how in the Haitian community ... it's an occasion. There's a funeral. We're going. My mom knew I wasn't one of those kids who were into it ... I wasn't one of those kids, so It's

> it … interesting as our family members started to pass. I just had this desire to be like; I want to be near everybody. I want to…. Go and lead and support with them. Now this is coming from somebody who's never … doesn't … and everybody knows, and now I've gone to So many Zoom funerals…. Um…. It's…. It's surreal. You know, I just…. (voice trails off).

Clearly, Edine could not participate in her customary cultural and religious mourning rituals with her extended family members due to the lockdown. This sense of surrealness fueled her longing for spiritual support that she normally would enjoy in fellowship with an inner circle of family and friends. Her retort that "I want to be near everybody. I want to…. Go and lead and support with them" may indicate that she holds a certain standing within that relational space that holds value for her and her family. This may be a profound loss for her.

Ginette, a social worker, having had no one from her immediate and extended family dying from the pandemic, tried to be emphatic for those who have suffered losses. Moreover, she acknowledged tremendous frustration in her spiritual sense of good, which she felt was being challenged by this pandemic. She offered:

> I felt like I saw a lot of denial in our community. And, and, you know, it's like, for some people, until it hits home for them, then they don't believe it's true. You know, I remember it was a lot of frustration in the beginning it was…. A lot of frustration, so I had to do a lot of self-care … to not even or even convince your aunts like don't go to church. It's, you know, it's tough. And you know I'm Haitian, they say I don't know, everything is "Se travay satan … it the devil's work … blame the devil. So, it was a lot of frustration, trying to explain to them like, listen, even in the Bible. God says, you know, stay inside until it's safe to come out, you know, trying to speak their language kind of bridge the faith with their beliefs…. You know, jobs are closing. It's not an attack against the church, per se. And, you know, you can still go to church online, you can still do a lot of things online. So, kind of bringing things home to my community. It was hard at the beginning, and not taking it so personal. So, like, you know, when you're watching somebody you love, not listening to you. It can get frustrated…. But that's what I was fighting. It was the faith with what's going on, you know, either. God is punishing you, or this thing is not real until it's real…. I mean, I am thankful. My parents are obedient are not like those hardheaded.

From the above, we can get a clear sense of Ginette's frustration. She is struggling with her sense of good and God being torn apart by this pandemic from what she perceives to be evil and the work of Satan. Ginette, like Edine, shares an understanding that a cornerstone of their family life is their spirituality. They simply expressed it in different manners. Edine lost the sense of fellowship while Ginette lost her spiritual barometer in fear that the pandemic's evil was overtaking good. So, both have been dislodged from their spiritual connections and long to be reconnected.

3. Embracing Uncertainty

The notion of embracing uncertainty and maintaining autonomy during COVID-19 was evident from the participants. This lack of control and autonomy was pervasive with all participants during the focus group. For example, four participants in the study were parents raising school-age children or adolescents. They expressed a sense of tremendous loss and lack of control over their children because they did not have the answers. Their absolute authority as parents, given in the Haitian household, was being threatened because of the uncertainties and lack of answers. Besides the chaos and mortal threat posed by COVID-19, two of our parents expressed that they felt at risk of not being able to parent effectively because they had no finite explanation to provide to their children about the COVID-19 pandemic.

Seranie, a family therapist, recounted an incident that was emotionally debilitating to her and her family. It involved one of her children who has a chronic medical history. She described herself as "they say that I'm a hippie at heart. I just, you know, go with the flow type of person I don't worry so much about things," but after taking two of her children with her to a supermarket she shared:

> Um, and the other day we went out ... she wanted to come with me because she's been in the house. This whole time because I don't let them do anything. They'll go in the backyard and play volleyball and come back to the house. We don't go anywhere with them. So, I decided, you know what, okay, you can come with me, her and her sister, all three of us. We went, of course, ... they had their mask, their face shields, gloves everything.... And then, a few days later, she started coughing, and I just lost it. And I started blaming myself like, oh my god; I should have never taken her ... you know, what if, what if, what if, I had all these thoughts going in my head.... And I didn't realize how much I was affected by this because I'm just not ... I'm not a person who cries. I'm not a person who shows emotion, no matter what's going on in in in my life. It takes a lot to break me, so break me so ... it made me realize that you know, it (pandemic) has been affecting me in more ways than then I even notice.

The participant group grew silent and attentive, allowing Seranie to emote without interruption. She went on to passionately share how this loss of control weakened her, making her doubt herself:

> I wasn't careful enough. I didn't … mm I should have been, you know, the parent, you know I shouldn't have just listened to her because she was bored at home to take that risk. So, it was a lot of blame, you know, coming from, from my end. And I didn't know how to handle that. I didn't know how to process it. With. You know what I was feeling, so I just had a had a moment where I didn't care. I didn't want to be strong. I didn't want to, you know, show people that I can handle stuff. I just let it go. I just lost it.

Jeanne also shared an account of how she had to embrace uncertainty with her children. She shared:

> I have a six-year-old. Every day I have to kind of look for new ways, a new word to describe it (pandemic) to her or explain it to her. And now, every sentence that she says questions when the corona's gonna be over. Can we … when corona's over. Are we going to win over corona? This is how she is communicating, and I, as a parent, I can't even say, oh, you know, August will do this September will do this. The uncertainty, it's…, it's hard.

Both Seranie and Jeanne felt the uncertainties of being a parent under lockdown during COVID-19. The uncertainties of this pandemic threatened their traditional role as the absolute providers. They did not have an answer their children's many questions, nor could they relieve them of the anxieties for the future. Although it weakened Seranie and robbed Jeanne of her parental voice, both participants unknowingly embraced the uncertainties of this pandemic.

4. Adapting to Change in Life Rhythm

Participants acknowledged this is an adjustment, and it helped to refocus and allowed them to embrace corrective measures to change their life courses during this COVD-19 pandemic lockdown. After surviving the first three steps of this process, participants acknowledged that change was necessary for life to continue. They reframed their experiences to recognize that growth accompanies change even during the epidemic. Jeanne expressed:

> We should be grateful because I complain so much about us (family). My husband and I, we worked opposite shift … we would literally Pass by each other in a parking lot, like this and stop and have a conversation in our car…. We came from that to me saying … we're having lunch at 12 together and kind of just be thankful, just for that.

Similarly, Edine and Seranie, respectively, articulated:

> You know immediately after the earthquake. like, Well, you know, a lot of people were like, it happened. Okay, this is, this is what happens to Haitian people, and then we're just going to move on, and we're going to build, and a lot of Non-Haitians were amazing. They were just like, how, how is that even possible like these people lost everything you see the even parts of their bodies, but there's just up, you know what, we're just, this is what happens. So, let's get up and re-built, and it.... Never processed. Anything. It was just like, Okay, well, we gotta go. We gotta feed the kids. We got to do this. We got to do this. You gotta keep moving. Just keep moving ... you know it's almost like the little fish in Finding Nemo, just keep swimming.

> This is something that I like I this is something that I've learned at a young age. I have to continue to keep pushing forward. Keep moving. That time to cry, that time to scream, that time to do whatever. But once that's over. You pick yourself up, and you keep going. So, um, this is something that I've experienced in within my own, you know, family than my own culture. That's We don't give up easily.

The participants discussed their growth from the COVID-19 lockdown experience and how they had to create new paths toward establishing a new normal. Remarkably, all the participants acknowledged taking this big step forward; they attributed this growth as revealed from the four themes detailed above. Even after experiencing personal grief and loss and uncertainties in their daily lives, the participants intuitively tapped into their cultural history to demonstrate their resilience. They rationalized, we have been through much worse, and we are still here, and this pandemic too, we shall overcome. As one group member stated, which echoed with observable head nods, "Haitians bounce back, we are not easily broken" and "so every day. I think we just start to kind of create a new normal."

CONCLUSION

The COVID-19 pandemic crash-landed in African diaspora communities like a wrecking ball leaving grief and loss as its signature imprint. For the Haitian community, this pandemic has unearthed some deep-rooted psychological wounds suffered from the traumatic disaster of all time, the earthquake of 2010 (Giuseppe et al., 2012; Shultz et al., 2012). During this epic natural disaster, the need for mental health services became much more pronounced in Haiti, as well as among the diaspora (Messiah et al., 2014; Kobetz et al., 2012). What was previously ignored in Haitian customs has been demystified and become relevant to psychological discourse. Haitian mental health professionals were sought after the earthquake, and they responded to the call as cultural brokers, community educators, advocates, and practitioners. Similarly, during the COVID-19 pandemic lockdown, these same professionals and their respective roles are once again summoned to support the Haitian diaspora communities.

This study highlighted seven Haitian American Mental Health clinicians' voices and contributes to the literature by offering an intimate snapshot into these clinicians' reflections during the COVID-19 pandemic lockdown in South Florida. Moreover, it speaks to the clinicians' perception of their emotional responses during this crisis and reinforces a collective experience of a healing process that some scholars surmise is culturally bound (Nicolas et al., 2010). Many within the group invoked their ethnic identity and pride as a testament to their resilience. This was evident when one participant stated that Haitians have a "stick to it-ness" that she described as innate and passed down as a core survivorship value. This notion of survivorship is said by some to be part of the cultural DNA of Haitians.

Nicolas et al. (2010) indicate that Haitians weather the storms of life like bamboo, which bends but never gets uprooted. Here these clinicians not only acknowledged their flexibility during stressful life events but offered a context from which it manifested. They noted their initial response was one of emotional shutdown and paralysis or "Séizisman" (Nicolas et al., 2006, p. 704). This state of temporary shock created a protective cocoon for these therapists to begin their ascent to life's equilibrium.

The cocoon became visible as each participant shared their story. At the forefront of these clinicians' recollections were past traumas and the similarities to this present crisis. Delving and sharing, they were able to find a cultural pattern of perseverance. They had reached deep into their past, gain clarity, and understood that "giving up" was never a viable option. Resulting from this recognition, they recounted a four-step process. First, defining their experiences and bearing witness to each other's story of loss and healing. During the loss, they also experienced a loss of spiritual connection due to being forced to deal with life's uncertainties at a crucial time. However, by embracing the uncertainties, they learned to adapt to changes and find a new life's rhythm. This ultimate step of change is accompanied by signs of personal growth and emotional equilibrium.

Another result of the study was to bring together a diverse group of Haitian American clinicians to engage in meaningful dialogue, both personally and professionally, regarding COVID-19 and beyond. These clinicians seemed receptive and enthused by such a process which may create room for future professional collaboration and support amongst clinicians from the Haitian diaspora. Unintentionally, the focus group process triggered a group response that seems to mimic a lakou system familiar to all Haitians. Désir (2011) explained that the "lakou system" is a social framework where cultural and spiritual knowledge is transmitted. This speaks directly to the intentional and unintentional benefits of this virtual focus group that provided a safe space for not only fellowship between these clinicians but self-renewal.

This focus group also served as a source and a mechanism by which the clinicians could reconnect and renew their professional commitments to help serve the Haitian diaspora communities during this crisis. They seemed eager to share freely with one another and share their hopes and expectation of the work ahead. Clinicians were once again committed to work with clients helping them tap into their cultural reservoir for sustenance during and after this pandemic. The clinicians also noted that they are gaining strength in knowing that other Haitian clinicians are heeding the call to heal the Haitian diaspora communities. This notion of strength in numbers reminds the authors of the national motto seen on our Haitian Flag, "L'Union Fait la Force," translated as in Unity, there is strength.

ACKNOWLEDGMENT

The authors wish to thank the clinicians who were so gracious to share their stories. We acknowledge Dr. Charlene Desir for her unwavering support and guidance in preparing this manuscript; Georges Bossous, Jr. for his input in kickstarting this venture, and all the Haitian Healers Think Tank members for this incredible journey of exploration and the opportunity to learn from each other.

REFERENCES

Capps, R., Batalova, J., & Gelatt, J. (2020). *COVID-19 and unemployment: Assessing the early fallout for immigrants and other U.S. workers.* Migration Policy Institute.

Denis, S., Metayer, N., Paul, L., & Saint Jean, G. (2020, April 9). COVID-19 pandemic is a menace to Haitian American communities. *Haitian Times.* https://haitiantimes.com/2020/04/09/covid-19-pandemic-is-a-menace-to-haitian-americancommunities/

Désir, C. (2011). Diasporic lakou: A Haitian academic explores her path to Haiti pre-and post-earthquake. *Harvard Educational Review, 81*(2), 278–296.

Dorn, A., Cooney, R. E., & Sabin, M. L. (2020). COVID-19 exacerbating inequalities in the US. *Lancet, 395*(10232), 1243–1244.

Esnard, A., & Sapat, A. (2011). Disasters, diasporas and host communities: Insights in the aftermath of the Haiti earthquake. *Journal of Disaster Research, 6,* 331–342.

Fortuna, L., Tolou-Shams, M., Robles-Ramamurthy, B., & Porche, M. V. (2020). Inequity and the disproportionate impact of COVID-19 on communities of color in the United States: The need for a trauma-informed social justice response. *Psychological Trauma: Theory, Research, Practice, and Policy, 12*(5), 443–445.

Goosby, B., & Heidbrink, C. (2013). Transgenerational consequences of racial discrimination for African American health. *Sociology Compass*, 7(8), 630–643.

Guensburg, C. (2017). *US Homeland Security inquiry into Haitians spurs fears about TPS*. Federal Information & News Dispatch. http://ezalumni.library.nyu.edu:2048/login?url=https://search-proquestcom.alumniproxy.library.nyu.edu/docview/1896866062?accountid=33843

Grudens-Schuck, N., Lundy Allen, B., & Larson, K. (2004). *Methodology brief: Focus group fundamentals*. Extension Community and Economic Development Publications. https://dr.lib.iastate.edu/server/api/core/bitstreams/4b1b9b74-3d16-416e-83aa-edff9dadd60/content

Ho, C., Chee, C., & Ho, R. (2020). Mental health strategies to combat the psychological impact of COVID-19 beyond paranoia and panic. *Annals of the Academy of Medicine Singapore. 49*(3), 155–160

Hollenbaugh, M. (2015). Working with Haitian immigrants during the grief process: Considerations for counselors. *VISTAS*. http://www.counseling.org/knowledge-center/vistas

Hutton, R. (2020, June 28). Lack of collective mourning compounds COVID grief. *Star Tribune*. http://e.startribune.com/Olive/ODN/StarTribune/shared/ShowArticle.aspx?doc=MST%2F2020%2F06%2F28&entity=Ar00103&sk=1075B082&mode=text

Kobetz, E., Menard, J., Kish, J., Bishop, I., Hazan, G., & Nicolas, G. (2012). Impacts of the 2010 Haitian earthquake in the diaspora: Findings from Little Haiti, Miami, FL. *Journal of Immigrant and Minority Health Center for Minority Public Health, 15*(2), 442–447.

Lai C., Liu, Y., Wang C., Wang, Y.-H., Hsueh, S.-C., Yen, M.-Y., Ko, W.-C., Hsueh, P.-R. (2020). Asymptomatic carrier state, acute respiratory disease, and pneumonia due to severe acute respiratory syndrome coronavirus 2 (SARS-CoV-2): Facts and myths. *Journal of Microbial Immunological Infections, 53*(3), 404–412.

Lai, C., Shih, T.-P., Ko, W.-C., Tang, H.-J., & Hsueh, P.-R. (2020). Severe acute respiratory syndrome coronavirus 2 (SARS-CoV-2) and coronavirus disease-2019 (COVID-19): The epidemic and the challenges. *International Journal of Antimicrobial Agents, 55*(3), 105924.

Laster Pirtle, W. (2020. Racial capitalism: A fundamental cause of novel coronavirus (COVID-19) pandemic inequities in the United States. *Health Education & Behavior: The Official Publication of the Society for Public Health Education, 47*(4), 504-508. https://doi.org/10.1177/1090198120922942.

Lazarin, M. (2020, June). *COVID-19 spotlights the inequities facing English learner students, as nonprofit organizations seek to mitigate challenges*. Migration Policy Institute. https://www.migrationpolicy.org/news/covid-19-inequities-english-learner-students

Lindskoog, C. (2018). *Detain and punish: Haitian refugees and the rise of the world's largest immigration detention system*. University Press of Florida.

Lyons, D. (2020, July 12). It could be years before Florida's jobs recover from COVID-19. *Sun Sentinel*. https://www.sun-sentinel.com/coronavirus/fl-ne-coronavirus-leisure-hospitality-south-florida-achilles-heel-20200712-odkt3oq2lfgxppidwohaeis2ry-story.html

Man, A. (2017, June 2). With population growth, Haitian community in South Florida sees more political clout. *Sun Sentinel.* https://www.sun-sentinel.com/news/politics/fl-reg-florida-haitian-political clout-20170601-story.html

Mc Lafferty, I. (2004). Focus group interviews as a data collecting strategy. *Journal of Advanced Nursing, 48*(2), 187–194.

Messiah, A., Acuna, J., Castro,G., Rodríguez de la Vega, V., Pura, G., Shultz, J., Neria, Y., & De La Rosa, M. (2014). Mental health impact of the 2010 Haiti earthquake on the Miami Haitian population: A random-sample survey. *Disaster Health, 2*(3–4), 130–137.

Millett, G., Jones, A., Benkeser, D., Baral, S., Mercer, L., Beyrer, C., Honermann, B., Lankiewicz, E., Mena, L., Crowley, J., Sherwood, J., & Sullivan, P. (2020). Assessing differential impacts of COVID-19 on black communities. *2020 Annals of Epidemiology, 47,* 37–44.

Moore, S., Jones-Eversley, S., Tolliver, W., Wilson, B., & Jones, C. (2020, July). Six feet apart or six feet under: The impact of COVID-19 on the Black community. *Death Studies,* 1–11.

Nicolas, G., DeSilva, A., Grey, K., & Gonzalez-Eastep, D. (2006). Using a multicultural lens to understand illnesses among Haitians living in America. *Professional Psychology: Research and Practice, 37,* 702–707.

Nicolas, G., DeSilva, A., Subrebost, K., Breland-Noble, A., Gonzalez-Eastep, D., Manning, N., Prosper, V., & Prater, K. (2007). Expression and treatment of depression among Haitian immigrant women in the United States: clinical observations. *American Journal of Psychotherapy, 61*(1).

Nicolas, G., Schwartz, B., & Pierre, E. (2010). Weathering the storms like bamboo: The strengths of Haitians in coping with natural disasters". In A. Kalyyjian & D. Eugene (Eds.), *Mass trauma and emotional healing around the world: Rituals and practices for resilience and meaning-making, Vol. 1. Natural disasters* (pp. 93–106). Praeger.

Raifman, M., & Raifman, J. (2020). Disparities in the population at risk of severe illness from COVID-19 by race/ethnicity and income. *American Journal of Preventive Medicine, 59*(1), 137–139.

Rowley, J. (2002). Using case studies in research. *Management Research News, 25,* 16–27.

Samuels-Staple, S. (2020). The state of COVID-19 in Florida and South Florida: An early look at disparities in outcomes. *Florida Health Justice Project.* https://www.floridahealthjustice.org/the-state-of-covid-19-in-florida-and-south-florida.html

Sapat, A., & Esnard, A. (2013, February 20). *Transboundary impacts of the 2010 Haiti earthquake disaster: Focus on legal dilemmas in South Florida.* https://papers.ssrn.com/sol3/papers.cfm?abstract_id=2221282

Shadmi, E. Chen, Y., Dourado I., Faran-Perach, I., Furler, J., Hangoma, P., Hanvoravongchai, P., Obando, C., Petrosyan, V., Rao, K. D., Ruano, A. L., Shi, L., Eugenio de Souza, L., Spitzer-Shohat, S., Sturgiss, E., Suphanchaimat, R., Villar Uribe, M., & Willems, S.(2020). Health equity and COVID-19: global perspectives. *International Journal of Equity & Health, 19,* 104.

Smith, J., & Judd, J. (2020). COVID-19: Vulnerability and the power of privilege in a pandemic *Health Promotion Journal of Australia, 31(2),*158–160.

Shultz J., Besser, A., Kelly, F., Allen, A., Schmitz, S., Hausmann, V., Marcelin, L., & Neria, Y. (2012). Psychological consequences of indirect exposure to disaster due to the Haiti earthquake. *Prehospital Disaster Medicine, 27*(4), 1–10.

Shultz, J., Marcelin, L., Espinel, Z., Madanes, S., Allen, A., & Neria. (2011). Haiti earthquake 2010: Psychosocial impacts. *Prehospital Disaster Medicine, 26*(5), 353–366.

Sonmez, S., Apostolopoulos, Y., Lemke, M., & Hsieh, Y. (2020). Understanding the effects of COVID-19 on the health and safety of immigrant hospitality workers in the United States. *Tourism Management Perspectives*, 35.

Tai, D., Shah, A., Doubeni, C., Sia, I., & Wieland, M. (2020). The disproportionate impact of COVID-19 on racial and ethnic minorities in the United States. *Clinical Infectious Diseases*, *72*(4), 703–706.

Task Force on Inequality and American Democracy. (2004). *American democracy in an age of rising inequality.* https://www.apsanet.org/portals/54/Files/Task%20Force%20Reports/taskforcereport.pdf

Tongco, M. (2020). Purposive sampling as a tool for informant selection. *Ethnobotany Research & Applications*, *5*, 147–158.

Wilder, J. (2020). The disproportionate impact of COVID-19 on racial and ethnic minorities in the United States. *Clinical Infectious Diseases*, *72*(4), 703–706.

Williams, D. (2012). Miles to go before we sleep: Racial inequities in health. *Journal of Health and Social Behavior*, *53*(3), 279–295.

Wright, J., & Merritt, C. (2020). Social equity and COVID-19: The case of African Americans. *Public Administration Review*, *80*(5), 820–826.

Zhou, D., Zhang, P., Bao, C., Zhang, Y., & Zhu, N. (2020). Emerging understanding of etiology and epidemiology of the novel coronavirus (COVID-19) infection in Wuhan, China. *Preprints.* https://doi.org/10.20944/preprints202002.0283.v1

CHAPTER 6

TELEHEALTH IS NOT "THAT BAD"

LaTasha Russell

In this chapter, I highlight multiple speedbumps that have been present in my field since March 2020, when clinicians were forced to see their client caseload through telehealth. My hope is to bring peace and tranquility to therapists, social workers, psychologists, and mental health providers who may have been having difficulties maintaining boundaries, being consistent, avoiding burnout, and staying mindful. Being afraid of change is okay, yet we have to adjust and not resist it during these uncertain times. This chapter will encourage different clinical and practical tools for managing crises, including paying attention, being creative, holding discomfort, and finding true serenity. My goal is to assist mental health professionals to plow through the virtual obstacles that, at times, feel impossible during this COVID-19 pandemic. Our effectiveness does not have to be compromised because our work is now through a computer or telephone.

MAINTAIN BOUNDARIES

I remember the first virtual teletherapy I had with a patient who decided to smoke marijuana during our session. I asked myself, "How am I going to

Coronavirus and Vulnerable People: Addressing the Divide in Harm and Responses and Exploring Implications for a More Peaceful World, pp. 111–120

address this?" Of course, everything that comes up in a therapeutic setting means that there is always something to process. So, I proceeded with, "Has it been difficult to meet with me for an hour in my office without smoking? I never knew how often you smoked." The patient explained, "Oh no, should I put this out, or is it okay?" I responded with, "Let me ask you. Do you think it is okay?" I found it productive because she did not notice her change in behavior with the therapeutic hour online. I did. During the session, we discussed the shame that coincides with her hidden habit and her partner's desire for her to quit.

Let us talk about another patient who started our video session lying in bed with the covers up to her neck. Before asking her to sit up in the bed while we met, I had to first check to see if she was clothed, asking, "Do you have a shirt on?" The patient replied, "No, I am naked." Before terminating the call, I asked her to please get dressed, then call back. According to David Gruder (2010), a boundary is any limit needed to be honored so that we can work without resentment and with integrity. After following my instructions, my patient and I addressed how frequently she prematurely exposes herself in a relationship before the other party is ready. Through the laughter and tears during this session, this patient was able to recognize how she has always used her body to relate to others.

BRING THE CONSISTENCY

After the first week of my full-time telehealth practice, I quickly realized that I needed to create rules to maintain the integrity of the therapeutic hour with all of my patients during this transition. Switching to telehealth, clinicians have to decide who calls who, when does payment take place, and how many individual or group sessions we can maintain a day. After determining this, we need to evaluate how lax our dress code will be and what space will look like where we meet with our patients. Another pointer, please do not have the computer facing anywhere that will reveal more than your career. "What do you mean, Dr. Tasha?" I am glad you asked. When determining your safe space to provide a therapeutic hour, make sure you do not provide microwaves in the kitchen, pillows on your bedspread, laundry on the couch, and/or spouses walking in the door. Make sure your background is uniform to who you are and what your brand stands for.

Oh, and please do not text during the session. It is rude. I hope you did not do this before the pandemic. Let me tell you why. Your patient will think he or she is not a priority, even if it was only for five seconds to respond to a text you received. I know a millennial would be used to being dismissed by a text. However, no one should feel that way, especially someone who is paying for your time and expertise. Remember to be seated and ready to start promptly on time. This may seem to be of minimal importance to you. Nevertheless, it is not professional when you are moving around when the patient calls. Lastly, let us talk about logistics. Please have your charger nearby or even plugged in already. Of course, I learned this the hard way after my computer powered down in the middle of a session due to my battery's life expiring before my eyes.

AVOID BURNOUT

Many clinicians have told me that telehealth has been more exhausting on the body than face-to-face therapy. I have heard one lady say that she had "Zoom Fatigue," something that, of course, is not in the DSM-5. But we all have felt it. At times, virtual sessions can feel monotonous and not as engaging as meeting in the office. However, "telehealth is not that bad." There are several ways for it to feel intimate. Think about it. You are actually now inside of their home, and they are inside yours as well. The key is making sure your space where you sit for hours on end is comfortable. Find your "sweet spot," which is your daily maximum of patients to see before your words start running together. According to Monroe (1998), caring for others without feeling cared for yourself is a recipe for burnout.

In fact, the way to find your sweet spot is to determine how many patients you can see consecutively in a row without looking at the clock to take a break; if that is three, then your sweet spot may be six patients with a break in the middle. If you are one of those clinicians who think you do not need a break, I will encourage you to get up to stretch after five hours. Clinicians, you may be able to meet with seven or eight patients on a Thursday. However, Friday, you may feel burned out. Stay mindful of the stress that we are all under in our new normal. Take a break if you are getting mentally drained. After sitting for three or four hours, my favorite thing to do is to listen to stand-up comedy to turn my brain off and laugh. Whatever it is for you, give yourself a buffer. It is called self-care; it is not a crime.

STAY MINDFUL

During this time of quarantine, many people are looking for coping skills. I have found that my patients have appreciated the meditative techniques I have given, especially the gratitude list. Learning to remain grateful during a time of uncertainty is difficult because it is easier for us to complain. To find gratitude amid chaos is a skill because a common way to distract ourselves from the present is to focus on our egos (Woldt & Toman, 2005), what we want and need. Writing a gratitude list is helpful and reciting the list aloud is transformative. This gives your patients permission to focus on what they have and less on what they lack, which is huge during this time of loss of plans and routine. Through the screen, I have been able to challenge ungrateful personalities to think about how many barren parents wished they had kids running around the house or getting on their nerves, how many single people wished they had a spouse to argue with, how many homeless people wished they had a home to clean, and how many foster children wished they had parents to give them rules to live by.

Telehealth also gave me a channel to teach families how to spend time together and be creative, like how families used to spend time without television or phones. Over 50 years ago, families did not have television to distract themselves from each other. The telephone was a landline, and we all remember there was no privacy on there. As much as I believe in the introvert needing time and space to themselves, I think in 2020, we could all learn to be less individualistic, especially while living in the house together. Also, I have found homework to be effective between sessions. Giving family homework between sessions, such as playing a board game, cards, dominoes, or going for a walk without technology for an hour one night per week, can bring laughter in a tense environment.

DO NOT FEAR CHANGE

Dear vulnerable mental health workers, it is okay if you are struggling with this type of change because this pandemic has forced us to accept it without permission. In this same vein, many of our vulnerable patients actively sabotaged closeness when they felt rejected from the idea of losing the face-to-face encounter on the couch. They have an unconscious imperative not to allow themselves to feel vulnerable (Delaney, 1998). In fact, the fear of change and the fear of the unknown are two common fears affecting many of the populations we work with. Ironically, some patients have not had seen their mental health professionals since March because of the transition. Many of my patients with schizophrenia or schizoaffective disorder declined to have a session. It is not personal. They had a choice between continuing services online or not. Can you imagine meeting with your therapist regularly, then not meeting with him or her for five consecutive months? I cannot. I cannot even imagine those quarantined in their homes without any privacy and with major distractions that cannot make telehealth an option.

EVERYONE'S CRISIS IS NOT YOURS

As a clinician during the pandemic, the referrals have been nonstop because most people are in a crisis mode. Death, finances, and relationships were the most prominent problems presented in sessions over the past few months. For example, from April to May, I recognized patterns such as couples who were contemplating divorce. "Dr. Tasha, when can we see you? We are not going to make it." Many of the couples did not appreciate waiting four to six weeks for a session. However, they were grateful after the wait to work through their frustration, their annoyance, and their irritability after the stay-at-home order was placed. Another population that pushed my practice to grow exponentially was my suicidal and depressed patients. I began meeting with this population around 6 A.M. or 7 A.M., an hour or two before I usually started my workday until they were more stabilized.

Even though our country achieved the greatest unemployment rate since the Great Depression, the number of patients calling did not cease. However, specific groups of people called more frequently: nurses (male and female), single progressive women, parents with teenagers, and Black males. It was not surprising that Black males had unresolved grief and loss issues that they needed to address. Unfortunately, many of these of men started to fear their own mortality and wanted to discuss it with a therapist. I have been honored to work with this population. Acknowledging the pain, the invisibility, and the Black male's numbness daily, I believe, is my obligation. I am helping them to process their anger alongside their fears seemed overdue for 400 years. As for the nurses that called, they were mainly experiencing compassion fatigue and grief. Many of them also needed to process how their medical teams were becoming more competitive and deceitful with scarce equipment, such as masks and gloves.

PAY ATTENTION

I found it unfortunate that parents were finally paying attention to their children's mental and emotional well-being after everyone was ordered to stay home. I will never forget when a father called, stating, "Dr. Tasha, I need your help. I didn't know my teenager hated me." Obviously, the hatred that this father was feeling was exaggerated, however, not far-fetched. Many parents asked me to facilitate family interventions with their children to assess the anger, avoidance, and sadness that their teenagers were experiencing. According to Erikson (1968), the primary task for youth in adolescence is identity development. Many teenagers were losing their identity with their peers' absence at school, which plays a crucial role. An adolescent needs to have a positive self-concept to move smoothly into their next developmental stage—young adulthood—in which they must confront the dual possibilities of intimacy versus isolation (Erickson, 1968).

Providing family interventions through telehealth has had its challenges, yet the younger generation has embraced it, especially if allowed to stay in their room. The single, independent women often called after a month of no affection, no happy hours, and no late-night visits from their romantic interest(s). What I heard most frequently from the women was disappointment in their life's choices. Their main concern was that they had focused on achieving their dream career with "no one to share it with." I found it interesting that their single status did not change due to the pandemic, yet they felt their singleness "differently" after everyone had to quarantine. One female CEO expressed that she did not previously consider that she has been more career-driven than driven to select a romantic partner, which "felt lonely now."

BE CREATIVE

Being in the same physical space often makes it easy for therapists, especially Gestalt therapists, to read subtle cues such as body language and eye contact. However, since the COVID-19 pandemic, clinicians have had to be more creative in how we read the verbal and nonverbal cues of our caseloads without losing the connection to our clients. Connectedness can be best described as an individual's positive perception that causes him or her to feel genuinely accepted, comfortable, and valued (Lee et al., 2001). Seeing patients in the office with a mask on taught all clinicians to value listening with both our ears and eyes. We have taken many things for granted when meeting in the same office, which has seemed inorganic and unnatural through a screen.

For example, when your patient becomes tearful, your conditioned response may be to offer a tissue. However, I have learned to verbalize the gestures that I would have liked to have done in telehealth. Such as, "I wish I could give you a tissue right now. However, I am here to process whatever is bringing up this emotion." Another example, I have said, "I can see the tears welling up in your eyes," when I see that they are trying to hide their emotions or "I can feel your anger building up," which permits them to allow themselves to feel it and express it. Lastly, any clinician that uses humor in session has also had to become more creative. One of the characteristics that set me apart from some of my colleagues is my sense of humor, and there is nothing worse than a joke that does not land well. Ask any comedian. Through the laptop or the phone, there are times where the Wi-Fi connection will create a delay in the session that does not allow for the call and response for a joke. At times, both the clinician and patient will speak simultaneously, which can feel like a loss of attunement in the therapeutic relationship. Every human being has a powerful need for connectedness (Lee et al., 2001).

HOLD THE DISCOMFORT

During the pandemic, the racial climate of our country was unveiled. Why do I use the word unveiled? We viewed the images on our televisions of Black men and women getting gunned downed and kneeled on. Those cannot be unseen. From April to June 2020, the world witnessed systemic racism and implicit biases without immediate justice. Langston Hughes (1945) said it best:

> I am afraid the nerve of some white folks has gone to their heads and affected their brains so that they can't think right—only white—which is too bad, because this is our world too, so they had better get over that.

This anger that surfaced was not new to Black clinicians, yet it felt brand new to corporations and individuals who told themselves that our country was equal. Not only was it challenging to manage my angry reactions during this unveiling, but everyday functioning also became such a visceral experience. In my practice, I saw Black clinicians, Black attorneys, and Black law enforcement officers having difficulty working and managing their professional reactions while staying sane.

The truth is that a clinician can determine which patients with whom they want to work. For any patient who causes stress, I believe you can refer to or process with another colleague or supervisor. Of course, the stress reveals some sort of transference that can be brought up in supervision or consultation. Yet, hearing "All Lives Matters" from a patient identifying as White was tough. According to Page (1996),

> Racism is a sensitive word. Americans often avoid mentioning it, even when it is relevant ... it exposes so much, both institutionally and personally. It is a Rorschach word, a linguistic inkblot test. How you define it reveals something important about you: how you see the world and your place in it.

What do we do with specific projections involving race, gender, and class inside the therapeutic hour? Reframe the question and see if what surfaces is related to the presenting problem or do not respond because their dismissive language became an emotional trigger? Hmmm ... needless to say, whatever "comes up" on the couch can always be addressed.

TRUE SERENITY

Providing grief work while grieving will teach you quickly how to accept the things you cannot change. Managing our reactions to deaths reported on the news, learning how to disconnect from our work, tolerating our local and national government while encouraging others who are fearful that "the end" of the pandemic is near is difficult and, at times, impossible. However, during this 2020 pandemic, according to Dr. Dobson (1980), if your heart stays pure as a healer, you can honestly become more effective, more intentional, and more productive. Let me take you down my pandemic timeline. Through telework, I shared with my patients ways to find true serenity in March, April, May, June, July, and August.

(March) ***Teaching Endurance.*** Because my brother and his family lived in Beijing, China (teaching English), I had an interesting perspective on how long the coronavirus was going to "hold us hostage" in the United States: at least three months. My brother and his family had been told to wear masks and leave the country since January. Even though clinicians were bombarded with the same news headlines of people dying around the world, we still had to encourage and contain our patients. During the first month of coaching people back to health, irritability surfaced in many homes as people struggled with the inability to leave the house during the pandemic. These patients appreciated just having a safe place to vent.

(April) ***Adrenaline rush.*** Encouraging my community as well as my colleagues to complain less and abide by the rules seemed to be my new role as a clinician. However, I believe a true healer is stimulated by pain or suffering around them. It did not come as a surprise when a friend of mine, a pastor, called with an idea to provide a safe space online where leaders and clergy could go to vent or process their experiences due to the pandemic. Then, with all of the free time I now had, I started to record videos weekly to share, through social media, ways to manage frustration, lower anxiety, and eliminate depression. I remember one of the podcasts that I recorded was solely focused on taking the virus seriously. Although there was a bit of a pushback from my patients who did not want to meet through a screen, my practice did not suffer from the shift.

(May) ***Podcast overload.*** As rewarding as it was to speak to populations, like the local Board of Education, sororities and fraternities, the Bar Association, Mayor's Offices, and medical clinics, my favorite Zoom workshops were when I was able to celebrate people of African descent and give them a space to verbalize their emotions of feeling forgotten, overlooked, and separated from each other. Celebrating the Haitian Revolution alongside the African American experience through a much-needed healing circle was transformational and powerful. Said best by Delaney (1993), "If you had to decide: am I going to change the world, or am I going to change me? Or maybe the world a little bit by changing me? If I can get ahead, doesn't that help my people." It was beautiful seeing people of the African diaspora as proud and collectivistic people. Although we usually come together by breaking bread with one another, we could "eat at the table" in a virtual healing circle.

(June) ***Pace yourself, Dr. T!*** All things that go up must come down. And boy, did they ever. With more exposure came more referrals. I had started to see 10–12 patients a day with a nightly podcast in the evening before having dinner. My self-care was out the door. This is when I found my own sweet spot to work until 7 P.M. instead of 9. Let me share a phrase that I learned from a young adult patient who was taught by her mother that "no is a complete sentence." Saying the word "no" without apologizing is a skill. Scheduling people on your time and not on theirs is the most organized self-preserving characteristic you can have as a clinician. After learning to pace myself, I strategically accepted three workshops to facilitate with three vulnerable populations: High school senior girls without fathers, entertainers, and artists who were out of work; and the most fulfilling was a Juneteenth celebration conducted online to commemorate over 150 years of slavery ending in Texas. It was a bittersweet holiday for most Black Americans because it sheds light on a false excitement of something that should have never happened.

(July) ***Lost my favorite guy.*** After George Floyd's death shifted the nation's racial climate, many therapeutic opportunities happened, such as corporations seeking diversity seminars through Zoom with their staff. Nationally, many Black and brown people witnessed major corporations start to second guess our American history and look for an understanding of what is right and what is wrong to do. This shift made some white folks vulnerable in their desire to not present as racist, and I was honored to provide telehealth in this specific area of privilege. After landing a few corporate trainings that my father and brother supported heavily, I received the phone call about my father's positive test for COVID-19. After returning to my hometown in Michigan, my father was put on a ventilator, and three days later, I lost my favorite guy.

Interestingly, I was booked through September with patients from 7 A.M. to 9 P.M. daily. However, I had to tell each of them that I would need to take some time off. Clinicians, grieving while working is dangerous. Be honest with yourself and take time off. Real strength submits during times of weakness.

(August) ***Do not bleed on the patients.*** Because I think we have the best job in the world as mental health professionals, I missed providing telehealth and started seeing patients after three weeks of not working. Clinicians, whenever you take a leave of absence, some patients will be concerned about your well-being. However, my father's death was none of my patients' presenting problems. To eliminate their awkwardness of wanting to ask how I was doing, I told them that I appreciated their patience with my grieving process and that I am "back in business and looking forward to meeting with them regularly." Clinicians, please do not talk about your loss extensively with your caseload or boast about your vacations or share your medical leave; it is not your patient's concern. Take care of yourself. There are a lot of vulnerable people that need us. Telehealth is not "that bad." Healing can take place anywhere!

REFERENCES

Delaney, R. (1998). *Fostering changes*. Wood "N" Barnes.

Delany, S. (1993). *Having our say: The Delany Sisters' First 100 Years*. Hill Hearth.

Dobson, J. (1980). *Emotions. Can you trust them?* Revell.

Erikson, E. (1968). *Identity, youth and crisis*. W.W. Norton.

Gruder, D. (2010) *Nice boundaries*. Thriving Now.

Hughes, L. (1945). *Essays on race, politics, and culture*. DeSantis.

Lee, R., Draper, M., & Lee, S. (2001). Social connectedness, dysfunctional interpersonal behaviors, and psychological distress: Testing a mediator model. *Journal of Counseling Psychology*, *48*, 310–318.

Monroe, L. (1999). *Nothing's impossible*. PublicAffairs.

Page, C. (1996). *Showing my color: Impolite essays on race and identity*. Norton.

Woldt, A., & Toman, S. (2005). *Gestalt therapy: History, theory & practice*. SAGE.

CHAPTER 7

THE VOICE OF THE NURSE

At the Very Front of all Frontline Workers

Mureen Shaw

While the world reacts to the astonishing changes that the coronavirus disease (COVID-19) has brought to all of our lives, nurses continue to do what they have always done. Nurses nurture and care for the sick and comfort those dying, hoping that they may experience a peaceful and dignified death. Physicians are often the ones seen at the podiums and in various media interviews issuing safety initiatives and spouting statistics. Yet, no one seems interested in the stories of nurses as a means of examining the authentic human experience and tremendous personal toll that COVID-19 takes on those affected.

The nurse is at the very front of all frontline workers. The nurse is the first to break the personal space barrier to perform the nasal swabs from those who must be screened at testing sites. It is the nurse you see covered in personal protective gear for endless hours outside in varying temperatures, triaging all potential persons who arrive at the acute-care facilities, and determining if the symptoms they present must be followed up with greater scrutiny. The nurse must spend endless 12-hour shifts at the affected patients' bedside and enter the isolation rooms when their spouses, families, and friends are forbidden to visit. The nurses comfort

Coronavirus and Vulnerable People: Addressing the Divide in Harm and Responses and Exploring Implications for a More Peaceful World, pp. 121–129

the patient moment by moment when they have been intubated and can no longer breathe independently. The nurse knows the importance of tying a spouse's wedding band to their palm or ankle as a significant personal touch in their caregiving, a tactic that no clinical textbook can teach. Yes, physicians and various other important and respected colleagues care for these patients on a 24-hour day, but only the nurse stays for every moment of that patient's direct care.

Nurses see hourly what the hardships are within the healthcare system, and they experience firsthand what the needs of the patient and their families are when they are being affected by a crisis such as COVID-19. Nursing's focus has *always* been caring for patients and implementing health promotion and teaching interventions for better health outcomes. Yet, at the front of this frontline, nurses seem relegated to being only a background voice. Nurses are virtually absent from being selected as expert guest analysts about health prevention and health promotion on nightly news programs. They are generally overlooked when key health committees and task forces are being formed.

More than ever, the nurse's voice needs to be heard as much as those of other frontline healthcare professionals. What are nurses behind the medical-grade mask thinking and feeling? What are nurses witnessing in these acute care, outpatient, public health, and long-term care facilities as it relates to care and treatment of COVID-19? How are they and their nurse colleagues dealing with the challenges that COVID-19 has brought to their lives?

This chapter will explore nurse's thoughts, feelings, experiences, and views related to COVID-19 and how the pandemic has impacted their lives professionally and personally. These nurses will share their views of the crisis from their vantage point. Direct excerpts will be shared from a diverse selection of professional nurses working in the diverse nursing field. The nurses who participated are from various cities in the southeastern region of the United States. Readers will not only learn their firsthand account about the conditions nurses face as frontline workers, but their anecdotes will reveal that their heroism comes with a profound emotional toll worthy of society's attention and admiration.

THE VOICE OF A PUBLIC HEALTH NURSE

Nurse D. Hawkins (personal communication, August 11, 2020) is from Baltimore, Maryland. As a public health nurse, she has a unique community perspective on the personal changes that have taken place in her life since the pandemic began. Hawkins reports that nightly, she has been working extremely long days, often not leaving the Department of Health until after

9 p.m. She states that "I am still not the last one to leave." It has been this way for Hawkins since January 2020, when this pandemic began to take on greater urgency.

Hawkins states that she and her public health colleagues are "tired, [and] exhausted but have a sense that we must keep going." The COVID-19 crisis has taken a tremendous emotional toll on this dedicated public health nurse's life. "I've listened to people cry tears of anguish because they've lost a colleague or a patient." Yet there are times the tears are not from personal loss but from the receipt of items that not so long ago seemed inconsequential. "I've listened to people cry tears of joy because they were going to receive 50 disposable gowns from us, meaning they wouldn't have to use rain ponchos to protect their staff." Each day on the frontlines of treating patients affected by the virus and preventing the spread to others in the population brings its own set of new challenges. The public health sector has limited resources that must be allocated with great thought, including trained public health nurses that are available. "There is no one to replace us. So, we work, grateful this week was only a 50-hour week and not a 60- or 70-hour week," says Hawkins. She goes on to say that the end goal is to see this pandemic end, but she knows that it will only end if [nurses and healthcare workers] continue to work at their current pace. "Like a soldier marching on, I pull up into my driveway, wipe away the tears and resolve that tomorrow will be another battle and that one day this war will end" (D. Hawkins, personal communication, August 11, 2020).

THE VOICE OF A NURSE-MIDWIFE AND MOTHER

Before this pandemic, nurse-midwife "L.O" (personal communication, August 8, 2020), who wishes to remain anonymous and works in the South Florida area, would ordinarily be sharing the special moments that accompany caring for mothers and babies through the maternity cycle. The pandemic has changed these once joyful times of anticipation, as expectant and birthing mothers and their families have increased anxiety and fear. The experienced nurse or midwife shares the realities of maternity care during this pandemic, noting that it both challenging and rewarding.

L.O reports that her practice facility started receiving notifications in March 2020 regarding patients diagnosed as positive for COVID-19 at their delivery time. Still, their positive COVID-19 status was unknown during their previous prenatal visits. L.O reports that administrators developed a policy that she and her colleagues were to wear masks when seeing and treating patients in their busy facility shortly after that practice. She reports that within a short time frame, more patients screened positive for COVID-19. These patients were abandoned from their providers' care and advised to "just go to the hospital" if they thought something was wrong or they were in labor. For nurse practitioner L.O, this advisement was unacceptable, as she felt that telemedicine could have been utilized for these patients. "I was frustrated that our patients were left to their fate without support. My conscience would not allow me to treat COVID patients any different than the other patient population.L.O reports having strong feelings about this decision in practice protocol. She expresses that "if you have ever helped someone have a baby, you are able to understand that the presence of the birth attendant is significant in the progress of the patient and the birth process." L.O conveys the vital bond of support that she forms with these women and the families. She feels she must "support these women by meeting their needs and being present in their journey." As both a nurse and community member with a family of her own to care for, L.O reports that she "stands on all sides" of this COVID-19 pandemic. She feels that she has a high risk of exposure from her professional role as a bedside clinician with risk from patient exposure. Yet, she also has the added risk as "a person exposed to COVID by the actions of another, a person who has cared for family members with COVID, and a person who has seen lives taken by COVID." Like so many other nurses and healthcare providers, L.O feels that this virus has brought so many changes to how we live and care for those we treat in the clinical settings.

It is uncertain how long these new changes and challenges that healthcare workers are facing will last. However, one thing is clear. As L.O so poignantly states, "our lives will never be the same" ("L.O," personal communication, August 8, 2020).

THE VOICE OF A NEUROSURGICAL NURSE

Nurse S. Marks (personal communication, August 8, 2020) has many years of experience in the acute-care setting with her neurology specialty. She is a resident of South Florida. This pandemic has changed her thought process, professional practice, and approach to rendering patient care. Marks reports that during this months-long COVID-19 pandemic, she has mentally struggled during the performance of her patient's physical exams, especially while inspecting their eyes, nose, and mouth. Things have changed, and they are quite unlike the way they were before this pandemic. Every close encounter is seen as "a potential choice between life and death for us both." Marks works in a busy neurosurgical environment, but the always challenging and busy work setting has taken on a heightened set of challenges since the start of the pandemic. Work now includes the need to "gown up, mask up, and go to battle with an invisible enemy." Marks reports that her clinical environment's new normal requires temperature checks at the hospital employee entrance. There is also the donning of a paper-thin, grade one mask required for entry. In her opinion, the distributed masks at her facility "provide the lowest level of protection against droplet viruses or bacteria."

Nurse Marks finds herself questioning the rationale for such interventive actions as she feels that "carriers of this deadly coronavirus can be feverless, and only level 3 or higher- grade facial coverings protect against airborne transmission." Still, she takes her "free mask" and places it over the N95 mask she brings from her home. Mark's clinical duties take her for rounds and consultations to various areas of her acute-care facility, including designated COVID-19 units. She reports that these units are "interesting places" to visit. After stepping off the elevator, one is surrounded by purple respirator masks "like some apocalyptic movie scene where human-like aliens have taken over the world with unidentifiable faces." It is clear from Mark's account that a lot has changed in the hospital settings. The changes have influenced how nurses must physically prepare to take care of patients, and some fears and worries enter their thoughts as that care is rendered to those in need. But healthcare does not have a start and end time. The vocation of nursing in acute-care facilities is 24/7, so Marks recounts that "after I complete orders and documentation related to my plan of care, I take a breath and brace for the next call" (S. Marks, personal communication, August 8, 2020).

THE VOICE OF A NURSE AND DOCTOR OF NURSING PRACTICE STUDENT CANDIDATE

Nurse A. Joseph (personal communication, August 5, 2020) has been nursing for many years and faces the challenge of balancing her nursing career with returning to school to pursue a doctorate during COVID-19. She shares her unique perspective on the pandemic's current effect on healthcare and her South Florida community. Joseph feels that the current pandemic has been "really stressful for those in healthcare as frontline workers" and that after many months of trying to manage and fight the virus from the frontlines, the stress is increasing. Joseph feels that there was a great deal of support from so many people at the start of the pandemic. She expresses her thought that "the government, the hospitals, frontline workers, and the community, all sprang into action, hoping to contain this deadly disease."

Nurse Joseph recounts that during the initial phases and at the height of the pandemic, "normal routines [were] suspended and everyone focused on being safe and keeping others around us safe. Support and resources poured in for healthcare workers, reminding us that we are essential, and our work is being appreciated." However, now six months into the pandemic, she feels that things have started to change as people are trying to go back to a familiar "normalcy." But the one thing that has not changed is the virus causing the pandemic. It remains in "full swing or even worse." Joseph feels that people follow local legislative mandates to prevent the spread of the COVID-19 virus in many communities. Yet, there are others who " seem like they are letting their guard down and eager to go about their normal life."

Joseph shares a sentiment felt by many nurses and frontline workers of being "worn out and exhausted." The public cannot fully understand all that nurses and other healthcare workers experience daily in the trenches during this crisis. "The stress is real for healthcare employees. Besides working an incredibly stressful and challenging shift at the hospital or the clinic, they are afraid to go home for fear of carrying this deadly virus to their loved ones." Nurse Joseph sees what many nurses and healthcare givers are seeing–that "the whole healthcare community is in crisis." In the United States and globally, new cases of COVID-19 continue to emerge, and every day brings an increase in the number of people who are dying from the virus. Joseph expresses her closing sentiment saying that we can "only brace ourselves with courage, and hope and pray that the worst is over" (A. Joseph, personal communication, August 11, 2020).

THE VOICE OF AN EMERGENCY ROOM NURSE AND A NEW MOTHER

Nurse B. Rodriguez (personal communication, August 7, 2020) is a young nurse and a new mother residing in South Florida. She expresses hopeful optimism during these difficult times when she returns to work from maternity leave during a new post-COVID environment:

> After maternity leave, it was time to go back to work as an emergency room nurse, which happened to be smack dab in the middle of this pandemic. Upon return, the halls felt gloomy; the patients had a scared look in their eyes, but the one thing that never changed was my coworkers' upbeat attitudes. Now being back for a little bit, you can tell we are tired, over the process of wearing PPE for long hours, and beyond sad for the patients who are severely ill or dying alone.... If there's one thing that every nurse wants, it's to continue spreading love, not germs! (B. Rodriguez, personal communication, August 11, 2020)

THE VOICE OF A NURSE MANAGER

Nurse C. Williams-Emanuel (personal communication, August 8, 2020) has more than 25 years of experience as a nurse. As a busy nurse manager for an outpatient facility in the state of Texas, COVID-19 has presented many challenges for her and her nursing staff. "As a healthcare leader, you're expected to be the role model, the fire putter outer, the know-all. COVID-19 has changed everything for everyone. I usually have the answers or know where to get the answers." Williams-Emanuel admits that this viral pandemic "has knocked me on my butt." As a nurse manager, she has been offered the option to work remotely and manage the daily facility services. However, she has declined the offer, choosing instead to be present in the clinical setting where her colleagues and staff are, stating, "I expect my staff to get up and come to work every day, so I do the same. They are there, so I'm going to be there."

Nurse Williams-Emanuel faces challenges with the influx of changing information that healthcare providers are inundated with daily. She reports that she does her best " to keep [staff members] as up to date as I can." The experienced nurse manager admits that this pandemic has been difficult to endure and that she is:

> physically and [emotionally] exhausted, but I need them to keep giving.... I've always believed in leading by example, so I'm going to be right there with them." Although Nurse Williams-Emanuel's work environment is not in the acute-care setting of a hospital where death and dying are a daily reality, she reports that she still faces challenges. There are anxieties and fears among patients who come in for testing or [for their] appointments. Nurses are pondering a similar thought expressed by Williams-Emanuel as she questions, "when will we really know the whole story, and if we are all doing enough. (C. Williams-Emanuel, personal communication, August 8, 2020)

THE VOICE OF A NEONATAL INTENSIVE CARE UNIT (NICU) NURSE AND PhD CANDIDATE

Nurse L.T (personal communication, August 14, 2020), who wishes to remain anonymous and works at a hospital in Southwest Miami, has been an experienced neonatal intensive care nurse for many years. She expresses her experiences in her work environment since the start of the COVID-19 pandemic and reveals the influence that it has had on her professional and personal life.

Nurse L.T shares that she clearly remembers the morning meeting when she and her colleagues were told in the neonatal intensive care unit (NICU) that they needed to "take all necessary precautions against the spread of this new highly infectious and deadly novel coronavirus known as COVID-19." Like so many people facing the pandemic, L.T had to sort through the innumerous data that was presented from the news outlets and social media, advising us to "1) wear a mask, 2) practice infection control, and 3) take measures for social distancing." Nurse L.T feels that those in leadership positions, both the government and healthcare sector, "were late in implementing infection control measures to stop the spread of COVID-19."

Moreover, L.T voiced that the leadership at the acute care hospital where she is employed did not "get on board with protecting patients and employees against this global pandemic" until many weeks after the World Health Organization had released their recommendations. She states that the documented reports from the World Health Organization had been released months earlier regarding the severity of COVID-19, and it included the possibility of fatality. Although authorities from the Center for Disease Control ultimately advised the use of personal face coverings, nurse L.T reports that her facility advised the employees not to wear a mask. Nurse L.T has voiced that "the decisions that were being made were, to me, not sound, nor underpinned by evidence-based practice."

Additionally, L.T reports that recent information shared from administration to nurses working in the NICU has impacted how she is being asked to carry out her daily duties. She states that the policies shared during a staff meeting at her healthcare facility caused her to feel very "disturbed." The NICU staff members were told by management that they were forbidden to wear a face mask while on duty in the unit. L.T believes this directive was due to the administration being apprehensive about the possibility of running out of supplies in the future. However, she feels that policies such as this in a NICU will only harm those who are the most vulnerable: sick and premature newborns.

Adding further to her distress, L.T revealed that nurses in her hospital facility providing direct patient care are not permitted to wear their masks on her unit. Furthermore, the nurses were informed that they would not be provided with personal protective equipment in the NICU. Management rationalized that the NICU is a closed unit with a very sequestered newborn population, and therefore not at risk of being infected with COVID-19. In conclusion, this lack of a proactive response to best practice scientific data is of great concern for nursing professionals. For nurses on the frontline caring for all patients, there must be a demand that administrative leadership places nurses' health and welfare above all else.

L.T goes on to reveal that her NICU admitted nine infants born of mothers who were positive for COVID-19. This new normal work environment is having a disruptive effect on her coworkers as well. She recalls receiving a telephone call recently on her day off from an anxious NICU coworker and friend. She recounts hearing her friend's voice being anxious and afraid as she proceeded to the operating room to assist with delivering their first positive COVID-19 baby. L.T did what nurses often do for each other–provide support and encouragement to colleagues during challenging times (L.T, personal communication, August 14, 2020).

REFLECTION ON THE ANECDOTES OF THE SHARED NURSING VOICES

It is both inspiring and distressing to hear these collegial accounts as they experience the COVID-19 pandemic firsthand. During this unprecedented time in history, many nurses' experiences leave an indelible mark on these dedicated healthcare professionals. The daily experiences among nurses from such varied practice environments are worthy of consideration for inclusion among administrative discussions regarding policies and effective procedures for the management of COVID-19.

Nursing professionals are performing a vital role during this pandemic. The care being rendered to those affected in our community from COVID-19 would not be possible but for many healthcare workers' collective efforts, especially due to the thousands of nursing professionals' dedication at all levels of care. For the nursing profession, these voices and thoughts must be heard and considered. As nurse "L.C" so accurately stated, "Every NICU nurse and every healthcare worker's action, behavior, and decisions on how they practiced nursing during this pandemic warrants recording." Agreed. The voice of nurses, at the very frontline of this pandemic, must be heard.

CHAPTER 8

THE PRECARIOUS POSITION OF ADJUNCT PROFESSORS

Christian A. I. Schlaerth

INTRODUCTION

The COVID-19 pandemic has had an unprecedented impact on our society, one that has not been seen since the Spanish Flu of the early 20th century. However, while not as deadly (as of this chapter's writing), this pandemic has shown us how fragile many aspects of our society, and indeed ourselves, really are. Many institutions of American society have been impacted for better or worse.

The COVID-19 virus (also known as the coronavirus) has affected all people but has had a particularly detrimental effect on historically marginalized groups. The working poor are specifically impacted by the closing of the businesses that provided their income. This book will focus on many historically dispossessed groups: LGBTQ, racial minorities, the underclass, and so forth. One group that is not often thought about in those conversations are professors, specifically adjunct professors, or contingent faculty. For this chapter, adjuncts are anyone who lectures in higher education but receives an appointment from semester to semester and are paid per class that they teach while often receiving few benefits (healthcare, retirement, etc.).

Coronavirus and Vulnerable People: Addressing the Divide in Harm and Responses and Exploring Implications for a More Peaceful World, pp. 131–151

Adjuncts are often not considered vulnerable because of their status, as their education should make them solidly part of the middle to upper-middle class. Still, their wages and their job security do not match their class expectations. They deal with "status inconsistency" in their lives: prestige in occupation, but without the benefits that such prestige should afford them (Kalleberg, 2007). It is important to note that the numbers of adjuncts in academe have increased significantly since the 1980s. They make up more than half of the faculty at many institutions, and in some places, they constitute up to 80%. Despite their growing numbers, adjuncts are often left out of policy decisions and are viewed as being expendable—they can easily be replaced with the growing number of MA and PhD graduates every year.

A lot has been written about the future of higher education after this pandemic, as college classes were forced to go online right around the semester's midway point. Professors had to adapt quickly to using online academic management systems, distance-learning techniques, and other technological advances that have allowed the process of higher education to continue. Some see this pandemic as a test for colleges and universities: will they survive, and if not, what form will higher education take? Some might highlight Ivan Illich's *Deschooling Society* (1971) as a visionary in this context—schools are not necessary; education takes place in the community (or in the 21st century, online community).

Where do adjuncts fit in all of this? Are they the future of higher education, and if so, at what cost? They have had to shift to online learning just like their full-time counterparts, but in many cases, without any extra compensation. Adjuncts have faced the same challenges that average Americans have faced, but without the "luxury" of job security, as their wages are attached to receiving classes each term, including the summer. This chapter will seek to explain the unique challenges of the contingent faculty in this time of pandemic and show how their experience may become endemic of higher learning institutions.

THE PRECARIOUS POSITION OF ADJUNCTS

The COVID-19 pandemic has wreaked havoc on the economy across the board. While the news has covered the impacts on major industries, such as the automobile, airline, and real estate industries, a lot of the coverage has been at a macro level. If one of these industries fails, then many people will lose their jobs. This type of coverage largely deals with corporate profits, liquidity, and other advanced economic principles geared towards their stock and dividends' health, rather than their employees' health and future job prospects. Indeed, the government handed out trillions of dollars to keep these companies afloat. Yet, some corporations still announced that they would be laying off workers, such as a recent United Airlines announcement (Gilbertson, 2020).

Another area that has been impacted more immediately has been the retail and service industries. Many stores, restaurants, and bars have had to close to prevent people from gathering. These businesses rely on customer traffic and turnover. Without customers visiting their establishments, sales, and profits (which are relatively thin and unstable, to begin with) have plummeted, causing them to furlough or layoff their employees. Many places have had to outright close for good, considering the instability of the economy now.

With the United States seemingly coming out of The Great Recession of 2008, it is hit with a pandemic that has pushed the unemployment rates from record lows (3%) and full employment to a skyrocketing unemployment rate of 15%, officially, with a real unemployment rate approaching 25% (Hoeller, 2020). Those who largely lost their jobs working in the service industries were already working paycheck to paycheck, with little chances of advancement, no sick leave or paid vacation time, and often without health insurance (Ehrenreich, 2011). These were already the most vulnerable workers in the United States, and this virus has exposed many of the country's failings. Adjunct professors can be added to that list of vulnerable workers.

The everyday struggles of adjuncts across the United States have been well documented in publications devoted to higher education institutions, such as *The Chronicle of Higher Education* and *Inside Higher Ed* as well as in the regular news cycles, such as in *Bloomberg News* and other news outlets. They are contingent faculty members, which means that they are employed contingent on their institution's needs. If enrollment rates go up, then so do their chances of getting a course offered; when enrollments are down, they are the first to be cut. Likewise, each semester, there is no guarantee that an adjunct will be offered a class regardless of the institution's health. Adjuncts are also paid in a piece-meal fashion, where they are paid a fee per course that they teach, meaning that their total compensation is directly related to the amount of work they do, which has to be offered to them. Adjunct teaching is the sweatshop work of the institution of higher learning. One will see that compensation and continued employment will become more precarious with the COVID-19 pandemic.

Another issue that is faced by adjuncts and exacerbated by the pandemic has been that of healthcare. Most adjuncts do not receive health insurance as part of their compensation. The lack of healthcare leaves them at greater risk of the virus due to other existing conditions' complications. It makes their access to treatment for infection either more difficult to obtain or more expensive.

METHODS

The internet, and particularly social media, has become a new avenue for research, both in terms of a source of research and connecting people who may otherwise never have crossed paths (Mann & Stewart 2000). Social media has allowed adjuncts from all over the world to connect with one another, commiserate, share their stories and struggles, and ultimately share their successes in the battle for better pay and working conditions.

The internet has also allowed for a wealth of new research strategies and topics to develop, such as researching new groups that exist solely online, virtual lives, and impression management (Chester & Bretherton, 2007). One of the new research methods that has been developed using the internet is virtual participant observation. The researcher observes activities online and participates in those same activities. With the pandemic shutting down most in-person research activities and many other social activities, combined with the connections that can be made with other people online, this method seemed the best-suited choice to research the COVID-19 pandemic.

For this chapter, a simple solicitation for stories was posted on Facebook in groups devoted to adjuncts: *Adjuncts United for Justice* and *Con Jobs: Stories of Adjunct and Contingent Faculty*—both of which the author of this chapter is a member. They have 1,298 and 1,843 members, respectively, with many members overlapping, as of July 2020. Since April, members have been posting in the groups regarding the struggles that they have been facing since their schools have gone online. These postings have been included as data points for this chapter. They were unsolicited, public postings meant to engender conversations with other adjuncts, allowing them to commiserate on their similar situations.

To better focus on the issue at hand, the author also posted a request in both groups soliciting adjuncts to share the unique struggles they have faced with the ongoing pandemic. The post read:

> Hey all:
>
> I'm writing a book chapter on the struggles that adjuncts have faced during this pandemic. The goal is to bring light to our struggles. I know what some of the things we have faced, but I would like to put a more human face to the problem rather than rely on *The Chronicle* or *Inside Higher Ed*. If you would like to share, post below, or send me a private message.
>
> If this post violates community rules, I understand. I should note that I am not making any money off the book or chapter. Thank you in advance.

The post was also made on the wall of the author's own personal Facebook account. It was posted to each group twice, as new members have been added to the groups since the first posting. The posts were approved by moderators, who promoted and encouraged members to respond.

There were many responses to the post, mostly regarding economic hardships and health issues in general. Those posts that were specific to the COVID-19 pandemic were used in the analysis for this chapter. Some respondents did not want to post a response to the solicitation out of fear of retribution from their institution(s) or of not being offered any classes in the future. Instead, those individuals sent a private message (email or through Facebook Messenger) directly to the author regarding their situations during the pandemic. No identifying information is reported beyond the United States region, the number of schools the person works at (as many adjuncts teach at multiple institutions to make a better salary), and other broad information when applicable.

Another source of data was personal communications with union organizers regarding adjuncts' state and their respective unions. This source was meant to get a pulse on what their members have been facing. The process of unionization and collective bargaining requires a lot of face-to-face work and cooperation. The pandemic has disrupted all of this, and the health of those efforts us indicative of the particular situation that adjuncts across the country have faced. Notes were taken during these conversations, with the conversant having been made aware of the data collection efforts for this chapter. For this part of the data, only the country's state or region was discussed to protect the participants' identity and prevent any harm to their bargaining or unionizing (depending on their stage).

Each of the posts and the field notes were copied into Microsoft Word and then analyzed for commonalities and grouped in search of repeated themes, consistent with the research method of grounded theory espoused by Glaser and Straus (2008) and Kathy Charmaz (2021). While unique aspects of a person's situation are important, they were not the focus of this chapter. If, for instance, a medical condition was mentioned by one person, it does not indicate what many adjuncts faced while that is important. The goal was to find commonalities that were shared amongst adjuncts, as well as ones that are unique to them as a group. However, many adjuncts face health problems and a lack of healthcare access, which are important themes in many of the responses.

FINDINGS

This research yielded some interesting findings concerning inequities that are not often associated with those working in higher education, specifically those doing the educating. Again, a college professor is not typically the type of person one pictures applying for public assistance or on the verge of homelessness. Yet, the reality of the lived experience of a growing number of those teaching in higher education is quite a bit different from the romanticized ideal.

From the data arose five themes that came through each of the responses that were given on Facebook, in emails, or in communications with union organizers. They were Extra Work without Extra Pay, Confusion and Uncertainty, New Roles for Adjuncts, The State of Unions, and Bright Spots. While low pay and health insurance are common issues faced by adjuncts, those became multiplied by the pandemic, as prices have risen, and health concerns became more drastic and seem to permeate all responses. These issues underlie all adjuncts' conditions and become focal points for any battles against their respective employers. It should also be noted that there is some overlap between the themes; they are not mutually exclusive. For instance, when it comes to extra work, which references the work professors had to transition to online classes effectively, it can also mean the new roles professors had to take on during the pandemic.

At this time, what many adjuncts are experiencing is despair. This has been expressed in many news articles that cover adjuncts and the pandemic, as well as by adjuncts themselves in the stories they have provided. For instance, an adjunct expressed in one of the groups on Facebook:

> Do I have any recourse? I am thinking, as an adjunct, I do not. Legal recourse? Suing wouldn't be worth the time and energy. Sigh. Sad. Frustrated. Angry. Broken system.

This professor was at her school for close to 20 years. She had her class taken away at the last minute and given to a full-time faculty member. The only explanation given to her was that she had used the wrong format for the class. While the loss of classes at the last minute has been documented in many complaints in unionization efforts, it points to adjuncts' frustration, something made worse by the pandemic.

Some subjects may be deemed unsafe to teach due to Centers for Disease Control and Prevention guidelines. As a chorus and singing adjunct expressed:

> (Singing has been deemed unsafe at this time). I'm not sure what I am going to do. I'm sure I'm not the only one facing these circumstances. I'm wondering if I might be eligible for unemployment?

Here, because the subject she teaches is singing, her classes are at risk of being canceled because, as she states, singing is not safe in these conditions. Her entire career, even as an adjunct, is at risk due to this pandemic.

Becoming an academic, for many, is more than just a career; it is their sense of identity and self-worth; hence the frustration and expression of despair during this pandemic—many are not sure what they will do, not just to survive and deal with the daily tasks of living, but also what they will be after this pandemic.

Another professor posted something similar but was given the notice that courses may not be offered in the fall due to low enrollment from the pandemic (Hoeller, 2020). For instance, the University of Massachusetts—Lowell is laying off around a thousand (1,000) employees, including one hundred (100) already low paid adjuncts due to budget cuts related to the pandemic (Reed, 2020). While being provided a reason for such layoffs may lead to some closure for professors, it does not lessen the sting of losing income from not being offered classes.

The three cases above demonstrate the overall environment that adjuncts are dealing with during the COVID-19 pandemic. They already knew that their respective colleges and universities' positions were precarious; they always step away from losing classes the following semester. Adjuncts receive contracts on a semester-to-semester basis, but often with the understanding that they will be offered classes indefinitely, barring unforeseen circumstances or poor evaluations. Well, this pandemic is an unforeseen circumstance. The remaining findings in the various themes should be read with the lens that adjuncts are usually in despair to begin with, but it is worse during this time in history.

Extra Work Without Extra Pay

In conducting the data analysis, the low wages earned by adjuncts often came up, even outside the pandemic. Adjuncts are paid on a per-class basis, where the average across the United States is around $2,600, varying by type of school and region of the country (Rodriguez, 2020). The pay is usually for a three-credit class during a semester, quarter, or summer session. What is left out of that pay is the time that professors spend preparing for the class, grading, traveling (between institutions, as adjuncts will teach at more than one school), and answering student and administration emails. When calculated, an adjunct may make less than minimum wage—not something one expects of those who teach in higher education.

The pandemic has caused a dramatic shift in how higher education is conducted. Across the country, classes were rapidly moved online around the period of spring break. This meant professors had to convert their classes to synchronous (learning happens in real-time) and asynchronous mediums to accommodate their students. As one of the participants asked:

> Did anyone get any additional compensation for the additional work they did in Zoom during the spring term?

This professor uses "Zoom University" to facetiously refer to all schools going online for the spring and summer semesters. There is a recognition that extra work was required for this transition. The question garnered a lot of conversation and elicited responses from many other professors, such as:

> I spent countless hours converting my classes to online (no easy feat when those classes are music ensembles and other applied music classes), in person and online trainings, learning new technology, fielding questions and supporting students beyond what I would typically do, responding to emails, attending additional meetings.... Adjuncts don't get paid enough as it is.

Converting in-person classes to distance learning was a very labor-intensive process for many faculty members, but especially so for adjuncts, who are already underpaid, as the respondent rightly pointed out. The process entailed working from home, recording lectures (both for synchronous and asynchronous learning), posting lecture notes, and posting assignments in their schools' respective academic management systems, such as Blackboard, Canvas, and Moodle (to name a few). It is a very time-consuming process. One professor broke it down by the numbers as to how much s/he made:

> This spring, I was bringing home $60/week for teaching 100 students in 2 sections. Commuting an hour each way three times a week. So certainly below minimum wage.... Going online during the pandemic meant no commuting but added many hours of work, putting the course online. I made about $2/hour some weeks.

In essence, with the already low pay of adjuncts and their piecemeal work, the take-home pay after all of the hours of work converting classes to an online format was less than the minimum wage for many adjuncts. As another professor put it:

> I can't afford to do more work without being paid for it. I know everyone is in the same boat, but some of us (adjuncts and contingent faculty) are in the part of the underwater boat.

Essentially, many of these adjuncts simply cannot afford to do more work. It is physically and emotionally taxing on them, for sure, but there is a financial cost neglected in these wage calculations. Many adjuncts have to use their computers and the internet to convert to distance learning, and they are not being compensated for it.

Over the last five years, one of the developments in higher education has been adjuncts' move to unionize for better pay, benefits, and working conditions. There have been many recorded successes across the United States with various schools, with Miami-Dade College being the largest and most successful union campaign to date. One may be wondering about the schools where the adjuncts are unionized—would the circumstances be better, or at least different? The results coming from adjunct unions are mixed. According to a union organizer at Miami-Dade College, where the adjuncts are in the process of bargaining for their first contract, the school has been quite aware of what adjuncts are currently facing and will not be challenging their claims for unemployment (a topic covered in another section). In other cases, however, many have expressed frustration with their unions. For instance, as one adjunct put in response to a Facebook post:

> Is there additional compensation for Spring, for all the additional work we did to bring students, online classes, and just off the fucking table? What the fuck?

Unions for many adjuncts represent the hope that their status quo will eventually change for the better through collective bargaining efforts. They are viewed as a panacea for adjuncts' ills, but unfortunately, unions are bureaucratic organizations and move slowly, working and compromising with management (Sutherland & Rainbird, 2000). With a union contract that governs for a period in place, it is difficult for unions to argue for greater compensation during this pandemic when (a) the colleges and universities are (claiming) to be financially strapped from these circumstances and (b) pay raises are often built into the structure of the contract. Again, these are unprecedented times where no one expected the global pandemic to wreak havoc across so many social, cultural, and economic institutions.

While low pay combined with extra work has been a dominant theme with adjuncts during the spring semester and summer terms, many have faced another problem: layoffs from their schools. This situation, unemployment, represents a whole set of problems for adjuncts that most have never faced before. Layoffs also present adjuncts with a new battle to fight with their government.

Confusion and Chaos

This section is called "Chaos and Confusion" because that is what many adjuncts have expressed since COVID-19 became a pandemic in the United

States during the spring 2020 semester. This virus has disrupted everyone's lives, and it hit very quickly, causing a dramatic shift in the American way of life. While those were the feelings when the pandemic was developing, the aftermath for adjuncts is the same: uncertainty about the future of their employment and how to deal with the impending unemployment. The coming job losses and position cuts were expected by some, as one professor put:

> Our president and provost have said they will cut adjunct positions, but we are paid less for teaching online beyond that. So we have to move courses for the fall online, and we will be paid nothing for developing online versions of these courses, in addition to taking a pay cut. If we still have positions.

As discussed in the previous section, adjuncts are expected to complete more work in transitioning to online classes and distance learning modalities. They can now also expect to be paid less if they are offered classes at all. The administration at this professor's school announced that job cuts would not only be there by job cuts but for adjuncts to also expect a cut in their wages after moving online. Administrations know that online classes do not provide the same quality of education as face-to-face classes, and they know that they can pay professors less because of that fact. Many administrations have also used adjuncts' precarious position, knowing that they need classes to make a living, to force them back into the classroom when it is not clear that it is safe for face-to-face meetings. As one professor expressed:

> The fact that so many adjuncts are being given "teach face-to-face or we get someone else" from their institutions.

Indeed, many adjuncts are being given the option to teach in the classroom in the fall or not have classes given to them at all. It has been offered as a "take it or leave it" option for adjuncts.

Aside from the fear of not getting classes, many adjuncts have expressed anxiety over whether in-person classes will happen during the fall semester, even at a lower pay rate. Currently, most schools are planning to go "on the ground" for the fall, with various plans in place to do their best to protect their employees and their students. Yet, with the virus spiking in many states during the month of July, there is also the fear that schools will go online at the last minute:

> We may see tenured professors push back, but it hasn't happened yet. Everyone seems to hope on ground will be canceled at the last minute.

Here, the professor mentions the word "hope" in what seems to be a hopeless time. S/he uses the word hope because there is an acknowledgment that going back to school in August will be dangerous for students and professors. That same professor also explained:

> During a recent interview for an adjunct gig, I was on the line with the dept chair and dean. They're planning to be "on ground," but I was less than enthusiastic about taking a job that would be risky for very little pay and no health insurance. They understand the situation but don't think they can change anything.... The pandemic should make it unconscionable to ask someone to work without health insurance.

Adjuncts already have to deal with low pay, and many are without employer-based health insurance. Now, they are being asked to expose themselves to the risk of viral infection at work while not covered by their school's health insurance policies. Certainly, some schools are providing professors who feel uncomfortable going back into the classroom with accommodations. Still, adjuncts are afraid to ask for them, as they may not be offered classes (Rodriguez, 2020). One adjunct, who asked that her class be moved online due to her health issues and health issues of her ailing parents, said:

> Unfortunately, both my parents have now contracted COVID. My stepfather is in the ICU on a ventilator, oscillating between critical and grave condition; my mom is currently doing OK with mild to moderate symptoms. As a result of this, I asked my dean if the one class for the fall could be transitioned online. I was told she'd look into it. However, my contract was immediately revoked, with the reason being listed as "instructor declined class."

She also contracted COVID. This particular professor communicated her story via email. The courses are used as the stick to get the professors to accept low pay and adverse working conditions. Many feel compelled to take the classes that are offered, regardless of accommodations, as otherwise they face unemployment. Yet, there have been stories of adjuncts being offered classes, only to have them taken away at the last minute and given to a full-time professor to fulfill the teaching load. As one professor put it in response to the Facebook posts:

> Online courses are taken from adjuncts who had been teaching them for decades and given to full-time faculty.

Earlier, a professor who had worked at an institution for 20 years lamented that she had her class taken away; this is what she wrote regarding the chaos behind her situation:

> I just got into my course to grade papers and found an announcement from another professor there. Literally, they put another professor in my class to take it over and to take my fall courses without any notification to me. I have taught successfully at this school for 20 years. I will not name them because I am not vindictive, just confused. 20 years. I hate to think about what is coming. I am thinking they have a full-time person they need to give my classes to, if they would tell me that, I would be ok with it, but their actions feel sneaky and underhanded.

The lack of communication from the administration and departments to adjuncts has been worrisome and added to the overall chaos. Like many others who have responded to the Facebook post, this adjunct is unemployed, which presents a new set of problems.

The unemployment system in many states is complex and difficult to navigate. Some could say that seeking unemployment is a full-time job in itself. Like those in the south, certain states actively discourage people from seeking unemployment benefits by allowing for website designs to fail, such as what has happened in Florida (Milberg, 2020). Many states have implemented algorithms that are purposely designed to keep people off the unemployment rolls (Eubanks, 2018).

While the United States' unemployment system is already labyrinthine, it is doubly so for self-employed or contract employees. Adjuncts are often considered contract employees, so they are not considered unemployed when their contracts are up. In addition, the definition of adjunct professor makes them part-time, and therefore they are rarely eligible for unemployment benefits. One problem that adjuncts face in this area is that they often work multiple jobs in academia and elsewhere to make ends meet. As one professor who also works in retail wrote:

> Because of these low wages, I also work a retail job. At first, I was furloughed but then went back to work after three weeks of stay at home. So, converting four classes and a lab online, working retail, homeschooling an 11-year-old. I'm the only wage earner in the house because my spouse doesn't work and can't qualify for Unemployment (*sic*). I also cant (*sic*) qualify for unemployment because of a minimum wage retail job.

This particular professor is being faced with many of the same problems that others are dealing with during this pandemic: moving classes online, homeschooling a child, and so forth. However, this person has the added complication of working at multiple institutions (according to another post) and working a retail job. S/he has been let go from some of her classes, yet because she is still employed at another institution and at her retail job, she is not eligible for unemployment benefits. For this individual, it is a major drop in income. This type of situation is one of the traps of being an adjunct.

In the end, adjuncts are left with a dearth of answers regarding their situations. Most answers to their questions regarding either next semester's employment or if they are able to collect unemployment begins with the very unsatisfying response of "It depends." All chances depend on the state, institution, length and continuity of employment, and other means of employment, among other factors. To confound matters, schools are not forthcoming with helping adjuncts get unemployment benefits and often challenge their claims—they were not rehired for cause. In a conversation with one union organizer during contract negotiations, a college was told that adjuncts were going to apply for unemployment, and the school agreed not to challenge their claims.

New Roles for Professors

Educators have always taken on multiple roles, especially with the rise of two-earner households. However, higher education was largely insulated from that. College is a time when young adults begin to explore being independent from their families— the students are treated largely as adults where they are expected to be self-directed. The college process had traditionally been simple: students show up to class, the professor lectures, work is exchanged, grades are handed in at the end (a very simplified version of higher education).

Granted, students have often looked to professors for more than just their classroom needs. They are seen as mentors in the field, guides for educational journeys, advocates, and other necessary roles. These are the parts that make higher education exceptional and worth taking on as a vocation. Many professors revel in these experiences, often citing that they make up for the lower pay compared to what they could make in the private sector or in a corporate job. Adjuncts are often left out of those experiences due to the nature of their positions: show up, teach classes, and hand in grades on time. That is not to say that they avoid the greater higher education experience. It is more or less deprived of them as their jobs are not stable, and they are relegated to teaching introductory classes with little chance of seeing students in subsequent classes.

The pandemic threw adjuncts into roles that they have rarely, if ever, had to deal with before. For instance, many would have thought that this current generation of college students, those who have grown up with the internet and smartphones, would be the most technologically savvy ever. That has simply not been the case:

> Students had to learn the new rules, procedures, protocols, and mechanical techniques of e-learning as much as teachers. And this was often *not done* because there's a false assumption that "young" = "digitally adept." Not true.

One thing this pandemic has shown is that the techno-generation is not all that technologically savvy. Professors had to answer more emails and troubleshoot more problems than they have ever had in the past. As another adjunct expressed, besides extra trainings, s/he also had to engage in:

> learning new technology, fielding questions, and supporting students beyond what I would normally do, responding to emails, attending additional meetings.

The move to online and distance learning modalities forced many adjuncts to become information technology specialists on the fly. With the move to online, it seemed as though students were just as confused as their less technologically adept professors. If the problems were not related to the academic management systems, then there were problems with the students' home situations, especially regarding internet access. As another professor described:

> Many of the students struggled with the technology as much as I did. Although the department chair encouraged Zoom, many did not have enough bandwidth at home for that to work well … I also had an international student who had only intermittent internet access. I made alternative assignments for her, but there was no way to make an equal experience for such students.

The pandemic has exposed class differences for students, even with things as basic as the internet. Many students rely on their residences (at college) for their internet access when in college, as some may not have it at home with their families. Students may go to a public library or a coffee shop for their internet needs in those times, but the pandemic cut off access to those as well.

While access to the internet was a common subject among adjuncts, even the more basic access to proper technology was also a problem for less affluent students. It has been widely reported that students from disadvantaged backgrounds face more challenges in college than many of their better-off classmates (housing, food, debt, etc.). Some professors expressed that their students had trouble gaining access to computers, in particular, as one professor put it, due to racial inequality:

> I noticed a racial disparity in technology access: several black students were sharing computers with siblings, but no white students. This affected their ability to Zoom and to take exams in the correct time slot.

Unequal access to resources while in college is nothing new, and neither is the racial component. Yet, the pandemic has brought these issues to the forefront and made them worse. It is difficult to do well in a class that has been moved online while you, as a student, have to budget time with siblings over internet access and computer time. At the same time, professors are aware of that and are pushed to be compassionate to these situations, thus creating even more work in the end. However, technical problems and lack of access to students' resources while not on campus are only part of the problem.

It cannot be stressed how chaotic the transition from in-person to online classes was for all involved. While it has already been discussed what adjuncts had to go through themselves during the process, they also had to deal with the emotional toll that it exacted on their students. Suddenly, professors were not just IT professionals, but they also had to act as counselors for their students. As one professor put it:

> Students were so completely scared and anxious. There was little guidance on how to adapt to expectations. I talked with a teacher friend, and we discussed what was fair. But I wish the college had given feedback on outcomes because our usual outcomes no longer fit.

Everyone's expectations had to shift once the college experience was moved online. Students were no longer sure how to succeed in their classes, and professors were given little guidance as to how to alter their outcomes. The earlier professor who had the international student also expressed worry for his/her students:

> I'm just worried about our students because I was flooded with anxiety-filled students. If it wasn't health-related, it was financial and or work issues. Time issues. Pressure.

Professors were not only doing the intellectual labor and moving their classes online; they also had to engage in a lot more emotional labor with their students (Ashforth & Humphrey, 1993). This work is not accounted for when discussing teaching compensation, but it is an essential part of the job. It also tends to take a detrimental toll on educators over time, who are often faced with burnout prospects.

State of Adjunct Unions

It has been well documented that adjuncts were making lots of progress in terms of unionizing, collective bargaining, and negotiating contracts that presented them with a better work environment and more rights. These advances require a lot of contacts and physical presence. One of the issues that came up in conversations with union organizers and from the prompts on Facebook dealt with unions: what were they doing to help adjuncts and their overall health?

In some instances, unions have been hamstrung by the pandemic. As they were winning their newly negotiated contracts, it became difficult to ask for more once the pandemic hit, according to conversations with union organizers at Service Employees International Union. Once they had won raises and payment for canceled classes, it seemed excessive to ask for extra help during this time. Some unions did not know how to respond to the pandemic. As the professor who earlier called this the semester of "Zoom University" lamented:

> I just sent this to my union:
>
> So is additional compensation for Spring, for all the additional work we did to bring students, online classes, just off the fucking table? *What the fuck?* I can't afford to do more work without being paid for it. I know everyone is in the same boat, but some of us (adjuncts and contingent faculty) are in the part of the boat that is underwater. From the view here on the ground, it doesn't feel like our union accomplishes much except a self-congratulating self-justifying newsletter every couple of weeks. Bottomline (*sic*) is wages, hours, and conditions, of course. *This is a cry for help*. Or do we need to organize a wildcat adjunct strike across the system? Please forward this to the higher-ups in the union who always seem to be patting themselves on the back for a single-digit wage bump every four years. (Emphasis added)

It seems as though this particular union was unresponsive to its members' needs once the pandemic hit. This professor was not alone in criticizing his/her union's response to the pandemic. As discussed earlier, many professors reported having to go through many hours of training for online courses and making the actual move to online without receiving any extra pay. Participation in these training sessions was offered as a precondition for future employment opportunities, with the expectation that adjuncts would accept the unpaid training. Other adjuncts agreed that the unions seemed impotent in their ability to help with the pandemic beyond what they had already done.

Not all of the developments with unions were negative. Some adjuncts reported receiving extra pay, albeit not a lot (sometimes a couple of hundred dollars, others received an extra week's pay), but this at least served as recognition that extra labor was involved. In discussions with union organizers, it was learned that some schools were actively seeking out adjuncts to provide them with resources to succeed in the transition online, such as computers provided by their schools or help with internet access (or at times, just access to campus). However, those reports were exceptions rather than the norm.

In terms of unionization efforts and the health of unions, the evidence has been inconsistent. For instance, Broward College won its first contract providing adjuncts with greater employment security, raises, and a grievance process. Around the same time, the University of Southern Florida has won its right to collectively bargain making it the second-largest public college system in Florida to do so in a state that is traditionally hostile to unions (as it is a right-to-work state) (McCann, 2020). Union organizers and leaders at Miami-Dade College (the largest public college system not just in Florida but in the United States) have reported greater participation from union members and an increase in their membership numbers. At the same time, they go through the process of negotiating their first contract. However, in other parts of the country, the reports were not positive. In a phone conversation with one of the Facebook adjuncts groups' leaders, it was communicated that the move to online and the disruption to the process of higher education has led to a decrease in union activity and participation at his university located in New York. Of course, more research would be needed to determine the trends that have been occurring with the pandemic.

Bright Spots

Much of the research on the pandemic's effects, particularly those related to adjuncts, has been overwhelmingly negative. Again, this event happens once in a century—some could go a whole lifetime and never have to deal with a pandemic of these proportions. The last was the influenza pandemic in 1918 (also known as "the Spanish Flu"), and the world and science were much different in the early 20th century compared to today. When turning on the news, one is bombarded with negative stories about virus rates, death rates, unemployment, government deadlock, and so forth. There have to be some positive reports out there, even in the world of adjuncts, as one professor responded to the Facebook post:

> Guys, is there *no university* or *no administration* in a current university or college that decently, sensibly faces up to and deals with the struggles adjuncts face during this pandemic? .... Is the situation as 101%

> negative in US higher education as it sounds here? Or are you guys mostly just venting?........ Hey, not that venting is all that bad. :-)

It is true that the Facebook posts did allow many adjuncts to vent; that was sort of the point. Most of the responses and stories from adjuncts have been overwhelmingly negative, as can be seen from the previous sections. However, this individual brought up a good point. No college or university was prepared for this situation, and some have done better than others in communicating with and treating their employees. Most of the stories about the universities from adjuncts were more akin to the following:

> A school I work for announced that we all have to take 40 hours of training on Canvas to be considered for classes at all in the fall (online or otherwise). This time is, of course, unpaid, just like all the heck of the Spring semester. I myself have worked online for years; I will work through it if I choose to continue at the school, but this seems egregious to me. I am trying to contain my rage, so I figured I would look for peers in similar situations and get to a place of constructive thought.

Most reported having to do more work without pay and more training to be considered for future classes. Yet, there were some positive responses. As one professor reported:

> We got a wee bit, but nothing close to a fair amount for the actual work that went into the transition. And they shortened the time frame for reimbursement.

This individual's college did provide some compensation for the extra work they had to put in for moving classes online. S/he also reported that they could be reimbursed for certain expenses, as this person's laptop fan gave out after moving online. The college allowed him/her to get it replaced quickly. This was rare, as most adjuncts reported not being compensated for using their computers, internet, or printers.

Another professor provided a comparison between two institutions that s/he was teaching at, providing a little insight into how different institutions operate. S/he wrote:

> My community college job compensated us an extra paycheck since they extended the submissions deadline by two extra weeks. It wasn't part of my contract but was appreciated, nonetheless. My four-year institution did nothing.

It seems as though the community college was more in-tune with their employees where the four-year college/university was not. They went beyond the contract to compensate their adjuncts, and this person seems pleased with what the institution did. In addition, the extension of deadlines is also important, as it gives both the students, who were stressed about the move, and the professor, extra time to get their work submitted.

When a college or university is good about their relationship with their professors, it can inspire a sense of pride on the professor's part to be part of that institution. As a third professor, who earlier expressed concerns for students, wrote that she was extremely happy with her employer:

> I teach at two schools. One school has been excellent at providing training and even a stipend for a 3-week training I finished last week. I'm super impressed with the university, and I am proud to be a part of it.

Many adjuncts reported having to complete extra training to move to distance education modalities and do it without extra compensation or the guarantee of future class assignments. In this case, the college/university helped to encourage their professors to get the extra training by offering a stipend. These kinds of actions are expected when one enters into the vocation of higher education: a humane, respectful work environment, more of a partnership than a typical job; very much, unlike what a lot of higher education has become in the last 20 years (Schrecker, 2010).

While these were the exceptions to what was primarily reported, the readers need to know some schools are doing what is right for their professors, employees, and students. As the fall 2020 semester begins, these developments will play out as schools implement plans to fully reopen, remain virtual, or implement some hybrid version of the two. How the schools have treated the adjuncts in this section is also an indication of how they will approach the upcoming semesters and the future of higher education.

CONCLUSION

When it comes to considering vulnerable groups and the COVID-19 pandemic, race, class, and gender issues immediately come to mind. So do transgender issues and those who live with disabilities. It is widely reported that this virus is disproportionately impacting minorities and working-class people. The struggles that the institution of higher education has faced during this time have also been widely reported, as the pandemic uprooted the system and brought to light many of the underlying problems and trends. For that reason, this chapter dealt with adjuncts because they are the "academic underclass," a term coined by Herb Childress (2019).

Studying and writing about adjunct professors is becoming more common simply because they are starting to make up a more significant proportion of those who teach at the college and university level, at times making up to two-thirds of a college's professors. Simply, they are becoming more visible. This chapter should be taken as a small part of a larger project in studying the problems that adjuncts face. Surely, low wages and no benefits are problems, but those problems have become exacerbated by the pandemic. As one professor put it, concerning the reopening of campuses:

> One of my colleges is requiring f2f this fall ... unless one can provide medical documentation of a need to stay home. As an adjunct, I have no insurance and no longer have a primary care provider, so I can't provide documentation of my two health issues. So, even though I'm medium to high risk, I will be teaching f2f this fall. I'm a nervous wreck.

The reopening of campuses highlights a significant issue that adjuncts face: working in these conditions without health insurance is literally a life or death decision as Figure 8.1 shows. Many adjuncts in this research expressed this exact sentiment, which really sums up their plight overall, with few viable solutions on the horizon. In the end, adjuncts are a vulnerable group, especially during this pandemic.

Figure 8.1

Adjuncts Dying Due to Work

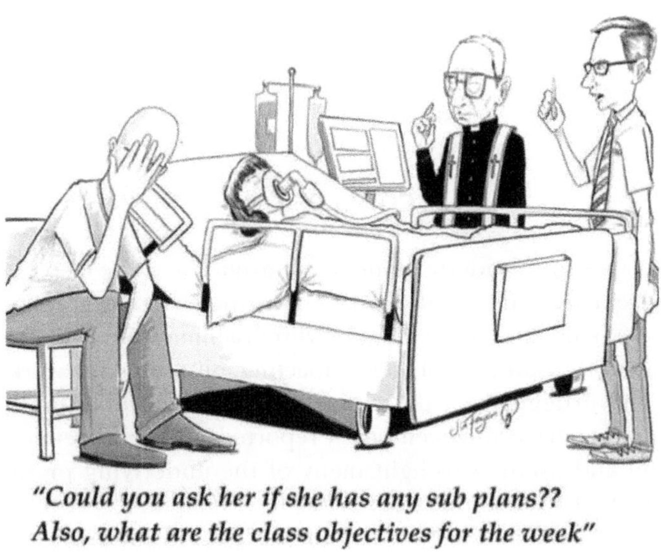
"Could you ask her if she has any sub plans??
Also, what are the class objectives for the week"

REFERENCES

Ashforth, B., & Humphrey, R. (1993). Emotional labor in service roles: The influence of identity. *Academy of Management Review, 21*(4), 986–1010.

Charmaz, K. (2021). *Constructing grounded theory: A practical guide through qualitative Analysis*. SAGE.

Chester, A., & Bretherton, D. (2007). Impression management and identity online. In A. Joinson, K. Y. A. McKenna, T. Postmes, & U.-D. Reips (Eds.), *The Oxford handbook of internet psychology* (pp. 223–236). Oxford University Press.

Childress, H. (2019). *The adjunct underclass*. University of Chicago Press.

Ehrenreich, B. (2011). *Nickel and dimed: On (not) getting by in America*. Picador.

Eubanks, V. (2018). *Automating inequality: How high-tech tools profile, police, and punish the poor*. St. Martin's Press.

Gilbertson, D. (2020, June 8). 'Gut punch': United Airlines to lay off up to 36,000 employees in October as travel remains depressed. *The USA Today*. https://www.usatoday.com/story/travel/airline-news/2020/07/08/united-airlines-layoff-up-36-000-employees-october-coronavorus-fallout/5396857002/

Glaser, B., & Strauss, A. (2008). *The discovery of grounded theory: Strategies for qualitative research*. Aldine Transaction.

Hoeller, K. (2020, July 22). Colleges layoff underpaid adjuncts then challenge their claim to unemployment. *Monthly Review Online*. https://mronline.org/2020/07/22/colleges-layoff-underpaid-adjuncts-then-challenge-their-unemployment-claims/#lightbox/0/

Illich, I. (1971). *Deschooling society*. Harper & Row.

Kalleberg. A. (2007). *The mismatched worker*. W.W. Norton & Company.

Mann, C., & Stewart, F. (2000). *Internet communication and qualitative research: A handbook for researching online*. SAGE.

McCann, N. (2020, June 30). *Proposed contract would give adjunct faculty minimum pay standards and other benefits*. The Crow's Nest at USF St. Petersburg. http://crowsneststpete.com/2020/06/30/proposed-contract-would-give-adjunct-faculty-minimum-pay-standards-and-other-benefits/

Milberg, G. (2020, April 27). Florida unemployment website is back online, but issues are still being reported. *Local 10 News*. https://www.local10.com/news/local/2020/04/27/florida-unemployment-site-is-back-online-but-issues-are-still-being-reported/

Reed, M. (2020, July 23). Empty chairs with pink slips: Group protests layoffs at UMass Lowell. *WCVB 5*. https://www.wcvb.com/article/empty-chairs-with-pink-slips-group-protests-layoffs-at-umass-lowell/33404587

Rodriguez, C. (2020, July 23). *Adjunct professors: Jobs are low on pay and health benefits with high risk of COVID risk*. Kaiser Health Network. https://khn.org/news/adjunct-professors-jobs-are-low-on-pay-and-health-benefits-with-high-covid-risk/

Schrecker, E. (2010). *The lost soul of higher education*. The New Press.

Sutherland, J., & Rainbird, H. (2000), Unions and workplace learning: Conflict or cooperation with the employer? In H. Rainbird (Ed.), *Training in the workplace* (pp. 189–209). Springer.

CHAPTER 9

PANDEMIC, PEDAGOGY, AND POSITIVE PEACE

Equity in Education During the COVID-19

Wim Laven

As of June 9, 2021, the COVID-19 pandemic has killed at least 3.75 million people globally. The global pandemic is caused by the coronavirus, SARS-CoV-2 and the disease has spread rapidly. Vaccines are available, though there are issues with global distribution and some disputes over the efficacy of this treatment along ideological and political grounds, the prognosis on the whole currently appears positive. This chapter highlights the relationships between COVID-19 and higher education among vulnerable populations in the United State of America. Many experiences and recommendations will be relevant to other contexts and groups, but the scope of this project is intended to be more limited. In January of 2020 COVID-19 was first identified in the United States. During spring 2020 the average number of new cases per day peaked at 31,000 (on April 10) and deaths exceeded 2,000 on multiple days during April 2020. The American geographical and political contexts were a significant part of the discussion and response. This chapter examines the disruptions that the pandemic caused as well as the conditions created by the threats to public

Coronavirus and Vulnerable People: Addressing the Divide in Harm and Responses and Exploring Implications for a More Peaceful World, pp. 153–177

health and safety, and the reactions to both. This is done through anecdotal experience, a review of available reporting, and a qualitative analysis presenting academic impediments and unique challenges. In some cases, the problems are predictable and still addressed with poor acumen and an absence of good problem solving. This evidence of cultural, structural, and systemic violence is alarming and clearly impacts equity in classrooms. It is also a reflection of broader cultural and ideological values that privilege some groups while providing disservice to others. The priorities within society undermined both a quality educational experience and safety for many vulnerable populations. Aid management, at points, clearly values the economy over the lives of some vulnerable populations, at other points higher education appears to suffer from deferred maintenance—the systematic defunding and underfunding of higher education has had consequences on opportunities for resistance and resilience to adversity caused by the pandemic. Strategies and recommendations for improving the function of higher education for both educators and learners is provided. These include coping strategies that are applicable in a wide diversity of cases and in repurposing classrooms to better deliver positive peace.

INTRODUCTION

Following in the tradition of Paulo Freire's (2000) engaged pedagogy I begin by acknowledging that *how* students learn is as important as *what* they learn. Pedagogy: the strategy employed in educational settings whereby educators aim to impact student achievement and learning outcomes. Education is a deliberate process, and inputs can dramatically impact outcomes. I aim for practices consistent with research showing the efficacy of engaged learning and student-centered learning (Ambrose et al, 2010; Davis, 2009; Svinicki & McKeachie, 2011). Deeper learning shifts consciousness and students solidify learning when they create plans and allow new information to change their behaviors. I offer practical skills as a supplement to theoretical knowledge and theoretical knowledge to supplement actual experiences. In my courses students engage in activities that are designed to impact their metacognition—how they think about thinking—in addition to increasing motivation, and improving study skills (McGuire & McGuire, 2015). This type of instruction provided significant data about student experiences and observations during the global pandemic and I reveal some of the takeaways and lessons from these experiences.

This chapter serves as a qualitative reflection of my experiences and observations in classrooms impacted by the global pandemic of COVID-19 from spring 2020 through spring 2021. It is hard in some ways to situate these observations into normal and abnormal expectations. In over a decade of teaching I have had over 1,500 students, taught on three different continents, and worked with students in a great variety of settings. I extrapolate from experiences when thinking about teaching plans and activities all the time, but this is admittedly guesswork. For example, my work coaching for the Special Olympics helps me think about different modes of learning and teaching for learners with different skills sets and my experience teaching in prison has made me more cognizant of contexts and environmental challenges than I would be otherwise. Normal is elusive; students are dynamic, and I do not want to suggest that I have figured out what to expect, but I do have a good sense of things that tend to work and others that do not. The global pandemic changed all of this, in that process there were new challenges and opportunities. I think these experiences can help classrooms to be more trauma informed. Hopefully there is not a return to viral threats, and the need to socially distance, anytime soon, but the lessons can help to create more safety in classrooms.

The observations provided showcase both violence and mechanisms for escaping the violent structures and systems. During this period, I taught classes on conflict resolution and peace studies and these classes provided interesting opportunities for catharsis; students were forced to deal with new challenges, and I was too. We were learning together. The lessons had greater utility because the skills were immediately applied to new environments and were part of students' deeper learning (Kuh, 2008). The following sections present deductive theory and inductive empirical observations about vulnerable populations during the pandemic. I begin the discussion by offering a model for vulnerability. This model helps to articulate the difference between the vulnerability—as risk—that everyone faced during the pandemic and the vulnerability—as a population—that some individuals and groups are more susceptible to adverse consequences. From this model of vulnerability, the conversation turns to violence in higher education, then student experiences, and lastly analysis, recommendations, and conclusion.

MODEL OF VULNERABILITY

There are two important features in defining vulnerability, in terms of student populations, for the purposes of this chapter. First, that vulnerability can relate to both physical and emotional harms or the threat of harm. Second, that vulnerability, as it relates to groups, describes those with special needs or special care required to confront expected risks and threats. The pandemic spread and many college and university facilities closed. Most of these campuses made adjustments, offering some version of online instruction in order to mitigate or limit exposure and the spread of the virus. In this process students experienced *vulnerability* and *dysfunction* (see Figure 9.1). It was rare in my experience, but some students were *resistant* to the challenges associated with the pandemic.

Figure 9.1

Stress Resistance and Resilience

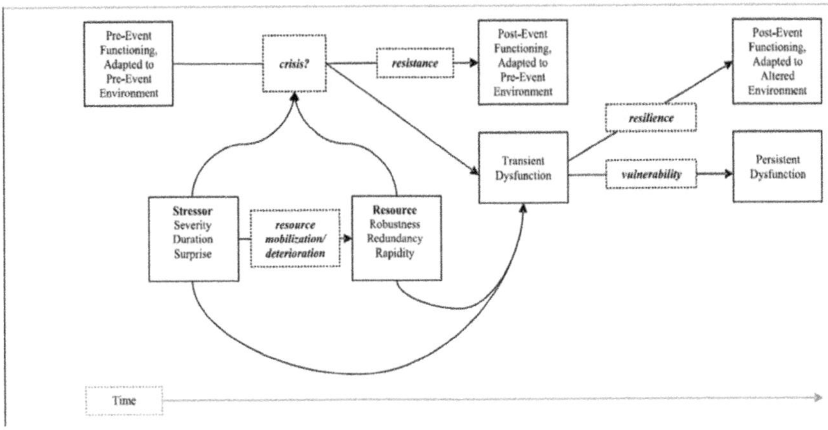

Note: Norris et al. (2008).

Model of stress resilience and vulnerability as described by Norris et al. (2008):

> Resilience occurs when resources are sufficiently robust, redundant, or rapid to buffer or counteract the stressor's effects such that a return to functioning, adapted to the altered environment, occurs. For human individuals and communities, this adaptation is manifested into wellness. The vulnerability occurred when resources were not sufficiently robust, redundant, or rapid to create resistance or resilience, resulting in persistent dysfunction. The more severe, enduring, and surprising the stressor, the stronger the resources must be to create resistance or resilience. (p. 130)

The chart presents two different sets of inputs. The first is the individual or group, they have their own capacities, faculties, and skills. The second set is external forces identified as resources and stressors. Greater detail on these features will be offered during the section on student experiences, but one main starting point is that the pandemic did not influence or impact individuals' lives in a uniform way. While many people realize the differences in capacities, both as internal and external forces, there is a tendency to miss the cumulative and ongoing impacts. Contexts lacking equipment for responding to crisis are also likely to have persistent challenges with addressing dysfunction. As an example: the system provided some relief in the form of stimulus payments. When the pandemic caused business to close many students who lost their jobs received some benefits. Those who were able to sufficiently pay their bills with the benefits found resilience during the pandemic, those whose needs were not met with the provided aid would face growing deficits as the pandemic continued. I refer to the costs of deferred maintenance at several points, students regularly pay large penalties for deferred maintenance (as we all do), delaying the more affordable visit to a dentist may lead to a more expensive procedure like a root canal or dental extraction, delays in repairing a minor water leak can lead to much more expensive water damage, or an inability to afford an oil change in a car may lead to an expensive engine replacement. Students have presented all of these examples to me, and they have identified that sometimes these problems have emerged as their own mistakes and in other cases as problems out of their control, frequently because they simply did not have the money.

The qualitative analysis of vulnerability is offered for theory development. I believe that there are important insights to be gained from the richness of student experiences and what these experiences tell us about what higher education is achieving and where it is falling short of desired goals. Much like I tell students that looking for abandoned cars on the side of the freeway can be an indicator of economic health (i.e., cars rarely breakdown/get abandoned when drivers can afford repairs) I believe that we have signs of clear shortcomings in higher education that are reflected in numbers and grades. Limited bandwidth and Zoom fatigue were common explanations offered by students who were dropping classes that they were otherwise interested in taking. I believe vulnerable populations frequently experienced increased adversity, and sometimes hopelessness. This chapter offers that there is great value in exploring these relationships.

PART 1: VIOLENCE IN HIGHER EDUCATION

Outlining all of the ways violence is experienced in higher education would be a daunting and seemingly impossible task. The goal here is not outlining the myriad and manifold operations allowing, condoning, enforcing, exercising, or promoting violence intentionally or unintentionally to operate within higher education, but to look at concrete examples and ways the pandemic created increased antagonisms and new opportunities for addressing violence. The contexts and nuances for each classroom or campus are complex and dynamic, but systematic analysis of these underlying mechanism and the relationships between these variables and outcomes provides sufficient grounds for considering the efficacy of strategic responses and problem solving. This section first defines the different types of peace and violence, then explores some of the different ways this violence has presented in higher education.

Thinking about human behavior, human nature, and social systems presents different ways to conceive of conflict, peace, and violence. The orientation of these concepts for this chapter aims towards praxis and thinking of management, problem solving, and social change. I begin with Houston Wood's (2016) accounting of peace: positive peace, negative peace, inner peace, and outer peace. I believe this presents a robust way of thinking about physical and psychological well-being (later in this chapter I present evidence on the role of trauma in learning). Johan Galtung (1996) is credited with coining the distinction between positive and negative peace; the absence of violence, is negative peace, and the presence of social conditions which prevent violence—equity and justice—is positive peace. In terms of violence negative peace is the absence of direct violence (intentional physical harm) and positive peace is absence of both direct and indirect violence (harm produced by cultures, structures, and systems). Nobel laureate Malala Yousafzai was famously shot (direct violence) by the Taliban in 2012 for trying to get an education, the Taliban demanded that girls not be allowed to receive an education (indirect violence). The following presents other conditions, like Malala's, which limit or prevent potentials for success by impacting physical and psychological wellbeing.

Inner peace is peace within the self—psychological well-being. Outer peace is wellness in the community—being healthy in our surroundings—and being able to provide for physical comfort and security. The relationship between these two goes in both directions; those who do not have inner peace are unlikely to experience as much opportunity in their academic communities, and conflicted academic communities will afford fewer opportunities for inner peace. Rachel MacNair (2002), an expert on traumas like post-traumatic stress disorder and participation induced traumatic stress, concludes that stress and trauma change and distort the way people process social information, learn, and problem solve; in the worst or most acute cases students may be too scared to learn (Briggs-McGowan et al, 2012; Terrasi & Crain de Galarce, 2017). There are linkages between a great range of psycho-social phenomena and the science on learning. Taking sleep as an example, not reaching minimal thresholds for a good night of sleep will reduce performance outcomes. Anxiety about the threat of COVID-19 can disturb sleep as much as gunshots outside can, but as I learned from students, some neighborhoods suffered from both.

The outer world impacts many of the determinants of peace and students frequently found themselves without much control over their environments during the pandemic. Students shared a large number of coping strategies, and efforts at creating inner peace, in efforts at exerting control over their environments, but, again, some communities had greater hardships than others and some students had greater access to resources than others. The promises of safety and security were met by greater suspicion in some communities and with greater acceptance in others, especially given histories of distrust with authorities, political figures, and governmental agencies. Those with previous or continuing vulnerability presented many examples to support their apprehensiveness. What, if any, grounds are there for believing a failed healthcare system will improve during a complex emergency?

Like Paulo Freire's (2000) engaged pedagogy says that students perform better when their needs are met and they feel comfortable in their communities, John Burton (1990) theorizes that people who have met their basic needs and have positive feelings about their communities are better positioned to respond to conflicts and problem solve. This chapter takes intuitive observations like sleep deprivation, hunger, and nutritional deficiencies make life harder and examines the ways these challenges are exaggerated for vulnerable populations in higher education during the pandemic. In many cases it is not merely a distraction, I allege, but a predictable byproduct of cultural and structural violence.

During the pandemic messaging of fear and insecurity was ubiquitous. The fomented dramas, however, were not universal; in some cases, groups were united in shared loss, suffering, and death, while others focused on the scapegoating of responsible parties or vigilance over responses. There were many "us" or "them" narratives and scientific accuracy was not always a necessity. In many ways the pandemic was a political event, and the crisis a political problem more than an expression of public health and safety. While the common practice of manufacturing or exaggerating threats is nothing new its role in the pandemic is not to be missed. Some groups were made particularly vulnerable by the blame they received or by conditions these narratives created. One person's existential threat was another person's hoax and so on.

The obstacles to access, like bureaucracy or red tape, can cause significant indirect violence. In the medical setting lack of access to care can produce negative consequences in health impacts including death. The violence is that people are harmed when conditions prevent their physical and mental wellness. The same is true for academic settings, though the links between education and wellness are not always made as clear. Education can provide access and is sometimes credited with being the most reliable pathway out of poverty (especially for minority populations) (Minton-Bedoes, 2012). So, while those of means are able to find academic resilience those without means experience academic vulnerability and persistent dysfunction. In turn achievement gaps will continue to cause disadvantages in the future. During the pandemic scarcity of resources was an emergent problem, but the burdens of resource scarcity were not shared equally. The unequal distribution of resources has dire consequences that result directly from cultural, political, structural, and systematic choices that explicitly or implicitly showcase the priorities of values.

Cultural violence is promoted and legitimized in practices and values for many different reasons. Where some groups seek to help those in need out of values in charity, compassion, and solidarity other groups seek to punish those in need for alleged laziness and/or other character flaws. Poverty presents a value struggle in the U.S. and much has been said of a "47% narrative." This narrative claims many people are too lazy to work for themselves, but this does not register that

> over half have jobs and pay payroll taxes but earn too little to be subject to income tax as well. Another 20 percent are retired. Only 8 percent of households pay no federal tax at all, usually because their members are students, disabled or unemployed. (Minton-Bedoes, 2012)

The principles of fairness (or lack thereof) emerged in bold relief in the discussions over healthcare and the costs associated with saving lives. It was clear to me that some students were threatened, or perceived threats, significantly more than others.

Education is a delivery system for delivering students opportunities for achieving their full potential. Healthcare is a delivery system for meeting the basic needs of wellness. Structures that prevent individuals and communities commit violence. Dr. Paul Farmer (2004) examines the Hippocratic oath: first do no harm, but he finds a glaring problem—many features of our healthcare system cause individuals to suffer from easily treatable conditions. I believe many educators are in a similar position. Affliction is embedded in our educational system and social determinants impact so much of what constitutes academic success. Social systems deny access to some groups while benefitting others, and this discussion highlights the multitude of barriers I observed. This systematic oppression places limits on individual potentials and also life expectancy. Identifying and acknowledging these harms creates opportunities for rectifying social policy, leveraging culpability and accountability in the negative consequences, treating the harms, and creating positive change. What I learned and observed is intended to stimulate thinking for those purposes.

Student Centered Learning Strategies

Hands-on and experiential learning is central to both the way I learn and teach. As mentioned previously, a significant part of the experience present here is the result of conversations I had during the pandemic, which arose directly from the material I was teaching in Conflict Resolution and Peace Studies courses. Rather than imagining conflicts I ask students to think about the challenges they face or witness in their own contexts. This is grounded in the pedagogy presented in "Experience and Education" (Dewey, 1938) and grounded in the work of Jean Piaget (1936, 1945), and David Kolb's (1984) "Experiential learning: Experience as the source of learning and development." I remember the details my students share because I care about them. My students remember the lessons from class because they directly impact and relate to their lives. Active participation and reflection on experience creates durable learning. In order to be effective, reflections need to be processed into concepts, and I design group-work and activities which involve problem-solving around those concepts. The details in and of themselves are not as significant as making sense of the key concepts and recognizing the prioritization of values in play. The truism I find most noteworthy in this regard: students who live in relative peace tend to focus on examining violence and students who live in conditions of elevated violence tend to focus on examining justice. These activities move students to more in-depth knowledge (Webb, 2005) contrasting with shallow or superficial activities like remembering or understanding; evaluating and creating (like making plans of action and problem solving) access the highest levels of knowledge (Kuh, 2008: Webb, 2005). In general, I offer the disclaimer that class will guarantee safety but not comfort, but during the pandemic I really questioned to what extent I was really guaranteeing safety. While I was comfortable that the problem-solving activities were not burdensome in the discomfort/anxiety/stress they caused, I really was not sure that the discussions on current events were not traumatizing or re-traumatizing students grappling with reflections on illnesses that still presented mortal (and other) dangers.

My Context

From spring 2020 through spring 2021, I taught courses for the Department of Political Science at Cuyahoga Community College (Tri-C). My classes on Introduction to Conflict and Peace Studies and Skills in Conflict Resolution are a part of their Conflict Resolution and Peace Studies Certificate program. Through Tri-C's various learning streams, the multiple campuses serve more than 50,000 students annually. Tuition at Tri-C is the lowest in Ohio, ranking 1st in Ohio and 25th in the nation among colleges conferring associate degrees. Tri-C's campuses are located in the Cleveland area of Ohio, and they serve a diverse population. These observations may not be broadly generalizable, though they are consistent with other experiences and observations shared by colleagues and students in other locations. Many student experiences have been publicly shared through a variety of social media and other public platforms. It is also worth noting that my courses' content leads directly to sharing experiences and additional aggregate information; around half of the final papers students submitted discussed conflicts caused or influenced by the conditions of COVID-19. I was lucky because I had a full 12 days to prepare my transition from face-to-face classes to online instruction and the adjustment was made early. I learned on March 11 that classes would be postponed until March 23 in order to accommodate changing the format and guaranteeing maximum public safety. I considered myself lucky by comparison.

Students' Struggles and Satisficing

Decision making and information collection in there most basic forms are operations directed toward the satisfaction of needs (Wilson, 2005). These processes involve reflecting on and considering alternatives when establishing or deciding upon an optimal solution (Stroh et al., 2002). Linear decision making looks at what option is best, provides the most utility, or fits within an individual's calculus for outcomes in satisfying underlying interests and needs. Teachers, I argue, did not have time to sufficiently prepare materials for teaching during the pandemic, and I do not believe student's (in most cases) were suitably empowered to make good decisions for themselves. Online environments require different strategies for both teaching and learning, and the time do so was missing. Everyone was forced to deal with the dilemma of *satisficing* (Simon, 1955): the "contrast between choosing what is satisfactory and choosing what is best" (Byron, 2004, p. 1). Decisions are rarely made from complete information, but the new context made it hard to form educated guesses. In normal circumstances an activity may work fantastically with one group of students and fail to adequately engage another. Educators and students are limited; they have imperfect and incomplete information about their subjects, and nobody can predict the future. Rational choice theory says that when provided different options people usually do what they believe will produce the best outcome (Scott, 2000) but the global pandemic forced people to make decisions without weighing options.

Satisficing During the Pandemic

Forced choices—a requirement to act—despite uncertainty about what are a predictable source of discomfort. The need for certainty is understandable, but during the pandemic it has been in short supply. At the time I was preparing for my online classes the health briefing focused on washing hands and indicated that wearing masks was unnecessary, a year later the opposite seemed true, in some cases people even advocated wearing two masks. Making plans in such a dynamic and fluid environment requires flexibility, but best practices in metacognition and teaching involve alignment, planning, and preparation in courses to embrace the totality of a class and delivering on learning outcomes and evidence for success. There is no good way to "wait and see" in higher education. The pandemic is just an exaggeration of the status quo. Policies and budgets often dictate insufficient capacity for best practices. This includes challenges with predicting the future, the impacts of current events on students, and change and uncertainty. During the pandemic it was unlikely important questions will have been answered when policy decisions are made (Freiman, 2020; Kesslen, 2020), but all the other issues were also in place.

Mistakes at the policy level also prove to have dramatic consequences beyond educators' control; for example, schools in Georgia with large numbers of students and faculty requiring quarantine after exposure to the coronavirus one week into the fall 2020 semester, and the closure of several high schools in one district (Fausset, 2020). The pandemic required many teachers to pivot and as the threats to public health persisted, teachers were/are required to think about teaching plans from different perspectives. Many had to consider questions like: Are face-to-face lesson plans suitable for the potential transition to online and asynchronous teaching in the event of another wave? Should the topic order be changed to accommodate possible changes and disruptions, or should other accommodations be made? What assignments and assessments will be feasible? In the next section the implications, both practical and moral, are explored. Each context presenting different capacities and definitions for success. Ultimately individuals decided to what extent "problems are considered resolved when a good enough solution has been found" (Choo, 1998, p. 49).

PART 2: STUDENT EXPERIENCES

All of the challenges relating to educators' planning and preparation should also be applied to students. Strategies for success change and students identified unique impediments in the online learning environment that they were otherwise insulated from. In some cases, these challenges may be undiscovered or unknown. Many students indicated additional roles and workloads caused by the pandemic. Incorporating student needs into teaching plans, understanding changes to their contexts are fundamental to hierarchies and taxonomies for student learning, which be considered in creating lesson plans (Anderson & Krathwohl, 2001; Bloom, 1956; Maslow, 1943, 1954, 1962). Students preparing for classes while distracted by their instincts for survival will experience the classroom differently. Students' learning processes during times of anxiety and stress are likely stifled by predictable psychological processes (Maslow, 1943, 1962). This makes all affected students vulnerable to some degree.

Before the pandemic at least half of the students in U.S. colleges and universities have recent experience dealing with, chronic stress, trauma, or the aftermath of violence (Jennings, 2019). Students have an increased need for social and emotional learning (Jennings, 2019). These conditions showcase student needs in academic support that connects their behaviors, performance, and struggles with the compassion and mindfulness that can increase their achievement, resilience, and retention (Cummings et al., 2017); neurochemicals and other reactions to threats (like fight, flight, and freeze) hinder student achievement in predictable ways (Statman-Weil, 2015), vulnerable students may be too scared to learn (Briggs-McGowan et al., 2012; Terrasi & Crain de Galarce, 2017).

Struggles and Violence in Classrooms

A popular metaphor in conflict transformation and peace studies ask people to think about dealing with parties in conflict like you would an iceberg. This iceberg theory (Cloke & Goldsmith, 2000) suggests that while some of the issues are present there is much more that is below the surface. Addressing conflict in this way requires an awareness that work is required to identify the roots to the dispute and the underlying interest, values, and needs. My experience in education is very similar. Students arrive with baggage as well as hopes and dreams that have been informed by past experiences. Part of the following discussion includes my evaluation and identification of interests and needs, some of this was self-reported but significant parts of it are assumptions (incomplete ones at that) that I made after the fact.

In class we examined strategies for addressing or responding to physical threats. One common example was of violence over physical distancing and/or mask wearing. There was a dilemma: if someone gets too close without a mask, they might risk infecting you with the virus, but if you say something about a mask or distancing it could turn into a physical altercation. Nearly every student was aware multiple events of violence over such disputes, and there was abundant speculation that such confrontation would have taken place on campus if there had not been a transition to online learning. The episodes of such violence that colleagues on other campuses identified were extremely rare, though shouting about masks seemed to be more common. The issue, most frequent, was not the absence of a mask, but masks being worn ineffectively (i.e., not covering the nose). The question of mask or no mask, while visible, does not necessarily reflect the issues or concerns below the surface. Students generally identified an apprehension to engage in such a conflict and could not imagine masks as central to constructive conflicts.

Most of the violence described here is cultural, structural, and systematic. This violence features in presentations of care, priority, and value. The lack of accommodation to needs and the presentation of privilege in access to resources was significant. Students on the whole reported exaggerated stress levels from academic demands. There were a large number of students who complained about access to services and a smaller group of students who wanted to drop out of classes for the term or permanently. There is a strong correlation between highest level of education completed and socioeconomic indicators like quality of life and life expectancy. In the U.S. there is a direct line between education—income—healthcare. Students were generally familiar with poor quality and lack of availability in healthcare services. Privilege tends to feature as an important predictor of academic achievement and opportunity.

Two first-generation college students describe increases in academic adversity. They were called upon to serve as caregivers for children when the childcare facilities were closed. They suggested that their families did not understand the academic demands they faced. They also identified that while challenges increase, they had responsibilities to chip in. Traditional college aged students and older students had different experiences in this regard. There was inequality in the maintenance of expectations between the different groups. There were dramatic differences in the duration, intensity, and proximity to individual's experiences of crisis. The lack of recognition of contexts and struggles did harm to student. The entire system was failing and even when instructors tried to align their classes to accommodate student needs there was no way to uphold the promises they made or the expectations of students. Some instructors, on the other hand, did not adjust expectations and placed students in impossible situations.

Persistent Vulnerability and Dysfunction

Several academics expressed a pandemic-productivity in which they were getting more work done by virtue of fewer distraction and interruptions. I only encountered two students who described something similar. Almost without exception students described increased adversity. One student understood it clearly, they were completely financially secure due to their parent's employment situations and had an appreciation for the online courses. This cut out commute times and left more time for completing assignments. The other student reported being an introvert who felt like classes were generally a waste of time and complained that students do not generally come to class prepared, so the discussions were not generally valuable. Even still the student said that for classes where discussion is helpful, the discussion can still be done online.

There were many different complaints from students. They did not feel like they were learning as much, and this was a source of concern and frustration. In some cases, they wondered if they should wait until things were back to normal, but they decided that nobody knew how long that will take either. Other students indicated that student loans had become their only source of income, so they were dependent on college in a way they had not expected. Many students became unemployed but those who work commonly found themselves work more overtime than they were used to, which left them less time to prepare for class.

Mitigating the impacts of crisis is *resistance*, and the speed of those adjustments makes a significant difference. For many students locating resources and identifying strategies for adaptation (to both academic and life changes) was slow. Adaptation is a way to think of *resilience,* but it is hard to conceptualize what delays in adaptation mean. In some cases, the costs of deferred maintenance can be very high because the delayed response allows the problem to get considerably worse. What does it mean, for example, for a student to have to wait two weeks to buy a computer in the middle of a pandemic, or to heal from a bad case of COVID-19 while trying to complete course work? In the first case the student was happy to be able to catch up quickly by watching the necessary videos, reporting that it was not so bad. In the second case the student reported that it was to painful to talk for almost a month, and not asking questions due to pain made understanding concepts significantly more difficult. Multiple students wanted to drop one or more courses. One student wanted to drop all of their classes because online was not meeting their learning needs. But they felt trapped when they discovered they could not afford to drop the course(s) due to financial aid obligations; a drop in credit hours would trigger immediate repayment of overpaid financial aid. In this regard students were required to adapt but the systems did not.

Technology was clearly a mode of adaptation. It provided the means for classes to be conducted without risk of transferring the virus, but it also created new challenges. Students dealing with inflexible instructors struggled with deadlines they could not manage and expectations that were not reasonable. Everyone instructor I spoke with was familiar of at least one student going to Herculean lengths to complete assignments like writing term papers on smartphones or using Wi-Fi while sitting parked in a car in a parking lot. Several students who were also parents shared computers with children who needed to use the technology during the day. Others had enough computers but not enough bandwidth for everyone to do class at the same time.

The corona virus was spreading, and it put people into difficult situations. Multiple students described facing symptoms without a clear treatment pathway. Those who tried to get tested either did not want to wait, did not qualify, or did not want to risk standing in line with people who looked really sick. One student said they were sure if they did not have COVID they would definitely have it after waiting. Many waits were long, and choices between health and academics were being made. Students reflected on the stigma associated with the virus, even though they were online they did not want to mention symptoms or being sick with or without positive test results. Over time this changed some, students did, on occasion, disclose their situations. As an instructor I did not know how to talk about it. Eventually I became concerned with issues of student privacy and disclosure and was told I was allowed to ask, "how are you feeling?" but not for disclosure of test results.

Testing shortages present a great example of transient dysfunction because it placed students in a kind of stasis (Firozi, 2020). Not knowing the truth about your physical health can make it difficult to choose the best course of action. An infected person might go into quarantine or self-isolation, but those steps would be burdensome for a person who does not risk exposing others. Students with jobs are challenged by moral and ethical choices. Should a person with a runny nose go to work or not? What about when they need the money? What about when the boss does not offer them the option of staying home? These were all questions that students raised, and they were clearly stressed about the conditions of their real lives. Stresses and anxieties, at least for some students, were simultaneously impacting performance and getting worse. They started satisficing, good enough would have to do.

A full third of the students indicated the pandemic had increased their workloads. A common problem was that instructors added assignments or content to make up for the changes. One of the worst examples was tests being changed from multiple choice answer tests, which would take around an hour, to multiple page essay tests that could take several hours. But there were other examples of class lectures being replaced with additional readings or documentaries. This form of compensation increased demands upon students. A number of these students reached out to instructors, deans, and other campus departments in efforts to receive relief from the increased demands. None of them reported a successful outcome, several dropped classes. They did not like being accused of being lazy and I was surprised with how many students asked for advice and also with how many instructors did not make accommodations.

Students identified a wide range of real-world issues. Many wrote their papers about these conflicts and other asked for help. I also received a large number of inquiries from former students: "I am about to graduate, and unemployment is going through the roof. Do you have any advice?" And "my daughter's ex was locked up for domestic violence but since this virus ... he was let out early. What can I do?" are two challenging examples. Their options for assistance were significantly more limited, and prior learning did not apply as clearly to the obstacles they were encountering. They were balancing academic needs with survival needs and they were as overwhelmed as the systems they relied upon.

Not all Coping Mechanisms Are Healthy

Quoted by *CNN*, Judith Butler says, "without a way to gather with others to mark a loss, to acknowledge the loss, we are left with an intensified sense of isolation and also, often, a heightened sense of self-reproach, anxiety, and what used to be called melancholy" as deaths in the U.S. approach 200,000 (the number is increasing with no end in sight), the number was 100,000 in late May 2020 as the spring term was finishing up (Sanchez, 2020). Over the last 15 months many people have gotten sick and died. The gravity of the moment needs to be clear. Few worries elevate to the magnitude of death, and it seems there has been a lack of a collective reflection of loss and grief—students, like the public at large, are alone in processing events. As a result, it seems, processing is not leading to personal healing, and an overwhelming number of students and instructors expressed some version of the following: they knew others had it worse than they did, so they did not want to complain, but they were having a hard time. Many students noted (or observed) increased use of intoxicants as a coping mechanism (self-medicating), but few describe effective (by their assessment) coping strategies.

Mood, anxiety, and alcohol use disorders are associated with significant costs to the individual and society including low levels of educational attainment, unstable employment, decreased work productivity, reduced health-related quality of life, and increased primary healthcare needs (Donovan et al., 2005; Kessler, 2012; Walley et al., 2012; Wittchen, 2002); these short term issues can turn into long term problems and are associated with other (sometimes severe) comorbidities (example: stress is a contributing factor in heart disease, the leading cause of death for adults in the United States). One study (Drabwell et al., 2020) worth highlighting observed the following:

> [I]t is common for young adults to report a change in drug or alcohol use after traumatic bereavement, whether by increasing their use to self-medicate aspects of grief, or restricting use as an alternative coping strategy. The former group described binge drinking, an awareness of addiction, and a range of harmful consequences to their increased use. The potential for negative health outcomes is apparent, and this analysis provides a means for clinicians to understand the context for this health behavior in young bereaved adults, and how best they might intervene. (p. 12)

They offered the following for clinical guidance on interventions:

> This suggests that a watchful approach may be more acceptable for some young, bereaved people, monitoring drug or alcohol misuse to ascertain whether it is self-limiting or if sensitive interventions are required to address emergent addiction. This more nuanced understanding helps clinicians move away from a paternalistic, punitive approach to substance use and understand where it might be a temporary phenomenon, used for a specific aim, and where brief alcohol interventions or referral to substance misuse services are indicated. (pp. 12–13)

My prior experience with behavioral intervention and behavioral response teams on different campuses has been quite varied. I have found very few faculty members have utilized such reporting services, and it is rare to find faculty members who know how to file reports if necessary. In prior experiences with reporting, I did not feel students' needs were adequately handled. During the pandemic I would not have known how to file such a report, or when to do.

One communication I had presented the intersection of substance use with the virtual format of online instruction. The professor indicated a student was visibly smoking a joint during class and asked if it was fine (Belcher, 2020)? Responses and suggestions to the tweet were quite varied. In some states, marijuana use is legal for medical or recreational reasons. Beyond the legal guidelines some, likely many or most, campuses have substance use guidelines in codes of conduct. While such cases are likely to be rare or isolated, they reflect something important that happens in every class. Students and faculty are turning on cameras and broadcasting from their personal spaces. One person's disruption is another person's home life. Have instructors developed plans for students who have not turned on their video? Is video required? Have instructors considered what a video may show or why a student may not want to be seen?

I relate in very personal ways and openly share with students. The day my father died, I taught my first class as an instructor of record, it was a class on Anger and Hatred. I started with a description of the intense emotions experienced when covering the subject, then I confessed about my feelings due to the loss of a loved one. In true catharsis and serendipity, every student in the room shared a story about losing a loved one. The one thing we had in common was that it was never convenient. The class was indeed my therapy that day. I share stories like this in class when they are appropriate for the material being covered, in part, because I get to remember and honor my father's memory, but also because it is important, to be honest with students. This prior experience contrasted dramatically with the coronavirus. At the same time, we all shared in generally similar experiences, and I noted students were increasingly disinterested and hesitant to discuss the pandemic as the spring 2020 and fall 2020 terms went on. Many students described conditions of oversaturation and feeling overwhelmed, accompanied by powerlessness—talking would not change things—and compassion fatigue. Other faculty members added sentiments that they could not let the crisis distract from coursework anymore because they were already so far behind.

Some students got sick, and some admitted they were scared. My response has always included some version of, "we will figure out a makeup assignment when you're healthy." I had a student who was sick, worried and did not appreciate this response. We talked, and I tried to avoid hyperbole, but I said, "your paper will not matter if you die, will it? So, I need you to worry about getting healthy first" it worked as a reframe, but it is not something I would recommend, but, like so many cases described here, I was unprepared for the magnitude of chaos and uncertainty. Other students had sick family members, and I found letting them know "none of my assignments are more important than your family" made more sense when I shared my own story. I promised to be a compassionate instructor after I was graded down for being distracted on a presentation, I gave the day my brother died. We suffer, struggle, live, and learn, but I am not sure it means anything if we do not share humanity. We remember those who have treated us with dignity differently than those who have not.

Several students identified being in one or more high-risk categories or living with those who were in a high-risk category. In some cases, risk factors were presented as age or ethnicity. My African American students were all aware that their communities were impacted more than other demographics. Indeed, a *Washington Post* poll in June 2020 revealed that "31 percent of Black respondents said that they know someone who has died from the virus, though overall only 13 percent of respondents knew someone who has died from COVID-19" a likely source of asymmetric trauma (Johnson, 2020). The experience of trauma appeared to be very divergent, impacting students, and the awareness of responses presented through the media. Those who described strong or extreme feelings of fear also shared concerns about social distancing behaviors and mask-wearing. They did not understand why anyone was calling the pandemic a hoax or refusing to wear masks. Several students were worried about insufficient personal protective equipment (or the complete lack of) at their places of employment. I do not know how all of these situations played out. I know several students and educators who quit jobs or started job searches to leave employment where they did not feel physical and mental health were taken seriously. Employment has been a higher priority than classwork for an overwhelming majority of my students at Tri-C.

Deterioration

Conditions appeared to worsen at all levels: local, county, state, nation, and global. In that process, systemic and structural violence emerged more clearly. The pandemic presented as a complex humanitarian disaster, with human-caused elements. Personal and social identity started shaping the disaster's experiences and politics (Tajfel & Turner, 1986). Experiences attached to "social locations" and identified in ordinary socialization via mores in cultural scripts, the experiences and value to them was debatable—is this really happening on purpose?—and also responsible for suffering and conflict; intentional or not, people were struggling, and it did not look like people cared or cared equally—a kind of existential crisis (Brubaker & Cooper, 2000; Conklin, 1997: Dove, 2006).

For some students, the conflict appeared as little more than political disagreement. For others, it was dishonest but no different from the typical—all politicians lie—narrative. For others, it was a threat to be taken seriously; some students used the word genocide to describe the seriousness and intentionality. In class, I tried to make this a teachable moment, and I made great efforts to validate and acknowledge all of my students' subjectivity and experiences. Still, I felt inadequate in responding to some of the objective details. While many experiences were unique to individual students, there were also objective details, trends, and recommendations though they were difficult to stay current with. There were stories from students who felt gas-lighted by instructors they said called the Coronavirus, a "hoax," or "scamdemic," and they felt expectations were inappropriate. From my perspective, it was clear that performance categorically diminished, from both students and instructors, despite significant efforts to maintain high levels of quality and achievement.

Positive Peace and Equity

I have examined conditions of violence impacting students during the pandemic of COVID-19. I have placed the concept of peace into higher education by exploring a range of relationships. I see equity, peace, and social justice as essential to a true liberal education. I experience the banality of my good intentions, but I do not feel I could deliver students with the value for which they paid. Individuals cannot deliver real equity; it needs to be built into the policies and systems. I could not provide positive peace without a system with robust attention, as a preexisting feature, to inclusive cultural diversity and awareness built into its principles and practices. "Positive peace focuses on the restoration of relationships or the creation of new relationships and peers deep into the societal structures to examine constructs such as social justice, human rights, equality, and well-being" (Lee, 2018, p. 1). Structural and systemic problems must be addressed at structural and systemic levels. I believe, however, that I was able to provide some level of equity to students. In the practices of tailoring assignments and expectations to students on an individual level and by leveling expectations with a modified version of pass/no-pass grading, I think I provided service to the development of social skills, critical thinking, and the linkages between humanities and human rights.

The culture of higher education is inconsistent in many of these features. What I saw as equity some would see as unfair. Some colleagues were critical that my practice contributed to grade inflation and was fundamentally unfair to students whose hard work was not fully appreciated. Others said that working to tailor to individual students' needs sets an unjust precedent for other faculty members. At some level, I could sympathize with this challenge, and I would not have been able to manage the same practices in prior terms when I had 150–200 students. Where does fairness to instructors fit into the calculus? In transitioning to online courses, I doubled or tripled my workload because I care about teaching. Still, I was not financially compensated for the extra work.

This showcases inequity between faculty members. While some people have time and resources that make such a transition and increased workload viable, others will struggle to manage expectations when confronted with increased demands and limited resources. In my case, I know many colleagues without as much discretionary time and disposable resources. Many people cannot afford to put in an extra 10 or 15 hours per class per week for free. Is it fair to compare performance evaluations or student feedback between faculty members during a pandemic? Higher education does not have a culture or design for equity, and the global pandemic exaggerated inequalities at all levels.

PART 3: ANALYSIS, RECOMMENDATIONS, AND CONCLUSION

The articulation of my experiences and data collection is admittedly small, biased, self-serving, and methodologically limited for broad specific assessments. I believe many of the themes identified were common, but it was clear that experiences varied dramatically both between different campuses and, also between different classes on the same campus. I like to think I did a good—better than average—job, but I know that I came up short of my desired outcomes despite my considerable efforts. In this regard, I have taken great effort to explain the causes of these shortcomings beyond the control of faculty members. I want to encourage examining lessons learned; how can these experiences be used to catalyze cultural, structural, and systematic changes that make managing crises in education more manageable?

Individual educators can pause and assess the ways their pedagogies are providing trauma-sensitive education. Including opportunities for self-care, healing, and processing anxiety and stress would likely benefit students in most terms but are not likely to have been scheduled into daily lesson plans or the term's schedule. Educators are familiar with taxonomies and hierarchies of needs but may assume survival needs are met before such a confirmation is present. Still, I believe human needs may serve as little more than keywords and catchphrases when confronted with squeezing more content into the curriculum. Acknowledging moods and collective consciousness can validate the experiences of students and normalize the importance of mental health—mental health cannot be an aspirational goal. Many of these metacognitive activities will improve short-term and long-term achievement, but they are experienced and presented as counterfactuals. It is illogical to pretend that classes could go on as normal during a global emergency, but, somehow, this was the standard of comparison that regularly emerged. I was even hesitant to admit that my classes did not go well and justify diminished performance outcomes when that should have been the starting point: students should not have been expected to achieve at the same high levels when they are experiencing high levels of stress during crisis.

There would appear to be utility in developing protections and steps for student advocacy for episodes with serious crises and disruption. Many dynamics offered show latent manifestations that privilege the protection of the institution over the needs of students. I feel that there is no malicious or nefarious intent so much as the system going into survival mode (austerity measures) when becoming overwhelmed by the crisis. But, again, this comes from my experience on a campus where I felt "lucky" with early strategic decision making and was simultaneously aware of preexisting budget shortfalls. Some efforts at "good enough" could quickly come up short given challenges with decision making. Anyone could, and likely would, make mistakes given the constraints; students needed advocacy to protect their interests in responding to mistakes that created excessive burdens and stress.

I believe this would all be well served with early acknowledgment of the mental and physical health impacts and how to mitigate them. Announcements to cancel courses or transition from face-to-face to virtual classrooms should have been accompanied by robust services to facilitate the adjustments and potential student needs. This begs bigger questions like, why education is not funded at a level where it can manage during a crisis? And, why education is not funded to do the best job it can, as opposed to a "good enough," which positions institutions in a struggle during good times and incapable of resisting dysfunction during crises?

Educators should be trained for and accept the responsibility of their roles as essential workers. Positions that are required as part of the backbone of our society and economy, which put educators on more even footing with mental and physical health professionals. This includes familiarization with the availability of services and identifying warning signs and trauma for crisis management and a sensitivity causing unnecessary harm to students. At the same time, to varying degrees, educators should be made aware (for better and worse) of the inequity built into the system and the impossibility of maximizing outcomes in some contexts. In such contexts, alignments with trauma sensitivity are likely to present increased value. It is never too early to identify opportunities to incorporate physical, social, and emotional safety for students. Educators can work with their departments and administrations to share their understandings about the impact of trauma and adversity on students. Whenever possible, culturally responsive, and restorative practices can be instituted, do not shy away from inequalities when they emerge. Increase capacities for behavioral, mental, and physical health services on campuses and in communities. Increase capacity and relationships for engagement and collaboration between campuses and communities.

Educators should rethink, revisit, and stress the impacts of economics and familiarize themselves with the potential impacts of poverty on their classrooms. Dr. Ruby Payne (2005) is one of pioneers of this terrain providing skills for bridging the gaps at the intersections of pedagogy and poverty. The sensitivity endorsed in this paper is one that understand the linkages between economic conditions and an individual's psychology and also fundamental differences in thought and behavior. Payne's (2013) cognitive approach provides even greater emphasis on the thinking, community, and learning patterns involved in learning, which I argue are antagonized in my observations of students' experiences.

COVID-19 should be a wake-up call on realigning pedagogies in service of trauma-sensitive education and repurposing classrooms to pursue positive peace. When the pandemic hit, most of the community was impacted, not just campuses. Classrooms and campuses could be a source of collaboration and an opportunity for combating the crisis, not another source of stress or location for chaos. Thinking about which elements of courses improve students' lives and resilience during periods of dysfunction can be conceived in terms of what is being done well. Those elements which would increase vulnerability during dysfunction should be questioned for their utility? Classrooms should be safe places though this is not a guarantee of stress-free-comfort. Stress should not be excessively or unintentionally elevated when it can be avoided, crisis or not.

REFERENCES

Ambrose, S. A., Bridges, M. W., DiPietro, M., Lovett, M. C., & Norman, M. K. (2010). *How learning works: Seven research-based principles for smart teaching.* Jossey-Bass.

Anderson, L., & Krathwohl, (2001). *A taxonomy for teaching, learning, and assessing: A revision of Bloom's taxonomy of educational objectives.* Longman.

Belcher, C. (2020, Sept. 1). Twitter Post, 2:03 PM. https://twitter.com/chris_belcher/status/1300856759016284161

Bloom, B. (1956). *Taxonomy of educational objectives: The classification of educational goals.* Longmans, Green.

Briggs-Gowan, M. J., Carter, A. S., & Ford, J. D. (2012). Parsing the effects violence exposure in early childhood: Modeling developmental pathways. *Journal of Pediatric Psychology, 37,* 11–22.

Brubaker, R., & Cooper, F. (2000). Beyond "identity." *Theory and Society, 29,* 1–47.

Burton, J. (1990). *Conflict: Basic human needs.* St. Martins Press.

Byron, M. (2004). *Satisficing and maximizing: Moral theorists on practical reason.* Cambridge University Press.

Choo, C. W. (1998). *The knowing organization: How organizations use information to construct meaning, create knowledge, and make decisions.* Oxford University Press.

Cloke, K., & Goldsmith, J. (2000). *Resolving conflicts as work: A complete guide for everyone on the job.* Jossey-Bass.

Conklin, B. (1997). Body paints, feathers and VCRs: Aesthetics and authenticity in Amazonian activism. *American Ethnologist, 24*(41), 711–737.

Cummings, K. P., Addante, S., Swindell, J., & Meadan, H. (2017). Creating supportive environments for children who have had exposure to traumatic events. *Journal of Child & Family Studies, 26,* 2728–2741.

Davis, B. G. (2009). *Tools for teaching.* Jossey-Bass.

Dewey, J. (1938). *Experience and education.* Macmillan.

Donovan, D., Mattson, M., Cisler, R., Longabaugh, R., & Zweben, A. (2005). Quality of life as an outcome measure in alcoholism treatment research. *Journal of Studies on Alcohol, 15,* 119–139.

Dove, M. (2006). Indigenous people and environmental politics. *Annual Review of Anthropology, 35,* 191–208.

Drabwell, L., Eng, J., Stevenson, F., King, M., Osborn, D., & Pitman, A. (2020). Perceptions of the use of alcohol and drugs after sudden bereavement by unnatural causes: Analysis of online qualitative data. *International Journal of Environmental Research and Public Health, 17*(3), 677.

Fausset, R. (2020, August 12). 1,193 quarantined for covid. Is this a successful school reopening? *New York Times.* https://www.nytimes.com/2020/08/12/us/georgia-school-coronavirus.html

Farmer, P. (2004). An anthology of structural violence. *Current Anthropology, 45*(3), 305–325.

Firozi, P. (2020, August 13). The health 202: Shortages are forcing Louisville's biggest hospital system to cut back on covid testing. *The Washington Post*. https://www.washingtonpost.com/politics/2020/08/13/health-202-louisville-biggest-hospital-system-is-cutting-back-covid-testing-under-shortages/

Freiman, J. (2020, August 10). Georgia school seen in viral photo temporarily closes after 9 students and staff members test positive for coronavirus. *CBS News*. https://www.cbsnews.com/news/georgia-coronavirus-school-viral-photo-temporarily-closes-positive-covid-19-tests/

Freire, P. (2000). *Pedagogy of the oppressed* (30th anniversary ed.). Continuum.

Galtung, J. (1996). *Peace by peaceful means: Peace and conflict, development and civilization*. International Peace Research Institute Oslo. SAGE.

Jennings, P. A. (2019). *The trauma-sensitive classroom: Building resilience with compassionate teaching*. W. W. Norton & Company.

Johnson, M. (2020, June 26). Nearly one-third of Black Americans say they know someone who died from Coronavirus: Poll. *The Hill*. https://thehill.com/policy/healthcare/504696-nearly-one-third-of-black-americans-say-they-know-someone-who-died-from

Kesslen, B. (2020, August 12). Coronavirus prompts closing of Georgia high school in district with over 1K in quarantine. *NBC News*. https://www.nbcnews.com/news/us-news/coronavirus-prompts-closing-georgia-high-school-district-over-1k-quarantine-n1236492

Kessler, R. (2012). The cost of depression. *Psychiatric Clinics of North America, 35*(1), 1–14.

Kolb, D. A. (1984). *Experiential learning: Experience as the source of learning and development*. Prentice-Hall.

Kuh, G. D. (2008). *High-impact educational practices: What they are, who has access to them, and why they matter*. Association of American Colleges and Universities.

Lee, V. V. (2018). A culture of positive peace: Counseling for structural and cultural transformation. In C. C. Lee (Ed.), *Counseling for social justice* (pp. 23–42). American Counseling Association Foundation.

MacNair, R. M. (2002). Perpetration-induced traumatic stress in combat veterans. *Peace and Conflict: Journal of Peace Psychology, 8*(1), 63–72.

Maslow, A. (1943). A theory of human motivation. *Psychological Review, 50*(4), 370–396.

Maslow, A. (1954). *Motivation and personality*. Harper and Row.

Maslow, A. (1962). *Toward a psychology of being*. D. Van Nostrand.

McGuire, S. Y., & McGuire, S. (2015). *Teach students how to learn: Strategies you can incorporate into any course to improve student metacognition, study skills, and motivation*. Stylus.

Minton-Bedoes, Z. (2021, October 13). Special report: The world economy—for richer, for poorer. *The Economist*. https://www.economist.com/special-report/2012-10-13

Norris, F., Stevens, S., Pfefferbaum, B., Wyche, K., & Pfefferbaum, R. (2008). Community resilience as a metaphor, theory, set of capacities, and strategies for disaster readiness. *American Journal of Community Psychology, 41*(1-2), 127–150.

Payne, R. (2005). *A framework for understanding poverty*. aha! Process.

Payne, R. (2013). *A framework for understanding poverty: a cognitive approach*. Aha! Process.

Piaget, J. (1936). *Origins of intelligence in the child*. Routledge & Kegan Paul.

Piaget, J. (1945). *Play, dreams and imitation in childhood*. Heinemann.

Sanchez, R. (2020, August 16). Few signs of collective mourning as the U.S. nears 170,000 coronavirus deaths. *CNN*. https://www.cnn.com/2020/08/16/us/coronavirus-pandemic-national-mourning/index.html.

Scott, J. (2000). *Rational choice theory*. University of Essex, Colchester.

Simon, H. (1955). A behavioral model of rational choice. *Quarterly Journal of Economics, 69*(11), 99–118.

Statman-Weil, K. (2015) Creating Trauma Sensitive Classrooms. *Young Children, 70*, 72–79.

Stroh, L., Northcraft, G., & Neale, M. (2002). *Organizational behavior: A management challenge*, (3rd ed.). Psychology Press.

Svinicki, M., & McKeachie, W. J. (2011). *McKeachie's teaching tips: Strategies, research, and theory for college and university teachers* (13th ed.). Cengage.

Tajfel, H., & Turner, J. (1986). The social identity theory of inter-group behavior. In S. Worchel & W. Austin (Eds.), *Psychology of intergroup relations*. Nelson-Hall.

Terrasi, S. and Crain de Galarce, P. (2017) Trauma and learning in America's classrooms. *Emotional Life and Learning, 98*(6), 35–41.

Walley, A., Paasche-Orlow, M., Lee, E., Forsythe, S., Chetty, V., Mitchell, S., & Jack, B. (2012). Acute care hospital utilization among medical inpatients discharged with a substance use disorder diagnosis. *Journal of Addiction Medicine, 6*(1), 50–56.

Webb, N. (2005). *Depth-of-Knowledge levels for four content areas* [Paper presentation]. The Florida Education Research Association, 50th Annual Meeting, Miami, Florida.

Wilson, T. (2005). Evolution in information behavior modeling: Wilson's model. In K. E. Fisher, S. Erdelez, & L. McKechnie (Eds.), *Theories of information behavior, information today* (pp. 31–36). Information Today.

Wittchen, H. (2002). Generalized anxiety disorder: Prevalence, burden, and cost to society. *Depression and Anxiety, 16*(4), 162–171.

Wood, H. (2016). *Invitation to peace studies*. Oxford University Press.

CHAPTER 10

A JOURNAL OF THE PANDEMIC YEAR

Teaching at the Margins in the Age of Novel Coronavirus

G. Michelle Collins-Sibley

"Here we may observe, and I hope it will not be amiss to take notice of it that a near view of death would soon reconcile men of good principles one to another ... Another plague year would reconcile all these differences; a close conversing with death,or with disease that threaten death, would scum off the gall from our tempers removed the animosities among us, and bring us to see with differing eyes thanthose which we looked on things with before."

—Daniel Defoe, *Robinson Crusoe and a Journal Of The Plague Year*

"There is just as much beauty visible in the landscape as we are prepared to appreciate—not one grain more."

—Henry David Thoreau, "Autumnal Tints"

Coronavirus and Vulnerable People: Addressing the Divide in Harm and Responses and Exploring Implications for a More Peaceful World, pp. 179–192

> "People saw what they wanted to see and wanted to see what they expected to see, and Paul could do whatever he wanted, like some sort of non-murderous Raskolnikov.
>
> —Andrea Lawlor, *Paul Takes the Form of a Mortal Girl*

An 18th century London merchant, a 19th century New England naturalist, and a 21st-century shapeshifting trans person: What might these individuals have in common? They mark the boundaries of teaching (and learning) amid a pandemic crisis that finds us caught in a paradoxical intersection of the old, the new, and an increasingly ambiguous future. The old: A lesser known early modern work by Daniel Defoe, *A Journal of the Plague Year* (1722/1948), its protagonist, the abovementioned London merchant. The new: Henry David Thoreau's naturalist writing and modern meditations on nature and culture, specifically, "Walking" (1862/2012), a posthumously published text grounded in both his journals, his lectures, and his own experience. The ambiguous future: A postmodern contemporary work of LGBTQ+ literature by Andrea Lawlor, *Paul Takes the Form of a Mortal Girl* (2019), in which Paul, the protagonist, who, like a postmodern Tiresias, lives as both a man and a woman but without the help of divine intervention. At the crossroads of this improbable intersection: One English professor and 12 students in an inaugural course offering about LGBTQ+ literature and theory, "Queering the Literary Landscape." In the postapocalyptic tradition established by Defoe, this chapter presents a pedagogical journey through a collective academic experience—in real and virtual space—of the pandemic crisis and how a potentially traumatic experience of a world turned upside down came to shape a safe space in which we were able to explore our own academically-framed and reinforced experiences of intersectionality. A quarter of the students in "Queering the Literary Landscape" also enrolled in Africana Literature, another student simultaneously enrolled in "Major Authors" reading Chinua Achebe and James Baldwin, and one professor taught all three courses. All emphasize race, gender, gender identification, and class, in the fragile aftermath of an "American Dream" that has been revealed as an illusion. It is an account of how we developed our own, if not trauma-pedagogy, reading practice that allowed for the working through of our various traumas (individual and collective), one memoir, novel, or poem at a time, three times a week, in a virtual classroom.

Daniel Defoe's (1722/1948) relevance to the current moment is immediately obvious; his *Journal of the Plague Year* is enjoying a renaissance of interest in light of the novel coronavirus. This account of an unnamed merchant and his experience with bubonic plague in 18th century London is today as topical in design and content as it was some 300 years ago at the time of its publication. This, as the narrator indicates early on, was his intention,

> I have set this particular down so fully because I know not, but it may be of moment to those who come after me if they come to be brought to the same distress and to the same manner of making their choice, and therefore I desire this account may pass with them rather for a direction to themselves to act by than a history of my actings, seeing it may not be of one farthing's value to them to note what became of me. (p. 351)

Indeed, Defoe's narrative became the model for apocalyptic plague narratives to come, just as he had intended. But for this chapter, I am less interested in its generic influence than in the process through which the novel unfolds and the merchant's perspective evolves. His protagonist shares his observations about the transformative impact of the plague on those who remain behind in a largely deserted London, largely the poor who lack the resources to flee. These observations are made on his walks through the city. As a man of means, he too could have fled the city—his newfound marginality derives in large part from more of a nondecision than a conscious choice as he ponders not so much whether to leave as when to leave and where to go. As readers share his internal monologue about how and when to leave, the source of his indecision presents as simultaneously complex and circumstantial. He is concerned with his business, describing himself as a single man but with "a family of servants whom I kept at my business"; these business concerns present as much as a desire to care for that family of servants and employees as to preserve his property. And, as he observes, "our part of town seemed to be spared in comparison of the west part" such that the need to flee seems less urgent than it might otherwise have been. He also has a brother who flees to the countryside with his own family, leaving his business in the protagonist's care. These dual business concerns and familial obligations provide initial motivation for his walks through London as he describes himself "going ordinarily about the streets, as my business required, and particularly went generally once a day, or in two days, into the city to my brother's house … to see if it was safe" (p. 359). But in relatively short order, these walks take on a new quality shaped at least in part from the desolation of the streets; his curiosity comes to the fore "[leading] him to observe things more than usual, and indeed," he says, "I walked a great way where I had no business"(p. 361) This shift in the merchant's perspective and attitude is key, I argue, to what he will describe as "of use hereafter to those unto whose hands these [observations] may come if they should ever see the like dreadful visitation" (p. 423); it is the manner of his observations rather than the observations themselves which is significant.

At the far end of this nexus is Paul Polydoris, the protagonist of Andrea Lawlor's (2019) novel, who shares the London merchant's "attitude of mortality." His story unfolds in the early 1990s against the backdrop of the AIDS epidemic. We first meet Paul in 1992, the year in which the eighth annual World AIDS conference moved from Boston to Amsterdam due to U.S. immigration restrictions (the HIV Immigration Exclusion Act became law in 1992), and AIDS becomes the number one cause of death for American men aged 25 to 44. A student of film studies and queer theory at the university, he tends bar in Iowa City's only gay club and has a rich and varied sexual life—the *New York Times* blurb on the back of the Vintage paperback edition characterizes the novel as "difficult to quote in a family newspaper." And Paul has a not-so-secret secret. The novel's title is a "spoiler." Yes, Paul *takes* the form of a mortal girl, and he does so at will. He is a shape-shifter, a restless walker like Defoe's London merchant, described in the opening paragraph of the novellas perpetually in motion: "[l]ike a shark, Paul had to keep moving.... He had business with the world, codes to crack, so many questions. Tonight, for example, Paul needed to know what f—king was like for girls" (p. 3). His attention to minute detail rivals Defoe's merchant's eye for everyday detail. And like him, Paul brings an attitude of mortality to his observations.

Interestingly, our discussions of Paul as a flaneur excited the students' interest in Defoe's (1722/1948) merchant. They identified with Paul as a reader and decoder of cultural texts; for one, the "shape-shifting" evokes gaming and the construction and customization of avatars in the virtual world. While not walkers like Defoe's merchant, they were already acquainted with the "cyberflaneur," one who "by definition, strolls through the Internet. Little purpose guides his journey.... How do you turn a corner into the unknown online? You click a link. You go places. Who cares where?" The cyberflâneur strolls more for the journey, the experience, the flow of the digital landscape" (Hendel, 2012).

A Journal of the Plague (Defoe, 1722/1948) year claims our attention by its link to our pandemic moment, and *Paul Takes the Form of a Mortal Girl* (Lawlor, 2019) comes straight from our LGBTQ+ reading list and leads us to Paul's contemporary counterpart, the cyberflâneur. Whence Henry David Thoreau and "Walking?" Like Defoe's merchant and Lawlor's Paul Polydoris, Thoreau was both walker and cultural observer; indeed, he was a cultural critic. More importantly, Thoreau can be read as a philosopher of walking as a practice and human relationship with the natural world as preparation for life by teaching us an attitude of mortality, both of which are necessary preparation for learning to *see*. Each of my opening epigraphs offers a position on sight and what it means to see. It is through the specific practice of walking that each character learns to see. I propose Thoreau and his philosophy as a theoretical lens through which we might understand the practice of walking as transformative, as an art; just as was the case with Defoe in writing *A Journal,* Thoreau (1862/2012) opens his essay with an assertion of his intent:

> I have met with but one or two persons in the course of my life who understood the art of Walking that is, of taking walks—who had a genius, so to speak, for *sauntering*, which word is beautifully derived "from idle people who roved about the country, in the Middle Ages, and asked charity, under the pretense of going *à la Sainte Terre,*" to the Holy Land … a Saunterer, a Holy Lander.… Some, however, would derive the word from *sans terre*, without land or a home, which, therefore, in the good sense, will mean having no particular home, but equally at home everywhere. For this is the secret of successful sauntering. (pp. 71–72, emphasis original)

Thoreau concludes this passage declaring his preference for the saunterer as derived from Holy Lander while I prefer the second derivation from *sans terre*. It is important to remember that Thoreau also understood himself to be living and writing at the margins of his cultural and historical moment. He was deeply concerned with the culture's increasing alienation from the natural world—his original title for this lecture/essay was "The Wild"—and he was also a passionate abolitionist who did not live to see the outcome of the Civil War. In many regards, he too was a man *sans terre.* But for the moment, let us focus on the art of walking, of sauntering, as he articulates it; in other words, on walking not as a means to an end but as an end in and of itself. Defoe's merchant and Lawlor's Paul Polydoris, like Henry David Thoreau himself, are not merely walkers but saunterers, of a specific disposition; they are *flâneurs*.

Midway through the opening chapter of the novel, Lawlor (2019) describes Paul using precisely that term:

> Chicago was only four hours away by Greyhound, and Paul didn't know anyone there, reason enough to make the trip, plus he missed starless nights lit by neon, the smell of sidewalks, rooms full of strangers. A *flâneur* [emphasis added], he walked from the bus station up North Halsted, looking for the gays.… Chicago was a grey ocean, all concrete, and big sky. (p. 48)

The trip is Paul's reason for being, Chicago s landscape as natural and compelling as Thoreau's woods. Several chapters later in the novel, while Paul is hiking on the beach with his girlfriend—himself in the form of a girl—Paul muses that "he preferred the term 'walking.' He was a flâneur, not a hiker; he still had standards. Plus, people killed lesbian hikers; that was a thing" (p. 166).

Paul, like Lawlor (2019), evokes the *flâneur* as a stroller (Thoreau's saunterer), an iconic, passionate, wanderer typical of 19th-century French literary culture à la Baudelaire and later Walter Benjamin. His landscape is the cityscape marked by "starless nights lit by neon, the smell of sidewalks ... a grey ocean all concrete and big sky" as described in the above-cited passage. Paul is "a city person, a bus surfer," and his cityscape is just as reminiscent of mortality as Thoreau's autumn woods (p. 93). Dancing at a club on this same trip, Paul encounters an enchanting, flirtatious boy who he trails from the club—taking on the appearance of a girl in the process so as not to appear too threatening—only to discover once he catches him "that the youth was now, without question, a girl. As surely as he had changed, so had the youth" (p. 54). The narrative takes on a hybrid character, that of a *flâneur* caught up in the monomyth, the hero's quest from this point forward even as it retains those elements of the *bildungsroman*, yet Paul continues to be motivated as a passionate wanderer, drawn to the city like "those idle people" Thoreau referenced, "who roved about the country ... under the pretense of going *à la Sainte Terre*"—first Chicago, ultimately San Francisco—Paul is drawn to cities in the same way that Thoreau describes himself as drawn to the woods, to walking.

Defoe's (1722/1948) merchant experiences a similar compulsion. Again, and again even as the plague comes to invade his neighborhood and he describes himself as "terrified by those frightful objects," telling us, "I would retire home sometimes, and resolve to go out no more; and perhaps I would keep those resolutions for three or four days" (p. 426); and while ultimately he will confine his "family" to quarantine, his "unsatisfied curiosity" drives him to walk the streets observing that "though I generally came frightened and terrified home, yet I could not restrain; only that indeed I did not do it so frequently as at first" (p. 431). The curiosity which compels him from his house and back onto the streets suggests a need to engage with the cityscape and its inhabitants; he manifests a kind of wonderous admiration for the poor who suffer most from the plague yet were, in his words,

> the most venturous and fearless of it, and went about their employment with a sort of brutal courage; I must call it so, for it was founded neither on religion nor prudence; scared did they use any caution, but ran into any business which they could get employment in, though it was most hazardous. Such was that of tending the sick, watching houses shut up, carrying infected persons to the pest-house, and which was still worse, carrying the dead away to their graves. (p. 441)

I cite this passage at length to demonstrate the transformative effect of Defoe's protagonist's experiences as *flâneur*. His narrative dutifully recounts the weekly "bills" through which deaths are indirectly reported by the number of burials, along with a calculation of an increase in burials over time. Early on, he describes rather differently scenes of the "richer sort people, especially the nobility and gentry" with their families and servants fleeing the city as "a sight which I could not but look on from morning to night. Indeed, there was nothing else of moment be seen" (p. 350). This sense of these people in motion as "nothing else of the moment" comes early in his plague adventure and precedes his accounts of his near-daily walks to attend to his business and watch his brother's house. Later, once he has been walking for some time, he comes to characterize his observations as stories, some of them diverting, all speaking a certain truth "or very near truth; that is to say, true in general" (p. 398). As his walks acquire an almost ritual quality, an embodied engagement with those who might otherwise have been invisible to him, and he is prepared to see what might otherwise have been invisible to him. He takes targeted walks after dark to the mass graves where plague victims are buried, observing that

> [a]ll the needful works that carried terror with them, that were both dismal and dangerous were done at night.... So that in the daytime, there was not the least signal of the calamity to be seen or heard of, except what was to be observed from the emptiness of the streets, and sometimes from the passionate outcries and lamentations of the people. (p. 398)

Along with the poor, who must take any work they can find, our merchant bears witness to the cycle of life and death otherwise nearly invisible in the desolate city. He actively seeks to see that which some of his fellow citizens would prefer to avert their eyes. His ritual walking has prepared him for the sight.

In his *Natural History Essays,* Thoreau (1980) speaks explicitly of a similar preparative process. In "Autumnal Tints," he asserts that,

> Objects are concealed from our view, not so much because they are out of the course of our visual ray as because we do not bring our minds and eyes to bear on them.... The greater part of the phenomena of Nature are for this reason concealed from us all our lives.... There is just as much beauty visible to us in the landscape as we are *prepared* to appreciate—not a grain more. The objects that one man will see from a particular hilltop are just as different as the beholders are different. (pp. 173–174, emphasis added)

If we chafe at Thoreau's conclusion that two persons walking up the same hilltop do not see the same objects or share the same perceptions, we assume the possibility of an objective perspective; Thoreau does not. Indeed, in citing the example of a botanist—objective, scientific observer *par excellence*—he asserts that the botanist "absorbed in the studies of grasses" will see only grass to the degree that he risks trampling other plants. Thoreau concluded, "I have found that it required a different intention of the eye, in the same locality, to see different plants" (p. 174). This follows from his discussion of walking as art in "Walking." Thoreau is careful to explain that he approaches the walk as an end in and of itself rather than a means to an end, insisting that as you walk, "you must walk like a camel, which is said to be the only beast which ruminates when walking" (p. 77). Walking is a contemplative practice and, as such, a transformative experience. His thinking echoes Ralph Ellison's (1995) observations on the subject of invisibility in his protagonist's introduction to *Invisible Man*,

> [t]hat invisibility to which I refer occurs because of a peculiar disposition of the eyes of those with whom I come in contact. A matter of the construction of their inner eyes, those eyes with which they look through their physical eyes upon reality. (p. 3)

Or, as Paul puts it more bluntly, "[p]eople saw what they wanted to see and wanted to see what they expected to see" (Lawlor, 2019, p. 144). Several students in "Queering the Literary Landscape" had also read *Invisible Man* with me before the university had sent students home and we pivoted to exclusively online classes. They remarked upon the resonance between Ellison's narrator's observation and Lawlor, through Paul, introducing the idea of an individual's choice: their declaration that "people see what they want to see" links back to the city fathers in plague-struck London. The dead are buried or even carted off to the pest houses in the dead of night, under cover of darkness. For us in 21st century America, my students observe that the cell phone video goes viral and makes its way onto the 6:30 network newscast, allowing us to bear witness to what authorities and institutions would prefer we not see. Or as one student put it, it is like the police officer who disperses—or attempts to disperse—the crowd with a "Move along, move along—nothing to see here." Thoreau's insistence upon walking as art recalls Baudelaire's essay about the flâneur, in which he characterizes him as "The Painter of Modern Life" (Baudelaire, 1993, pp. 390–436).

In his *New Stateman* article "Madness of Crowds," Will Self (2014) observes that it has taken two centuries to perfect the willed blindness to which Defoe alludes. "Perhaps the most essential attributed required to be an urban survivor is a strange visual impairment: a concerted ability not to look anyone in the face" (para. 4). This is for him a willed disjunction between appearance and reality, something most easily understood through our ability to distinguish between artists who capture the psyche of their subjects in contrast with those who "merely produce likeness." Like Thoreau, Self cites Baudelaire's characterization of the flaneur, asserting that this ability to see derives from *flânerie* by which we acquire this capacity, what Ellison might call "a disposition," or Thoreau "an intention" of the eye. Self concludes his column with this description:

> The flaneur stands apart from the crowd and is unafraid to see the individual rather than the functional stereotype imposed by mass urbanism—but it is a deeply uncomfortable perspective to adopt. Once you begin to analyze a stranger's face, she ceases to be a stranger: you feel the living oppression of her illnesses and neuroses, her joys and her sadness—she becomes part of a tightly knit community that takes up residence in your mind alone. (para. 6)

Perhaps you cannot touch a heart without telling a story, and if you look a stranger in the eye, she—her story—takes up residence inside your mind. That is what it means to *see.*

Christopher A. Dustin and Joanna E. Ziegler (2007), in *Practicing Mortality: Art, Philosophy, and Contemplative Seeing,* take up the question of what it means to see with an extended discussion of Thoreau, his practice of contemplative walking, contemplative seeing, and his attitude of mortality. For this essay's purposes, I will focus on their proposal that there is a practice of reading (and thereby seeing) that parallels Thoreau's practice of walking and seeing. For them, his practice of walking and seeing, what they also characterize as embodied engagement, suggests that

> [i]f what Thoreau preached, his practice of walking and seeing, is enacted in and through his writing, it could also be enacted through our reading of them. We would have to journey through his writing the way he journeyed through the landscape that brought it to life. (p. 19)

Their approach is particularly appropriate to teaching literature on the margins, as they describe this kind of reading as itself a journey, suggesting that "we would have to journey through [Thoreau's] writing the way he journeyed through the landscape that brought it to life. Its ultimate aim: for the reader to emphasize with protagonists and their experiences" (p. 423). Defoe's protagonist essentially identifies this as his purpose in writing and publishing his journal; he invites us as readers to join him—retrospectively—on his journey, expressing his hope that "I may be able to make an observation or two of my own, which may be of use hereafter to those into whose hands these may come" (p. 423).

The delight of reading Thoreau or Defoe or Lawlor, for that matter—according to Dustin and Ziegler (2007), is the invitation to locate ourselves within what he or she or they is writing about. So too is the delight for LGBTQ+ students in reading queer literature in locating themselves and their experiences; so too is the delight of reading literature by Black writers, or women reading women writers, relocating experiences and knowledge relegated to the margins. It helps us see ourselves and others as we really are, as "realization[s] of our human reality" (p. 32). This is Paul Polydoris's quest; as a shapeshifter, he thinks to himself, "[h]is body did whatever he wanted, so he belonged in all the genders" (Dustin & Ziegler, 2007, p. 20). Once he discovers that there is at least one other person out in the world like him, there's the possibility to see himself in a different mirror, one that reflects his reality rather than that he assumes or has been projected upon him. Midway through the novel, he's remained a girl—Polly—for almost a month straight; it would have been two months, he notes, but he had transformed himself briefly to demonstrate his ability for his girlfriend. He wonders, were he to stay in this form for longer than a month might he menstruate? He had the parts just like in *Our Bodies, Ourselves* (Boston Women's Health Book Collective, 1970), and thus far, his vagina did everything advertised except bleed. He wonders if there is anything unusual in his blood. Is gender merely performative, and if so, is it a question of the gaze—gendered or neutral—of a wardrobe, biology, or something else? Just as Paul begins to think that he likes being a girl, that he might stay a girl, his girlfriend dumps him. In the depths of vulnerability, he changed back, finding himself once again trapped in his old sense of inadequacy and unable to "muster the energy or the focus to become a more attractive version of himself" (Dustin & Ziegler, 2007, p. 197). He takes up his quest once more and relocates himself, this time to San Francisco.

Locating oneself under the best of circumstances is no simple matter, especially for those on the margins, those who are *sans terre*, to return for a moment to Thoreau (1862/2012)), "without home or country" (p. 72). Even Paul, for whom the subculture *is the culture*. However, complex the history of identities and relationships presented by the novels, Lawlor (2019) resists even the slightest of assimilative gestures. Paul only feels comfortable around people who like being queer. The challenge comes when he comes to his girlfriend as a shapeshifter and one who has lived the bulk of his life as a gay man. Once in San Francisco, Paul ultimately meets his alter-ego, Robin; each is the only other shapeshifter the other knows. The question is asked: "What are we?" His alter-ego's answer, "We're like everybody else, only more so ... we're just what we are. You're asking the wrong question, Polly" (p. 325). What's the right question? Robin doesn't say that, nor does the novel offer a definitive answer. Paul's temporary roommate—he is subletting a room—invites him to "stay on indefinitely." Paul responds, "My favorite word!" and thinks, "The universe was conspiring to keep him here" (p. 328).

Our classrooms and colleges often function for those *sans terres* as *La Sainte terre*, from which Thoreau derives his preferred etymology of "saunterer." The abrupt disruption and forced relocation this past March—while some students had gone home, others were literally traveling the country on spring break when the decision was made to move all teaching and learning online—and accompanying enforced isolation of a "stay-at-home order," which came hard on its heels, seems to have created conditions under which—ironically enough—this kind of close, empathetic and imaginative reading became more significant for my literature students across the board and a virtual lifeline for those subsets of students in reading queer literature who were also plunging deep into the work of James Baldwin. The quality of student writing submitted in the final days of the semester, literary writing, even when discussed in synchronous virtual space, is "real writing"; even the physical presence of fingers on the keyboard preserves enough of "the physical that real writing (and reading) also preserves the depth of meaning and the possibility of substantial 'communion' between real people" (Dustin & Ziegler, 2007, p. 326). Literary writing, real writing, provided a space for clear vision, if only briefly—an hour and five minutes three times a week. It is perhaps worth noting that this was my online class that routinely ran over our designated time

Much already has been written about those ways in which distanced online learning reimposes inequities of opportunity among students in both higher education and K–12 education, exposing their vulnerabilities. Broadband access has never been as widely available as many assume. True, but even if you do not have Wi-Fi at home, you can always go to the library, or a Starbucks, or a McDonald's, right? Yet under the stay-at-home order, we were not to congregate in those public spaces. Just as our Mount Union students lost whatever centrality they may have enjoyed while away at school, millions of Americans have seen themselves dramatically relocated from the "center" to the margins in this new normal. People who have always worked find themselves furloughed or laid off, struggling to file for or obtain unemployment, and discovering the inherent problems of a health care system in which health insurance is tied to jobs. Jobs have gone away, and with them, access to health care. In a pandemic, nursing home residents, the elderly and/or the infirm, are isolated from family and friends and are dying in droves. This apocalypse—true to its Greek etymological origins—brings with it an unveiling; pulling back the veil reveals the U.S. economy's brokenness, especially the so-called social safety net, as well as the fragility of our public health systems, not to mention our public schools. In this pandemic, those accustomed to seeing or imaging themselves at the center find themselves abruptly and violently shifted to the margins.

And if this were not enough, on May 25 of this year, George Floyd was murdered by a Minneapolis police officer, aided, and abetted by three other officers, one of them just a trainee. The murder was captured on camera, uploaded to the cloud, and millions, hundreds of millions, of people here in the United States and around the world watched as Derek Chauvin casually pressed his knee—the weight of his body—into Mr. Floyd's neck for over nine minutes. Hands casually in his pockets; he stared defiantly into the camera. By the next day, something amazing was happening, mass demonstrations for social justice and against police brutality began across the nation and worldwide. It was not the simple fact of the demonstrations that amazes—Black Lives Matter activists have been demonstrating against police brutality since the summer of August 2014 and the fatal shooting of Michael Brown in Ferguson, Missouri. It was their size, their depth, their range and the diversity of the participants. People marched in major cities on the East and West Coasts and in the Midwest and in major cities across Europe and the United Kingdom. People marched in small rural towns, including in virtually all-White towns across all parts of the country. Black LGBTQ+ people marched, declaring that Black Trans Lives Matter. According to an August 9 *CNN* report, as of mid-June, some 21 million adult Americans had participated in a Black Lives Matter or other organized protests against police brutality; demonstrations both in solidarity with Black Lives Matter in the United States and against Europe's racist colonial histories around the globe. And the demonstrations continue to this day, as I write this, even as the media coverage has primarily focused on the violent anti-police action. Remarkably, the overwhelming majority of demonstrations were peaceful. While most participants had not undergone the rigorous training in nonviolent resistance common across the Civil Rights movement, especially in the South, they came prepared with goggles, masks, anti-tear gas remedies and other first-aid supplies, as well as water bottles and hand sanitizers.

What happened? At a moment when videos of Black men, women, and children attacked and killed by the police go viral on a weekly, sometimes daily basis, to the point of banality, people *saw* George Floyd. They *saw* him die. People *saw* Derek Chauvin kill him. Whatever had been getting in the way of Americans seeing the visible realities of anti-Black racism as it really is, this murder, captured live on cell phone cameras, changed things that day. If what we see or do not see depends upon "a peculiar disposition of the inner eye," of a different intention of the eye à la Ellison and Thoreau,

> If a failure to bring out minds *and eyes* to bear on reality conceals the greater part of it from us *all our lives*, then it is fundamentally a matter not just of particular "perspectives," but of ways of living, of who we are and how we live as human beings. It is a matter of our nature. (Dustin & Ziegler, 2007, p. 39, emphasis original)

The answer is, no doubt, complex and nuanced, yet one thing is clear. The pandemic happened. Peoples' lives, *en masse*, were dislocated, their world turned upside down. Three centuries ago, Daniel Defoe, through his unnamed flaneur protagonist, noted that,

> Here we may observe, and I hope that it will not be amiss to take notice of it that a near view of death would soon reconcile men of good principles

> one to another and that is chiefly owing to our easy situation in life and in our putting these things far from us that our breaches are fomented, ill blood continued, prejudices, breach of charity and Christian union, so much kept and so far carried on among us as it is ... a close conversing with death or with diseases that threaten death would *scum off the gall from our tempers, ... and bring us to see with differing eyes than those which we looked on things with before.* (p. 538, emphasis original)

Death and the plague set off a similar unveiling. Defoe (1722/1948) invoked here the attitude of mortality of which Thoreau spoke, and Andrea Lawlor alluded to in her novel's title. Paul does not just take the form of a girl; he takes the form of a *mortal* girl. In his *Natural History Essays* (1862/2012), Thoreau approached mortality through tableau natural cycles of birth, death, and decay, which perennially demonstrated the interconnection of all life, shaping his sense of self as it evolved in community with others. And it is also death's invasion of spaces from which society had banished or from which it had averted its eyes in the form of pestilence: plague, AIDS, COVID-19, anti-Black racism, police violence, anti-LGBTQ+ violence; pestilence abounds. While it may be "evident death will reconcile us all," our 18th-century merchant was savvy enough to see that "as the terror of the infection abated, these things all returned again to their less desirable channel, and to the course, they were in before" (p. 539).

In the last, Defoe (1722/1948) reminds us that his *Journal of the Plague Year* is a retrospective. Will our post-pandemic, transformed vision last beyond the immediate pandemic crisis? Perhaps, like Paul, we are asking the wrong question. If it is true that beauty is visible to us, "as we are prepared to appreciate," it, might we consciously decide to build that capacity? I wonder. Thoreau's choice of the word *preparation* suggests that something is not necessarily an innate disposition as much as a capacity that can be built. Art appreciation courses teach us to see, as do studio courses. Martha Nussbaum (1998) reminds us that we cultivate our humanity through the arts and the humanities. But lastly and most significantly, re-reading my students' final reflective essays shows me how reading together this semester has taught them new ways of seeing. Hailey wrote that literature offered "a way to escape from our new normal and that in itself gives me a change to live a fulfilling life"; and Beverly expressed that "reading ... gives insight [into] the difficulties of a group you would otherwise have no compassion for ... can persuade you to give when you otherwise would not." Britt acknowledged "this pandemic was the single best and worst thing to happen to me.... It allowed me to write as I have never written before," because it prepared her "to simply be honest." Ren never missed a class but for a long while would only answer "terrible" to any question about how they were doing, seldom spoke but rather typed in the dialog box, and never turned on the camera until one day, midway through the "new normal," Ren turned on their camera, smiled, and once more became the student so excited to contribute to discussion that their thoughts outpaced their words. This class regularly ran well over our designated time because people just had so much to say and did not want to disconnect. Certainly, the collective experience of our little band of the marginalized—gay, straight, in transition, women, people of color, and *readers*—dislocated by the pandemic crisis bears witness to the power of art, as well as that of reading and teaching of literature to "create a space in which obedience to truth may be practiced" and the vulnerable find shelter.

REFERENCES

Boston Women's Health Book Collective. (1970). *Our bodies our ourselves*. New England Free Press.

Defoe, D. (1948). *A journal of the plague year* (Louis Kronenberger, Editor). The Modern Library. (Original work published 1722)

Dustin, C., & Ziegler, Z. (2007). *Practicing mortality: Art, philosophy, and contemplative seeing*. Palgrave Macmillan.

Ellison, R. (1995). *Invisible man* (2nd ed.). Vintage.

Hendel, J. (2012, February 8). The life of the cyberflâneur *The Atlantic*. https://www.theatlantic.com/technology/archive/2012/02/the-life-of-the-cyberfl-neur/252687/

Lawlor, A. (2019). *Paul takes the form of a mortal girl*. Vintage Books.

Nussbaum, M. (1998). *Cultivating humanity: A classical defense of reform in liberal education*. Harvard University Press.

Self, W. (2014, April 11). Madness of crowds. *New Statesman*. https://www.newstatesman.com/culture/2014/04/standing-packed-together-trains-studiously-ignoring-each-other-nothing-new

Thoreau, H. (1980). Autumnal tints. In R. Sattelmeyer (Ed.), *Natural history essays* (pp. 137–77). Gibbs-Smith.

Thoreau, H. (2012). Walking. In J. Elder (Ed.), *Nature/walking*. Beacon Press. (Original work published 1862)

SECTION II

CHAPTER 11

OVERCOMING INTERGENERATIONAL TRAUMA DURING THE PANDEMIC OF 2020

Healing Is Peace

Pamela D. Hall and Alexandra Lavado

My paternal grandfather was born in 1862, during American chattel slavery. Though many people state that the signing of the Emancipation Proclamation was in 1863, many slaves did not know they were free at that time. The proclamation was not enforced in many parts of the South for more than 20 years; therefore, my grandfather must have had a slave mindset because my father, his son, did. My grandfather grew up when the slave master held the Bible in one hand and the whip in the other, and when the slave master told slaves that God wanted them to be slaves. My grandfather received this love-hate message. The slave master could beat him, cut off his limbs, rape his wife or daughter, or sell him like he was a stock on Wall Street. These messages and actions had to be confusing to my grandfather, who saw his mother sold off when he was only five years old. That confusion was likely

Coronavirus and Vulnerable People: Addressing the Divide in Harm and Responses and Exploring Implications for a More Peaceful World, pp. 195–210

passed on to my father, who then passed it on to me and my siblings. This mental confusion created trauma in my family and many families who were direct descendants of enslaved Africans in America (Hall, 2001).

Many years after I wrote this passage, I copyrighted my yet published book called *Categories* (Hall, 2001). In *Categories,* I have a chapter whereby I discuss life growing up with a father who was a direct descendant of slavery. I also coined the term "Post-Slavery Syndrome" in the book. Recently, many mental health professionals have been referring to slavery as a form of intergenerational trauma. Dr. Joy DeGruy (2005), one of my "Sheroes," has outlined the characteristics of this trauma in her book *Posttraumatic Slave Syndrome.* The remainder of this chapter will focus on two areas. Area one will discuss the compound impact of the pandemic and intergenerational trauma on the lives of "Melanated Americans," a term to be defined later in the chapter. The second area of the chapter will discuss how Melanated Americans can begin to recover from the compounded impact of trauma. The principle of Sankofa, which in Kiswahili means "go back and fetch it," will be utilized as a central feature in the proposal for recovery. This recovery will include aspects of work done by researchers on Melanated Consciousness that discusses how Melanated Americans remain resilient through the Transatlantic slave trade, slavery, Jim Crow segregation, and current-day structural inequalities. In sum, the chapter will examine what makes Melanated Americans resilient and offer suggestions on incorporating Sankofa's philosophy to improve the mental, spiritual, and physical well-being of Melanated Americans. In sum, the goal of the chapter is to demonstrate that to heal is to have peace.

TRAUMA AND THE PANDEMIC IN MELANATED COMMUNITIES

To adequately discuss trauma and the pandemic's compound effect on Melanated Americans, it is important to address why I choose the phrase "Melanated Americans" to describe Blacks, African Americans, or direct descendants of enslaved Africans.

In 2017, I had the opportunity to go home—to Africa. My visit was to Ghana, West Africa. It is noted that enslaved Africans in the diaspora came from countries in West Africa, such as Ghana, Sierra Leonne, the Congo, and Benin. While in Ghana, I, and those I traveled with, including my niece, visited the Elmina Slave Dungeon on Africa's Gold Coast. This area consists of a museum and a slave river where captured Africans took their last bath before being branded and sold to the different would-be colonizers from many countries, including Portugal, Spain, England, the Americas, and the Netherlands. I was shocked because I never fully understood how I became a direct descendant of the Africans enslaved in

America. It became more apparent when I realized that even before my ancestors were placed on the slave ship, the country they would end up in was predetermined at the slave river. Upon leaving the slave river, the Africans were confined to the slave dungeons. At the dungeons, they were stored in cramped spaces with other "goods" for up to 60 days before they were shipped off to different parts of the world. The trip began at the Gulf of Guinea, and for those that reached the Americas, ended by crossing the Atlantic Ocean.

When I got to the dungeon, which was run by the Dutch, I went to *The Door of No Return*, located close to the female dungeon area. Stenches of the past could still be smelled. I stood at the gate with bars on it and looked out at the Gulf of Guinea. I could visualize the ships that must have docked there to pick up my ancestors. I could imagine how my ancestors felt when they went through this door. They must have been afraid and confused, perhaps even angry. I could also imagine the trauma my ancestors felt waiting in those cramped quarters for months, only to be escorted out bare naked to a courtyard where the "governor" looked down below to choose who he would have sex with that night. Yes, it was described as sex and not rape. My female ancestors had to stay in those cramped rooms without any care or consideration about their hygiene or mental state. *The Door of No Return*, where they slid down a ramp, led to the predestined ship that would take African ancestors to many destinations.

My ancestors came to the United States; however, it is likely that some of my 'ancestors' brothers, sisters, cousins, uncles, and aunties went to the West Indies, Haiti, and Brazil. The only thing that separated us was where we would be colonized. A great sadness overcame me and the group of friends that I was with on the tour. All of us, including my young niece, wept, and wailed at the treachery of this experience. "How could people be so cruel, so inhumane?" That was my first real trigger of slavery and connection to the trauma of those who were enslaved. I connected that experience with the trauma my grandfather must have experienced, the trauma he passed on to my father, and the trauma that my father passed on to me. I wondered if the trigger was genetic or learned, nature or nurture, or perhaps a combination of both. It makes me wonder if the coronavirus disease's trauma (COVID-19), triggers past trauma for Melanated people.

On the travel back from Ghana, I looked at the plane's television monitor. I looked at the GPS image showing the aircraft hovering over Ghana. It was then that it dawned on me that it was just an ocean that led to Melanated people's separation. The Atlantic Ocean is what those slave vessels crossed before they stopped in the countries, dropping off relatives in different locations. Since that trip, I have been engrossed in helping Africans in the Diaspora understand that we are from the same place. That is what led me to define those of us who have been kissed by the sun as "Melanated

Americans." The Atlantic Ocean separated us geographically, and slavery separated us mentally. Yet, when it comes to COVID-19, we are the same. We are suffering the same demise, the same trauma.

WHAT IS BLACK?

Many individuals do not think about the genetic connection that this trauma has on people of Melanated descent. Who are these people I refer to as Melanated? African American is a term that is used on the U.S. Census. The census forces Africans from the Diaspora, whose colonizer may have been from a country other than the U.S., to check the box "African American." Yet, these Melanated people may be Haitian, Jamaican, or Brazilian born. To be an African from the diaspora is to be kissed by the sun. This kissing by the sun gives us our melanin, our skin tone. Though all Melanated people who have to check that box on the U.S. Census are from America, they are all descendants from Africa. Some of us have a problem with identifying with Africa and do not wish to be called Black or African American, but what is a fact is that we are Melanated people living in the diaspora. For unification and clarification, I will refer to all Melanated people living in America who have been impacted by the trauma of African slavery and the current pandemic in the U.S. as Melanated people. It is that melanin and unfortunate trauma that unifies us. Whether we were born here and are direct descendants of Africans enslaved in America or came from another country, we are Melanated people; we have been kissed by the sun. That and our trauma (intergenerational trauma, historical trauma, and present-day COVID-19 trauma) is what we have in common.

The Association of Black Psychologists defines key terms related to trauma that has impacted Melanated people's lives. Trauma occurs when one experiences, witnesses, or is confronted with an event or events that involve actual or threatened death or serious injury, or a threat to the physical integrity of self or others and evokes intense fear, helplessness, or horror (Grills et al., 2016). Historical trauma "is cumulative emotional and psychological wounding, over the lifespan and across generations, emanating from massive group trauma experiences" (Grills et al., 2016, p. 336). Psychic terrorism has been defined as "any act or thought designed to immobilize and destabilize one's basic sense of security and safety (physically or emotionally) by assaulting 'one's sense of self or identity' " (Grills et al., 2016, p. 337). Examples include the intersections of psychological and economic residuals related to historical events such as American slavery, Jim Crow laws, apartheid, and global colonization.

It is important to note that what all Melanated people share is that we were colonized, and that colonization included the attempt to break our will.

This included stripping us of our identity, culture, language, spirituality, and religion. This separation and colonization made us think that we were different from one another because we came from different countries. It caused us to forget we came from the same continent. Yet, COVID-19 does not care about the country of origin of Melanated people. This is evident when we look at the impact that COVID-19 has on Melanated people in the U.S. The virus has produced higher rates of diagnoses and deaths for Melanated people, whether Haitian, Jamaican, Trinidad, Brazilian, or Afro Latinx, or African Americans. That is the commonality.

Since most of the country has been at home during the COVID pandemic, they have witnessed the death of Ahmad Arbury, Breonna Taylor, and George Floyd. The George Floyd event may have been the most traumatizing for Melanated people because the news media played it over and over, reigniting the trauma over and over again. Each time they showed the 8 minutes and 46 seconds, the police officer had his knee pressed in George Floyd's neck. It was likely to have compounded the trauma many Melanated people were already experiencing. Melanated people have lost family members from COVID-19. They could not visit family members while in the hospital or say goodbye to their family members who died from COVID-19. The trauma was magnified when individuals could not have a proper burial for their family members. In Melanated communities, like other racial and ethnic groups, the rituals and customs associated with family members' homegoing services could not be practiced. All of this is traumatizing.

Amid COVID-19 related deaths, Melanated people had to continue to watch more incidents of police killing innocent Melanated people even after George Floyd, such as Rayshard Brooks. This traumatization adds insult to injury as Melanated people deal with the fact that no police officers have been charged with Breonna Taylor's death at the time of this writing. Additionally, social media has exploded with Melanated males and females' incidents being targeted by "Karens" and "Chads" just because of their skin's hue. There are also numerous incidents of infiltrators pretending to be allies of the Black Lives Matter movement who are burning and looting to make Melanated people seem like violent criminals. The media and closed-minded insensitive people call those fighting for justice rioters instead of protesters as if the terms are interchangeable. The trauma of COVID-19 is rearing its ugly head in so many ways. The death rates and diagnosis of the pandemic amongst Melanated people are just a part of what is traumatizing us.

Another part of the compound effect is that many Melanated people are considered essential yet expendable workers. They stock shelves with food, work in fields picking food for the country to eat, and stock warehouse shelves while at risk of COVID-19 exposure. This is addition to the fact that in areas with high concentrations of Melanated people, such as Miami, Florida, people did not have access to testing as quickly as those in higher income brackets. These are examples of COVID-19 trauma. For example, in Weston, Florida, a suburban community in the South of Broward County, the first sites were set up months before they became accessible to areas that are highly concentrated with Melanated people. Weston has a population of 72,324 out of which 82.11% are White, and only 4.53% are Black or African American. Furthermore, Weston has a median household income of over $100,00 and a poverty rate of 7.51% (Weston, Florida Population, 2020). This differs remarkably from Miami, the second-largest city in Florida, which has a median household income of $36,638 and a poverty rate of 24.32% (Miami, Florida Population, 2020).

COVID-19 trauma is different from the usual trauma that Melanated people experienced pre-pandemic. The daily stressors come from microaggressions in the form of microassaults, microinsults, and microinvalidations. The term microaggressions weas coined by a Melanated psychiatrist from Harvard University named Chester Pierce. Dr. Chester Pierce and his colleagues stated that racial microaggressions are subtle and often automatic put downs that Melanated people experience (Pierce et al., 1978). Dr. Pierce's work was expanded upon by Dr. Derald Wang Sue and colleagues (2019), who said there were three types of microaggressions: (a) microassaults, (b) microinsults, and (c) microinvalidations (p. 122). Microsassaults are blatant, verbal, nonverbal, or environmental attacks intended to convey biased and discriminatory sentiments (Sue et al., 2019, p. 125). Microinsults are unintentional behavioral or verbal comments that convey rudeness or insensitivity, which can demean a person's racial heritage, while microinvalidations are verbal statements or behaviors that exclude, negate, and dismiss the psychological thoughts, feelings, or experiential realities of a marginalized group (Sue et al., 2019, pp. 125–26).

As the president-elect of the South Florida chapter of The Association of Black Psychologists, one of our current chapter president's practices involves facilitating microaggression confessions at the beginning of our meetings. This involves each member stating any microaggressions they experienced over the last week. We follow a round robin format, and without fail, each member has at least one major microaggression that has impacted their lives each time. As Reverend Al Sharpton stated at George Floyd's memorial in Minneapolis, we have always had a knee in our neck. This knee, which makes it difficult, if not impossible, to breathe, started with slavery.

POST-SLAVERY SYNDROME

I know that many people, especially Melanated people of all shades and colors from all socioeconomic statuses, refuse to discuss slavery. Some older Melanated folk believe slavery was in the past, and we should forget about it. I know my father and my mother did not talk about events that happened in the past. Yet, in his final years, my father did begin to share stories about the impact racism played in his life. He was born in 1921, so I can only imagine what life must have been like for him. He had to beware of those who might want to lynch him or imprison him because of his skin's hue. My father lived through Jim Crow and segregation. I remember my father sharing a story about not giving up his seat in the front of a bus and the police being called on him. He told me, "Rosa Parks was not the only one who refused to give up their seat in the front of the bus." Like George Floyd was the spark to start this new movement towards Melanated consciousness, she was just the spark that started the Civil Rights movement.

From stories such as my father's and some of the unhealthy ways he interacted with my siblings and me, we can see the need to address the impact that chattel slavery had on Melanated people in America. The notion that slavery is in the past and we do not need to talk about it allows our trauma to continue. This trauma has been magnified because of the pandemic and the racial injustices that have been rebirthed under "45's" presidency. Unaddressed trauma makes Melanated people more susceptible to illness and disease. Yes, slavery may be over, but its effects are ever-present in the Melanated community. Melanated people need to realize that they are treated differently because of their skin color. Melanated people must recognize that we must deal with the trauma from slavery passed down from our grandparents to our parents. The unhealthy thoughts, beliefs, and actions we engage in result from a traumatized and colonized mind. We must address Post-Slavery Syndrome by first identifying and acknowledging that it exists. Dr. DeGruy makes a great point in her book when she says we never received treatment or help after slavery ended, after Jim Crow and still to this day, we have not received treatment (DeGruy, 2005). I made similar points in the synopsis of Post-Slavery Syndrome in my book, *Categories* (Hall, 2001).

I describe Post-Slavery Syndrome as a group of thoughts and behaviors resulting from the way many people, Melanated people and White people, were told to think, feel, and behave regarding others' treatment from the same and different racial groups. The thoughts and behaviors of Melanated and White people are different. More than 100 years after the Emancipation Proclamation was signed, the relations between Melanated people and Whites are still tense. Whites had to get used to changing their language. They had to stop referring to Melanated people as "niggers," "my nigger," "porch monkey," "coon," and/or "boy" (Hall, 2001). Yet, telling someone comfortable with things a certain way that they can no longer do something may be easier said than done. It is like telling a leopard to change its spots. Post-slavery Whites had to comply with new laws that meant sharing space and resources with Melanated people.

In social psychology, theorists distinguish between compliance and acceptance. Both are forms of conformity. That is what we have been asking White America to do, conform. Compliance is when you publicly agree but privately disagree. Acceptance is when you both publicly and privately agree (Sowden, 2018). It seems that many Whites have complied but have not accepted Melanated people as their equals. They have not been willing to accept Melanated people's way of thinking or culture from Africa. They have told Melanated people that they could eat, shop, go to school, and church with Whites.

Such changes are examples of compliance. It was not until the 1960s that laws protecting the rights of Melanated people began to be enforced. This is almost 100 years since the Emancipation Proclamation. Affirmative action laws were created to get whites to conform. Again, if you make someone do something, that does not mean that it is in their hearts. There does not seem to be much love in the White man's heart for Melanated people. That is what is still dividing America, and that is what will continue to divide America. We see this now as we witness the disparities of COVID-19, and we witness how Melanated people are being treated by Whites when they try to have peaceful protests.

The United States now consists of more than two groups; the case is not Melanated people and White people only. However, the relationship between Melanated people and whites in America is unique because of this institution called slavery. This is not to say that the Post-Slavery Syndrome does not impact other racial and ethnic groups. They are impacted but not affected. These different groups were not the victim or the conductors of slavery in America. They were not those who tried to prevent people from being equal.

Many argue that Melanated people who still speak about the effects of slavery needs leave the past in the past. This is accurate. There is no way an individual can need to heal if he/she dwells on the past. This prevents new ways of thinking. Yet, the one thing that all those opposed to speaking about slavery must remember is that many past effects are still present. Such as trauma. Many Melanated people do not know their history or that the past is related to present trauma. They think they invent something new or do not realize the impact of the ways, customs, thoughts, wives' tales, and myths have influenced us just as our parents, teachers, the media, and so forth, influence us. Take spankings, for instance. The root of Melanated people spanking their children came from slavery. They would spank their children to keep them quiet because they knew that if the slave master or overseer heard them being loud or just playing, the punishment would be brutal; it would be a lot worse than what their parents did by spanking them. This residue from slavery has no benefit to Melanated people, and this practice should end. It would be if we realized that each time we spanked our children, we were triggering trauma from slavery. Intergenerational trauma has historical memory, and the spankings are like the whips and the 40 lashes our ancestors received. We may not know it on a conscious level, but the impact is the same. This also occurs when we identify with the oppressor by bleaching our skin or calling one another "nigger."

EPIGENETICS, OR TRAUMA TRANSMITTED TRANS-GENERATIONALLY

I believe that the fear and other unhealthy behaviors that many Melanated people experience and engage in are not learned but passed down intergenerationally from slavery (Hall, 2001). I have heard that for many Melanated people, the remnants of slavery could be passed down through their genes. I believe an individual's DNA can be altered, changed, or modified due to trauma. The trauma can be in the form of prenatal stress, it can be in the form of posttraumatic stress, and it can be in the form of intergenerational stress. In the 1990s, I was introduced to a Black science fiction writer named Octavia Butler. She was one of the first Melanated women I knew who wrote science fiction. Her book *Kindred* supported what I claimed regarding intergenerational trauma. This belief is now supported by research in the field of epigenetics.

Epigenetics pertains to gene expression changes, which do not result directly from mutations of DNA sequences. This leads to the formation of inherited traits intragenerationally and intergenerationally (Gomółka & Wszola, 2019). Epidemiological research suggests that inter/multigenerational nongenetic behavioral phenotypes are prominently or exclusively transmitted through the maternal line (Toth, 2015). Epigenetic research has been primarily embedded in Holocaust studies. It is based on the theory that individuals whose ancestors were in the extermination camps have something in their genes that makes them react to pain and violence differently (Dutta, 2018).

In Suchismita Dutta's (2018) analysis of Octavia Butler's *Kindred*, he demonstrates how this transportation in time is a common aspect of cultural memory and trauma. The main character Dana lives in present-day California during the 1970s. Throughout the book, she experiences confusion and dizziness that preempts her transportation in time to a slave plantation in the 1700s. There she is a slave and a witness to the trauma of slavery and experiences the trauma of slavery directly by having her left arm cut off. At the plantation, Dana meets Rufus Weylin, the young, white male inheritor of the Weylin plantation who forces himself on his concubine Alice, who is originally a free Melanated woman (Dutta, 2018). What brings her back to present times is the lived experiences through episodes marked with rape and merciless slave whipping. It causes her physical pain from the alternate World to get transmuted to physical and psychological anguish in her present-day California life (Dutta, 2018).

My niece, friends, associates, and myself who went through the Elmina Slave Dungeon had a transportational experience. We went back to the time where our ancestors experienced the trauma of being captured, branded, and sent to a foreign land—a land where their language, customs, values, and beliefs were beaten out of them. Yet was it? Epigenetics suggests that the hormonal, mental, psychic, and emotional memories have somehow been passed on to future generations. It often reminds me of one of the scenes from Octavia Butler's book, where the character Dana was transported in time from the 20th century to when she was a slave on the Weylin plantation.

Yes, I genuinely believe that epigenetics is real, and finally, the nation is starting to address the impact that slavery has on future generations. Reginald Byron Jones-Sawyer, Sr, a Melanated member of the U.S. House of Representatives, supported epigenetics awareness in 2018. Due to his support, The Assembly Concurrent Resolution 177 (ACR 177) was passed in California. It was the first resolution of its kind in the U.S. ACR 177 aims to highlight intergenerational trauma and propose methods on how to heal from said trauma (Grossi, 2020).

Why is epigenetics so essential and relevant for Melanated people in the United States? Because COVID-19 will likely have a long lasting effect on Melanated people. There is already buzz that those who recover from COVID-19 will have some long-term health issues. It is likely that the trauma from COVID-19 experienced by all people, particularly Melanated people, may have an intergenerational impact.

Yet, there is hope. I hope that Melanated people who survive this latest nightmare may be able to reverse the impact epigenetically or alleviate the impact. The effect of some of this trauma is already being reversed as more and more Melanated people realize that we must face our past directly and heal from it. As Dr. DeGruy states, Black, aka Melanated people, never received treatment from slavery, Jim Crow, or the trauma of seeing our ancestors lynched. We just pretended that not talking about it would heal us. Yet to forget is to remain wounded" (Setka, 2016, p. 115). Trauma still exists, and from an epigenetic perspective, those ancestral and cultural memories are again being passed on to future generations of Melanated people. From a social learning perspective, we are still engaging in harmful practices in the form of self-hatred and internalized oppression that we pass on to our future generations. We must heal, and in many ways, we Melanated people are healing. The healing comes in the form of both resiliency and raising our consciousness. To heal is to have peace.

MELANATED CONSCIOUSNESS AND RESILIENCY AS A ROAD TO PEACE

Melanated consciousness has been conceptualized as "an attitude of mind, a way of life, a search for Melanated identity, self-awareness, self-esteem, and the rejection of white stereotypes and morals" (Pityana, 2005, p. 70). The Southern Black Student Organization has stated, "the basic tenet of Melanated Consciousness is that the Melanated man must reject all value systems that seek to make him a foreigner in the country of his birth and reduce his basic human dignity" (Pityana, 2005, p. 71). Nyameko Pityan, a human rights lawyer, defined Black Consciousness "as an assertion and affirmation of the worth and dignity of the Melanated men and a positive confrontation of the self" (Pityana, 2005, p. 71).

The Black Consciousness movement was born in South Africa and is analogous to the Black Power movement in the United States during the mid-1960s civil rights movement. George M. Fredrickson stated that the Melanated consciousness movement's primary task was to "conscientize Melanated people, which meant giving them a sense of pride or belief in their strength or worthiness" (Fredrickson, 1997, p. 199). He asserted this would help overcome the psychologically harmful effects of white domination. The Black Consciousness movement and the Black Power movement instilled in many Melanated people a new sense of self-worth and competence that helped them cope with societal stressors such as racism. In the United States, Malcolm X became synonymous with the Black Consciousness movement. He argued strongly for the recognition and support of "Melanated history, Melanated culture, the Melanated-American heritage, and self-sufficiency" (Faragher et al., 2012, p. 1033).

Resilience is another construct that has been linked closely to the lives and experiences of Melanated Americans in the United States. The American Psychological Association has defined resilience as "the process of adapting well in the face of adversity, trauma, tragedy, threats, or significant sources of stress." It is characterized by "bouncing back from difficult experiences" ("Building your Resilience," 2012). Throughout history, adversity has been very present in the lives of Melanated Americans, starting with the forced migration and enslavement of Melanated Americans, the implementation and enforcement of Jim Crow laws, and the continuous perpetration of discrimination and inequality that has disadvantaged Melanated Americans at the individual, community, and societal level. An alternative conceptualization of resilience that focused on street-life oriented men's experience was proposed by Dr. Yasser A. Payne (2011), who argued for the consideration of the street "individuals" "personal or subjective constructions of resiliency" (p. 445). This definition considers race, gender, social class, and factors in the "structural inequality" in which street-oriented Melanated men are forced to live.

An example of the structural societal oppression and exploitation that Melanated Americans suffered is their experience in the post-slavery segregated South. Dr. Katherine Van Wormer and colleagues used a risk and resilience perspective to examine the personal narratives of three older Melanated American women who engaged in domestic service in the segregated South of the 1930s (Van Wormer et al., 2011). These narratives provided first-hand accounts of the forced labor of Melanated children, which negatively hindered them from receiving a proper education. Once they grew into adulthood, these women suffered harsh treatment and unfair payment by their white employers. The historical narratives gathered in their study provided a greater understanding of resilience during a Jim Crow Era. In their research, they identified six themes of resilience that were commonly found among older Melanated Americans: "respect for family and elders; community bonding; personal traits of optimism, self-efficacy, and moral integrity; strong religious faith; valuing education; and resistance to oppression" (Van Wormer et al., 2011, p. 416).

Present-day systemic racism continues to affect Melanated Americans' lives in different public domains, including education, employment, criminal justice, and health (Sue et al., 2019). For example, although Melanated Americans constitute 13% of the United States population, they account for 40% of the U.S. prison population (Sue et al., 2019). In a study investigating perceived sources of stress and resilience in Melanated American men, racism and discrimination were frequently cited as both specific causes of stress and as mediators of stress with various issues, including relationships, employment, and community (Chung et al., 2014). The researchers additionally found that in Melanated American men, family, friends, faith, and the concept of a "strong Melanated man" were personal resources of resilience (Chung et al., 2014, pp. 441–451). The study extended the literature on the detrimental effects of racism on Melanated American men and highlighted the multiple resources that promote Melanated American men's resilience.

Racial socialization refers to the process by which parents communicate both implicit and explicit messages about the meaning of one's race in the broad social context (Tang et al., 2015). Dr. Sandra Tang and colleagues (2015) stated that cultural socialization (i.e., messages about cultural heritage, cultural tradition, racial pride) is central to racial socialization (pp. 1141–1142). Racial socialization is an important factor associated with preserving resilience in Melanated Americans. Current research has examined racial socialization's moderating role in the racial discrimination-resilience relationship among Melanated American young adults (Brown & Tylka, 2011). More precisely, Dr. Danice Brown and Dr. Tracy Tylka (2011) examined whether racial socialization messages would act as a protective mechanism for Melanated American youth's resilience when facing racial discrimination. They found racial socialization moderated the racial discrimination-resilience relationship. Participants who reported "fewer racial socialization messages, greater racial discrimination was associated with lower resilience" and participants who reported a greater number of racial socialization messages, racial discrimination was no longer negatively associated with resilience (Brown & Tylka, 2011, p. 265). The researchers emphasized multiple racial socialization messages (e.g., expressing cultural pride; awareness of discrimination issues; understanding and appreciating cultural heritage) may be necessary for Melanated American young adults' resilience. Consistent with current research, the American Psychological Association's *Task Force Report on* Resilience *and Strength in African American Children and Adolescents* has also distinguished racial socialization as an important contextual protective factor that may help Melanated American children and adolescents cope with and navigate racism and be resilient in adverse conditions. The report also emphasizes the importance of parental engagement in the racial socialization process as parental racial socialization may buffer against racism and discrimination (American Psychological Association, 2008).

Prevalent systematic racism, police brutality, and a lack of justice and accountability has led to the rise of social activism. The Black Lives Matter (BLM) movement emerged in 2014 to address systematic and institutional racism. Since then, it has gained wide attention and recognition. Surbhi Godsay and Dr. Anne E. Brodsky investigated how BLM operates to "support, promote, and maintain resilience and empowerment processes among young Melanated men as they face racism (Godsay & Brodsky, 2018, p. 55). Their findings revealed that the BLM movement appeared to influence resilience and empowerment by "providing awareness of racial injustice, reinforcing racial pride, offering resources, and opening a window of opportunity for participants to enact change within their local context" (p. 55).

Though various studies have focused on resilience sources in Melanated Americans' lives, Melanated Consciousness may be a prominent mechanism by which racial socialization moderates the racial discrimination-resilience relationship in Melanated Americans. Current research has found racial pride as an important source of resilience in Melanated Americans.

Sankofa is a Swahili term that means "to go back and get it" (The Spiritual Project at the University of Denver, 2011). It pertains to Melanated people going back to their past and reclaiming their identity. This will be crucial to healing from past and present trauma, including COVID-19 trauma. This healing will be our road to peace and internal harmony intrapsychically and communally. There is no doubt that the healing is occurring and that we are a resilient people. That is an aspect of our identity that we must hold on to moving forward.

Melanated people are still here and, in many cases, thriving despite the obstacles placed in their way, despite the transatlantic slave trade, Jim Crow segregation, lynchings, racist policies and practices, police brutality, and mass incarceration, miseducation, housing disparities, daily microaggressions, and now COVID-19. How have they been able to maintain an existence of hope, harmony, and peace? Many believe it is due to our faith, music, artistic expressions, spiritual practices, and the raising of Black consciousness in our children, youth, families, and communities. We have always found peace amid the storm, and we will find it despite the many losses we have faced during this pandemic.

In conclusion, all Melanated people need to understand the importance of their history, culture, and identity to heal. This healing begins with the principle of Sankofa. The principle of Sankofa, which in the Twi language of Ghana, translates to "*to go back and fetch it.*" Fetch what? Well, the associated proverb answers this question, "*Se wo were fi na wosankofa a yenkyi,*" which translates as "It is not wrong to go back for that which you have forgotten" (The Spiritual Project at the University of Denver, 2011).

We have forgotten that what separates us is the Atlantic Ocean and the lies that we have been told about who we are as a family. We must stop the bickering among the different countries we were born in instead of focusing on our country of origin. Differentiating Haitian American, Jamaican American, Afro Latinx, and so forth, is divisive. We are all Melanated people whose ancestors came from the same continent. If embraced, that continent and our past will lead us all to find a rich history. This rich history will help us understand our true identity and reconnect us with Afrocentric principles such as harmony and balance with nature, paying reverence to our ancestors who provided us with guidance and strength, communalism, rhythm, verve, and most importantly, our spirituality (Belgrave & Allison, 2018). Forgetting and ignoring our rich history keeps us trapped and disconnected from one another. Forgetting prevents us from embarking on the path to peace and recovery. According to the concept Ubuntu, we must begin to live the South African philosophy of the Bantu people, meaning *I am because we are*. The late Bishop Desmond Tutu stated the essence of Ubuntu in the following way:

> A person with ubuntu is open and available to others, affirming of others, does not feel threatened that others are able and good, for he or she has a proper self-assurance that comes from knowing that he or she belongs in a greater whole and is diminished when others are humiliated or diminished when others are tortured or oppressed. (Reichbaum, 2008)

Yes, Melanated people are communal people. That is another principle we forgot. We not only need to go back and fetch our past, but we need to go back and fetch one another. Melanated people have to understand the notion that if one of us suffers, then all of us suffer. We witnessed it with the recent police killings that led thousands of Melanated people to protest our right to live and exist peacefully in this society. We protest and have a history of driving social change movements because something is triggered in each of us who have a spiritual and epigenetic connection to our home, Africa, when we see one of us suffering. What is triggered is the trauma and the wounds that have yet to heal. We have begun to heal, and we have begun to experience some justice, therefore, some peace. However, we still have ways to go. Let us Yola Up! (Love Up) on one another who are being devastated by COVID-19, and when the pandemic ends, let us not stop the work of healing. To heal is to have peace!

REFERENCES

American Psychological Association. (2008). *Task force report on resilience and strength in African American children and adolescents.* https://www.apa.org/pi/families/resources/resiliencerpt.pdf

Belgrave, F., & Allison, K. (2018). *African American psychology: From Africa to America.* SAGE.

"Building your Resilience." (2012). *American Psychological Association.* https://www.apa.org/topics/resilience

Brown, D., & Tylka, T. (2011). Racial discrimination and resilience in African American young adults: Examining racial socialization as a moderator. *Journal of Black Psychology, 37*(3), 274–275.

Chung, B., Meldrum, M., Jones, F., Brown, A., & Jones, L. (2014). Perceived sources of stress and resilience in men in an African American community. *Progress in Community Health Partnerships: Research, Education, and Action, 8*(4), 441–451.

DeGruy, J. (2005). *Post traumatic slave syndrome: America's legacy of enduring injury and healing.* Uptone Press.

Dutta, S. (2018). Indelible race memories and subliminal epigenetics in Octavia Butler's Kindred. *[Inter]sections, 21*, 88.

Faragher, J., Buhle, M. J., Czitrom, D., & Armitage, S. H. (2012). The civil rights movement. In *Out of many: A history of the American people* (6th ed., Vol. 2., p. 1033). Prentice-Hall.

Fredrickson, G. (1997). From Black power to Black consciousness. In *The comparative imagination: On the history of racism, nationalism, and social movements.* University of California Press.

Godsay, S., & Brodsky, A. (2018). "I believe in that movement and I believe in that chant": The influence of Black Lives Matter on resilience and empowerment. *Community Psychology in Global Perspective, 4*(2), 55.

Gomółka, M., & Wszoła, M. (2019, January 29). *Epigenetics-something that is not in the genes we can pass on to our children anyway.* https://fundacjabirn.pl/2019/01/29/epigenetyka/

Grills, C., Aird, E., & Rowe, D. (2016). Breathe, baby, breathe: Clearing the way for the emotional emancipation of Black people. *Cultural Studies ↔ Critical Methodologies, 16*(3), 335–336.

Grossi, E. (2020). New avenues in epigenetic research about race: Online activism around reparations for slavery in the United States. *Social Science Information, 59*(1), 102–103.

Hall, P. (2001). *Categories.* The United States Library of Congress.

Miami, Florida Population 2020. (2020). *World Population Review*. https://worldpopulationreview.com/us-cities/miami-fl-population

Payne, Y. (2011). Site of resilience: A reconceptualization of resiliency and resilience and street life-oriented Black men. *Journal of Black Psychology, 37*(4), 426–451.

Pierce, C. M., Pierce-Gonzalez, D., & Will. D. (1978). An experiment in racism: TV commercials. In C. M. Pierce (Ed.), *Television and education* (pp. 62–88). SAGE.

Pityana, N. (2005). What is Black consciousness?" In G. H. Muzorewa (Ed.), *Know thyself: Ideologies of Black liberation*. Resource Publications.

Reichbaum, J. (2008, April 7). *Desmond Tutu on ubuntu. Semester at Sea, Spring '07.* [Video] YouTube. https://www.youtube.com/watch?v=ftjdDOfTzbk

Setka, S. (2016). Phantasmic reincarnation: Igbo cosmology in Octavia Butler's *Kindred*. *MELUS: Multi-Ethnic Literature of the United States, 41*(1), 115.

Sowden, S., Koletsi, S., Lymberopoulos, E., Militaru, E., Catmur, C., & Bird, G. (2018). Quantifying compliance and acceptance through public and private social conformity. *Consciousness and Cognition, 65*, 359.

The Spiritual Project at the University of Denver. (2011, April 20). African tradition, proverbs, and Sankofa. https://web.archive.org/web/20110420131901/http:/ctl.du.edu/spirituals/literature/sankofa.cfm

Sue, D. W., Sue, D., Neville, H. A., & Smith, L. (2019). *Counseling the culturally diverse: theory and practice.* John Wiley & Sons.

Tang, S., McLoyd, V., & Hallman, S. (2015). Racial socialization, racial identity, and academic attitudes among African American adolescents: Examining the moderating influence of parent-adolescent communication. *Journal of Youth and Adolescence, 45*(6), 1141–1155

Toth, M. (2015). Mechanisms of non-genetic inheritance and psychiatric disorders. *Neuropsychology, 40*(1), 130.

Van Wormer, K., SudduthC., & Jackson, D. (2011). What we can learn of resilience from older African-American women: Interviews with women who worked as maids in the deep south. *Journal of Human Behavior in the Social Environment, 21*(4), 410.

Weston, Florida Population 2020. (2020). *World Population Review.* https://worldpopulationreview.com/us-cities/weston-fl-population

CHAPTER 12

RACISM, THE REAL CAUSE OF THE RACIAL INEQUITY OF CORONAVIRUS

Roni Bennett

Racism in the United States is a preexisting condition. It is embedded in all aspects of American culture and, more importantly, the country's socioeconomic system. It is primarily responsible for the uneven distribution of the nation's wealth, which grossly favors White people. Moreover, racism is also responsible for the uneven distribution of pain that is overwhelmingly inflicted on the nation's minority families. Therefore, as COVID-19 cuts a disturbingly unequal path across America, it should surprise no one who the disease is disproportionately killing: Black, Latinx, and Native Americans. People of color are dying at more than twice the rate of White people, according to Centers for Disease Control and Prevention (2020) data. The tremendous disparity in the death and hospitalization rates between Whites and people of color is striking. Although the infection data are less reliable than the data on mortality, the data show a disturbing disparity in infection rates even in this area.

The key reason for the disparities in COVID-19 infections and deaths is not biological but rather the result of racism. Systemic racism has a long history in the United States. It is deep-rooted, well-protected, and

Coronavirus and Vulnerable People: Addressing the Divide in Harm and Responses and Exploring Implications for a More Peaceful World, pp. 211–217

pervasive. At this very moment, White Americans are pretending to be searching for the underlying reasons for these disparities. Others argue that the disparities are caused by the infected people's lifestyles or choices. They assert that there could be no other explanation. Many of these people also contend that if George Floyd had not resisted arrest or held his neck in a different position, he would have prevented his death. As is obvious, they blame the victims.

Suppose we stop pretending to be searching for the true causes of the disparities in COVID-19's impact on people of color, as well as cease offering false explanations. In that case, we could focus on the key drivers for these disparities. People of color, as well as White people who seriously consider the racial disparities that exist in the United States, are not hard-pressed to identify the causes on which to focus.

First, one should focus on the disparities in exposure to the virus by people of color and White people. We should identify the underlying reasons for the varying risk of exposure. Second, we must investigate the healthcare and hospitalization experiences of the different groups, seeking to understand why they differ. And lastly, we need to investigate the reasons why Whites infected with the disease experience a better outcome than infected people of color, who are more likely to have a poor outcome or die.

PEOPLE OF COLOR ARE MORE EXPOSED AND LESS PROTECTED FROM THE CORONAVIRUS

People of color are infected with the coronavirus at much greater rates than White people simply because they are more exposed to the virus. People of color are overrepresented among frontline workers in the United States (Rho et al., 2020). These workers include low-level hospital and nursing home staff, grocery store workers, restaurant delivery workers, meat packers, public transportation workers, postal workers, warehouse workers, and construction workers. Many laborers are in contact with the public daily and can easily be infected by members of the public who are carrying the disease. Adding to their public exposure risk, frontline workers sometimes work in close quarters and cannot socially distance themselves. Many frontline workers are underpaid and unappreciated. Most occupy their current positions because of a lower education level and fewer other professional options. This is a result of their segregated living environments with poorly performing schools. These living conditions are driven by racism as well as a strong corporate desire to exploit workers to maximize profits.

When the coronavirus arrived in the U.S. last spring, frontline workers did not have the choice of sheltering in place as other (often White) Americans did. Their job positions were labeled essential, and thus they had to report to their jobs. Many essential workers commute to their workplace on public transportation in urban areas, such as frequently crowded buses or trains. Their commutes put them in an ideal environment where the virus can thrive. Crowded transportation environments that offer no protection from strangers who could be infected are likely to lead to elevated infection rates. Even if workers learn to protect themselves during the commute, exposure does not markedly improve while on the job. This is especially dangerous for nursing homes and hospital workers. Most people who are severely ill with COVID-19 are either in nursing homes or hospitals. This is the environment that essential health care workers must face every day. While personal protection equipment (PPE) helps protect healthcare workers on their jobs, low-level, frontline positions (i.e., nurse assistants) do not always access the proper PPE. Furthermore, lower-level health workers are seldom in jobs with paid sick time and access to excellent health care. This lack of protection and limited access to proper health care is demonstrated by a recent health-care work experience cited below.

This is the narration of the personal experience of a colleague in our organization. The story details the experience of a health care worker at a nursing home in South Florida. Our colleague's mother was a resident of a nursing home in the community. While at the nursing home last April, she was diagnosed with COVID-19. She was subsequently admitted to a nearby hospital and died of the disease two weeks following the diagnosis. The certified nursing assistant (CNA) who cared for our colleague's mother was very attentive. For example, after he had completed his daily work, he would arrange facetime calls with his patients and families. As a result, he was close to his patients' family members.

Following her mother's death, our colleague contacted the CNA to inquire about his health. To her surprise, the worker was not informed that his patient had died from COVID-19. Upon learning this information, he asked the nursing home to provide him the opportunity to be tested for COVID-19. The management refused to approve the test. He then decided that the risks were too high; the chance of not knowing if he was infected was too dangerous. He decided to get the test at his own expense. However, he was denied time off to get his test administered. He risked his employment, took time off, and completed the test. On the day he was tested, his office told him to promptly return to the job to care for other patients who needed his attention. He had not yet received his test results. However, he was instructed to return to his job to care for other patients regardless.

As is evident from this account, the CNA was put at risk, and he possibly risked infecting other patients and coworkers as well. This is not an unusual experience. In fact, shortly after the World Health Organization declared the Coronavirus a pandemic, it was ordinary to see frontline workers interacting with the public and wearing no protection. There were no masks or gloves provided. Further, no glass enclosure separated customers from workers where possible. Actually, many types of unprotected encounters between workers and customers were commonplace. These unprotected interactions have been reduced recently, but many frontline workers were put at unacceptable risk levels in the pandemic's early days.

WITH LESS ACCESS TO HEALTH CARE, PEOPLE OF COLOR ARE MORE VULNERABLE TO COVID-19

People of color cannot access quality health care at the levels of White Americans. Moreover, access to quality health care is a crucial determinant of the outcome a person with COVID-19 will experience. For someone infected with the coronavirus, the success of fighting it depends on several factors. Among the important factors are age, gender, underlying conditions, early detection, prompt and effective treatment, and quality medical care.

Although age and gender contribute to a severe outcome from Covid-19, these risk factors are not impacted by racism. However, underlying conditions are most definitely a direct result of racism. People of color are far more likely to have underlying chronic conditions, which greatly increase the risk of a severe outcome for those with COVID-19. People of color have higher incidence of diabetes and hypertension than White people (Rodriguez, 2020). These two underlying conditions are high on the list of risk factors that lead to the poor outcome or death of COVID-19 patients. There are no biological reasons for these conditions to be prevalent in people of color. The high presence of these conditions stems from racism. People of color live in predominantly unhealthy communities with poor food choices, referred to as "food deserts." These communities have polluted air, toxic dumps, very few health care facilities, insufficient corporate investment, and many other disadvantages of a disempowered residential environment (Frederick, 2018). These living conditions, along with restrictions on their ability to monitor their health, are the causes of these chronic conditions. All are driven by racism.

When a person of color contracts COVID-19, the health care options available to him or her are less than those offered to a White person. It is harder for people of color to get tested from the start because most test sites are located in White neighborhoods. Further, many are organized as drive-through testing sites. People of color do not have access to test sites in White neighborhoods for obvious reasons. They do not always have cars, and they certainly do not have the time to sit in long lines of cars in neighborhoods far from their homes. The fact that people of color have limited access to testing for COVID-19 is certainly driven by the continued racist segregation of most neighborhoods in America. It is related as well to the uneven allocation of public health resources in favor of White neighborhoods.

When a person of color becomes ill with COVID-19, an entire spectrum of obstacles must be overcome to ensure successful recovery from the disease. First, numerous documented cases exist where a person of color was sent home from the hospital even though she has several symptoms and is a member of an at-risk class. Often, people who have experienced this kind of racism ultimately die at home from the disease. For example, the case below was widely reported on by the local news in South Florida and confirmed by the hospitals involved.

A 70-year-old grandmother in South Florida recently died from COVID-19 after being turned away by two hospitals. This grandmother, who suffers from diabetes and hypertension, went to a local hospital, and was turned away. After continuing to feel ill with a fever, she went to a second hospital. There she was admitted and initially treated. Despite her age and medical condition, she did not have medical coverage. Although quite ill, she was discharged by a doctor around 4 a.m. local time. Due to a lack of public transportation, she waited on a bench outside the hospital until 6 a.m. Her family was not notified that she was discharged. Days after returning home, she experienced nausea and struggled to breathe. She died shortly after at home.

The hospital issued a statement asserting that they never turn away patients. However, they would not discuss the details of this particular case. As a Hispanic person without medical insurance in South Florida, it should be expected that she would be discharged early regardless of her condition.

PEOPLE OF COLOR WITH COVID-19 RECEIVE A LOWER STANDARD OF TREATMENT THAN WHITE AMERICANS

People of color receive less than optimal care from the existing health care system in the United States. Most observers do not believe this statement to be true, however. It is generally believed that Americans can choose to live where they would like, and health care resources are distributed in a fairly equitable manner. This is far from the reality we face in most disadvantaged neighborhoods. Rural health care facilities are often less well-equipped and staffed. This is primarily because these hospitals must cover a large geographic area with a limited population. Local demographics greatly impact the kind of services rural health care facilities can provide. Thus, the quality of health care provided in rural communities is often not shaped by racism but location.

Urban and suburban hospitals have the advantage of large population bases and condensed coverage areas. Some facilities are well-equipped and staffed by outstanding health care professionals. These hospitals offer excellent services even though it is at a higher cost. These facilities are located in chiefly White neighborhoods and serve White residents. People of color live in segregated neighborhoods away from the best facilities; a few privately-run hospitals serve them, if any exist at all in their communities. However, mainly due to costs and accessibility, minorities are forced to use publicly run hospitals in their city or county. Many publicly run hospitals have good equipment and skilled staff. Unfortunately, these facilities are often overcrowded and lack adequate equipment and staff to operate effectively. Publicly run facilities strive to provide excellent service; however, these facilities must serve all who enter regardless of means.

Particularly at this time, with the pandemic rapidly expanding throughout the United States, many COVID-19 patients are admitted to hospitals that are stretched to the limit. Providing all patients with the highest quality care may be a goal that is not attainable at this time. As a result, minority COVID-19 entering overcrowded hospitals in disadvantaged neighborhoods cannot expect optimum care.

Added to the current risk of inferior care resulting from overcrowding, minorities face additional risks due to the implicit bias built into the training received by American medical students. Numerous studies have shown that even when corrected for differences in insurance status, income, age, and severity of condition, racial and ethnic minorities receive a lower quality of care from their physicians than the care given to White people (Bridges, 2020). Lower-quality healthcare means minorities are less likely than Whites to be given appropriate cardiac care, receive kidney dialysis, receive the best treatments for cancer or stroke, and receive organ transplants.

Another factor that leads to lower-quality care for minorities with COVID-19 is the higher concentration of underlying conditions (such as diabetes and hypertension) among this population. In many hospitals, decisions regarding which patients get access to the available health care resources are based on the expectation of patient survival. Even though health care organizations try to conceal this decision-making process, the underlying selection procedures are quite obvious. Therefore, due to a higher occurrence of underlying conditions, People of color will receive lower-quality care and, in these cases, will experience higher mortality rates.

CONCLUSION

As a society, the United States systemically devalues its non-White citizens. The narrative that we are a society of immigrants and that we believe all men are equal is far from the reality that people of color experience in this country. Ronald Reagan's vision of America as "The Shining City upon a hill," God-blessed and teeming with people of all kinds living in harmony and peace, is dramatically different from America today. COVID-19 has illuminated this fact. The pandemic shines a light on some fundamental facts. America consists of two separate societies, one White and the other non-White. These societies are not living in harmony; instead, there are moving apart. The pandemic vividly shows that non-Whites are devalued, oppressed, humiliated, and forgotten on every level. Minorities have little chance of closing the disparities that separated the society, and White people will do nothing to help close this gap.

As the coronavirus's presence continues to illuminate the uneven treatment of minorities in the United States, it has also forced many citizens to ask, "who are we as a society?" Although sparked by police brutality, the recent demonstrations in all 50 states are also being fueled by this nationwide self-examination. As is often the case, whenever a group of people is undervalued, abused, and their future seems ominous, hope must be embraced. Embracing hope has supported indigenous people through the attempted genocide, immigrants through the current atrocities being inflected by the Trump administration, and African Americans through slavery, Jim Crow Laws, and mass incarceration.

REFERENCES

Bridges, K. (2020). Implicit bias and racial disparities in health care. *Human Rights Magazine, 43*(3). https://www.americanbar.org/groups/crsj/publications/human_rights_magazine_home/the-state-of-healthcare-in-the-united-states/racial-disparities-in-health-care/

Centers for Disease Control and Prevention. (2020, December 10). *Disparities in deaths from COVID-19.* https://www.cdc.gov/coronavirus/2019-ncov/community/health-equity/racial-ethnic-disparities/disparities-deaths.html

Frederick, R. (2018, May 10). *The environment that racism built.* Center for American Progress. https://www.americanprogress.org/article/environment-racism-built/

Rho, H., Brown, H., & Fremstad, S. (2020, April 7). A basic demographic profile of workers ion frontline industries. *CEPR.* https://cepr.net/a-basic-demographic-profile-of-workers-in-frontline-industries/

Rodriquez, C. (2016, September 14). *Hypertension and hypertension-related disparities in underrepresented minorities.* https://www.intechopen.com/chapters/51907

CHAPTER 13

COVID-19, COLONIALISM, AND INDIGENOUS PEOPLE

Laura L. Finley

Already marginalized, indigenous peoples faced unique challenges from COVID-19. Access to healthcare was already limited, and indigenous peoples suffer higher rates of other diseases that made them more vulnerable to the pandemic. Some very isolated groups that have historically had little interaction with outsiders have poorly developed immunity to infectious diseases. Yet outsiders are increasingly entering these areas, such as in Brazil, where illegal logging and mining threatens not just the land but dramatically increased the risk for indigenous peoples. Some experts warned that "ethnocide" is likely (Marx, 2020). Poor sanitation, limited provisions of other necessary items like soap, disinfectant, and even clean water, inadequately staffed medical facilities, combined with existing poverty, large multigenerational families living together, unemployment, and reduced chances to retain work at home exacerbated the problems for indigenous peoples around the globe. This is all on top of tremendous discrimination, all of which are legacies of colonialism. Testing for COVID-19 was not widespread in areas where indigenous peoples live, nor was educational material about infectious diseases or protective materials like masks and gloves. Food insecurity, an existing problem, has

Coronavirus and Vulnerable People: Addressing the Divide in Harm and Responses and Exploring Implications for a More Peaceful World, pp. 219–230

worsened for indigenous peoples during the pandemic (United Nations, 2020). Indigenous women suffer higher domestic and sexual violence rates, both of which have been shown to increase during this type of crisis. The coronavirus is no exception, with rates of abuse and assault increasing yet reductions in services as shelters and other organizations had to enact social distancing requirements and people were less inclined to donate to these services. Access to help services was already sparse and jurisdictional issues on native lands has always meant police responses are slow if not existent. This has not improved during the pandemic.

This chapter will explore these issues in greater depth, showing how and why COVID-19 is disproportionately killing indigenous people and how stay at home orders and other responses are differently experienced. It will conclude with recommendations for the future. The focus is on the United States, but some outside examples will show similar things happening to indigenous people globally.

INTRODUCTION

Access to healthcare on reservations is limited, and indigenous peoples suffer higher rates of other diseases that make them more vulnerable to the pandemic. According to the U.S. Census Bureau (2017), 19.2% of single-race American Indian and Alaska Native people lacked health insurance coverage in 2016, compared to 8.6% for the United States The Indian Health Service, or IHS, is responsible for providing medical and other health-related services to enrolled Native American tribal members. But the money allocated to the IHS is insufficient for the size of the population it serves. Further, because so many Native Americans struggle with obesity, diabetes, asthma, and heart disease, healthcare systems on reservation lands are already taxed. These are some of the conditions that make one more susceptible to getting coronavirus and for having a more severe case (Morales, 2020).

Further, since reservations are often so large, hospitals and other resources are spread out, making it harder to get care. Navajo with the virus, which they call Dikos Ntsaaígíí, sometimes had to be flown to Albuquerque, Flagstaff, and Phoenix because there are only a dozen hospitals and part-time clinics on their land (Jones, 2020). This is not only very costly but also takes more time, an expense that can be deadly (Morales, 2020).

The federal government is involved in Native healthcare due to treaties negotiated with nations, although these have never been followed as they should have been. In exchange for their land, the federal government is supposed to treat Native Nations as "domestic" and "dependent," meaning they are sovereign, yet the government also has a duty of care. The Indian Health Service is one piece of that duty, and according to Nations like the Navajo, it has been failing to meet its obligations from the beginning. The IHS serves 2.6 million people who are members of the 573 federally recognized American Indian and Alaska Native tribes. Before the global pandemic, the federal government spent $2,834 per person on Indian country health care. In contrast, it spends $9,404 on veteran health and $12,744 on Medicare.

The Navajo filed a suit against the IHS, arguing that the $2 trillion Coronavirus Aid, Relief, and Economic Security Act (CARES Act), which included $8 billion to help tribes fight the coronavirus, was not ample. The Navajo Nation and 10 other tribes are involved in the suit. Next to New York and New Jersey, the Navajo, whose land is approximately the size of West Virginia, had the third-highest coronavirus infection rate in April 2020. Just 4.6% of Arizona's population, Native Americans constituted 16% of that state's coronavirus deaths at that time (Native American tribes reject coronavirus checkpoint threat, 2020). By May 18, 2020, the Navajo had surpassed New York to have the highest infection rate in the United States (Silverman et al., 2020). The suit alleges that CARES monies were going to for-profit companies rather than to Nations, and in late April, a federal judge halted the Trump administration's moves to do that (Jones, 2020). Jonathan Nez, President of the Navajo Nation, said, "We are United States citizens, but we're not treated like that. You can hear the frustration, the tone of my voice. We once again have been forgotten by our government" (Morales 2020). Jones (2020) also attributes part of the problem of the spread of COVID-19 among Native people to "centuries of broken promises." "Structural inequalities born out of the U.S. government's treaty-violating, trust-abrogating policy decisions have caused the disproportionate COVID-19 crisis in Indian Country today" (Doshir et al., 2020). For their part, the Navajo issued some of the strictest stay-at-home orders, requiring that residents not leave home unless of emergency or if they are essential workers. Even then, they required documentation on company letterhead (Silverman et al., 2020). With little help from state governments or the federal government, leaders on reservations took matters into their own hands in order to curtail the spread of the deadly pandemic.

Since the Navajo, like other Nations, are sovereign, they can negotiate on their own for equipment and supplies but still had to compete for the limited testing, protective equipment, and ventilators needed to stop the spread of the virus and help those who were sick (Sepkowitz, 2020). Native access to healthcare is unacceptably limited, and the fault lies with the U.S. government, which continues to fail its treaty obligation to provide healthcare to Native peoples. "The conditions that are killing Native Americans now have existed for a long time, and have been unacceptable for a long time," said Shannon Keller O'Loughlin, a citizen of the Choctaw Nation of Oklahoma and executive director and attorney for the Association on American Indian Affairs (Deaderick, 2020).

Centuries of laws and court decisions have created a bureaucratic nightmare for Nations seeking any kind of assistance, so Nations must sometimes apply through state health departments, other times to the federal government, and often through varying agencies (Jones, 2020). The Navajo Area Indian Health Service must care not just for members of the Navajo Nation and San Juan Southern Paitue Tribe but also for Hopis, Zunis, and other tribes in the area. In all, it has 222 hospital beds to serve 244,000 people (Sepkowitz, 2020). When they have asked for help, it has not always been forthcoming or even included what is needed. When the Seattle Indian Health Board asked for coronavirus tests in mid-March 2020, they received body bags three weeks later. While clearly a mistake, it did nothing to help and obviously was macabre. Abigail Echo-Hawk, the health board's chief research officer, said, "This is a metaphor for what's happening," meaning that Native Americans were largely forgotten and left to die (Ortiz, 2020).

That the government has failed to take appropriate measures to halt the spread of coronavirus in Indian country is hardly a surprise to Native peoples. There is a long history of White people purposely spreading diseases to Native populations. Choctaw Shannon Keller O' Loughlin commented, "Time and again in our history, non-natives have spread disease among native populations, sometimes deliberately. Now, the administration continues that history by failing to consult with tribal nations, removing us from decision making on matters that affect our nations and peoples" (Deaderick, 2020). Some 90% of Native Americans were wiped out by smallpox, which was said to have arrived in the New World in 1520 on a Spanish ship from Cuba. While Europeans had suffered through bouts of infectious disease outbreaks, they had built up immunities. Native peoples had none. According to the PBS series *Guns, Germs and Steel*, "More victims of colonization were killed by Eurasian germs than by either the gun or the sword, making germs the deadliest agent of conquest" (PBS, 2005). There were also reports that colonists gave Native peoples blankets and linens they knew were contaminated with smallpox, although there is not much clear evidence the tactic was effective (Kiger, 2019).

Deep poverty has contributed to the spread of coronavirus. Due to it, many people living on reservations do not have routine access to clean water for handwashing, regular healthy food, jobs, savings, and other necessities that can help protect from the virus (Morales, 2020). Estimates are that among the Navajo alone, some 15 to 40% of homes lack clean running water (Jones, 2020). According to the U.S. Census Bureau (2017), while the poverty rate in 2016 was 14% nationally, 26.2% of single-race American Indian and Alaska Native people were in poverty. This is the highest of any racial group. Pine Ridge Reservation, home to the Oglala Lakota, a tribe of the Sioux, perpetually contains the counties with the highest poverty rates. Unemployment rates are 80 to 90%, and there are virtually no jobs. The reservation lacks critical infrastructure, and many children attend school only minimally or not at all. The reservation covers more than 2.8 million acres and has few medical facilities. Alcoholism rates are high, and a quarter of children are born with fetal alcohol syndrome. Life expectancy before the epidemic was 48 for men and 52 for women. Rates of tuberculosis and diabetes are eight times higher than the national average; diabetes is associated with more fatal coronavirus cases (Strickland, 2016).

Native and indigenous women suffered from disproportionately high rates of domestic and sexual violence before the global pandemic. One study found that more than half of American Indian or Pacific Islander women had experienced sexual violence in their lifetime. The same is true of domestic violence. These women are 1.7 times more likely to have experienced violence in the last year than White women and two times as likely to have been raped in their lifetime. Ninety-six percent of the perpetrators are nonnatives, which means that tribal justice systems are not allowed to address the issue due to previous court cases and laws that infringe on tribal sovereignty (National Congress of American Indians, 2018). These problems were exacerbated during stay-at-home orders. One survey of 250 indigenous women in Canada found that one fifth of respondents had reported experiencing physical or psychological violence in the past three months. Shelters are not a viable option now, as people are on order to stay home, in this case, often with their abusers. And, while the Canadian government committed $30 million in funding to Women and Gender Equality Canada for shelters and sexual assault centers and another $10 million to Indigenous Services Canada's network of 46 emergency shelters on reserve and in Yukon, many of these are not run by or for indigenous women so they will not seek help from them. Michelle Audette, who has worked on a national plan of action, ties the issue to colonialism. "Because we are facing the impact of colonialism, we are not a top priority, and we can see it with COVID right now" (Wright, 2020). Prior research has shown spikes in domestic and sexual violence during crises; for instance, there was a 35% increase in women reporting psychological violence during and immediately after Hurricane Katrina and an increase of 98% of those reporting physical abuse. U.N. Secretary-General Antonio Guterres said on April 6, 2020, that some countries have seen domestic abuse rates doubled. Even things like requirements to wear masks can trigger historical trauma related to colonialism (Hilleary, 2020).

Involvement with criminal justice is a risk factor for contracting COVID-19 that also affected Native peoples. Native Americans are four times more likely to be sent to prison than White Americans (The Sentencing Project,

2016). An April 29, 2020, report showed that more than 70% of tested inmates in federal prisons tested positive for COVID-19. Even still, prisons lacked ample tests to assess the situation or appropriate procedures to quarantine those infected (Balsamo, 2020). The cases of Andrea Circle Bear and Valentina Blackhorse are illustrative. Circle Bear was incarcerated for a nonviolent drug offense when she caught the coronavirus. Pregnant at the time, she was placed on a ventilator the day before her cesarean section. She died four weeks later, never having met her daughter. Circle Bear was just 30. Blackhorse, 28, died after contracting the virus from her partner, who worked at a detention center for the Navajo Department of Corrections (Jones, 2020).

One recommended method for curtailing the spread of COVID-19 is contact tracing, which involves following who an infected individual was in contact with to see patterns and quarantine or assist sick individuals earlier. Yet, contact tracing has been much more challenging on reservation lands. For instance, the Navajo employed 80 contact tracers during the worst phase of the pandemic, but many of their people do not have phones to make contact simple. To physically track down individuals is far more laborious and takes more time (Morales, 2020).

Stay at home orders were difficult for many but particularly so for Native Americans. As was noted, many lack clean water, electricity and live in homes full of black mold. Approximately one-quarter of Native Americans and Pacific Islanders were already food insecure, defined as not having regular, reliable access to the foods needed for good health. Not being able to go to get groceries, or doing so at huge risk, only exacerbated the problem of food insecurity. For instance, the Navajo have few grocery stores and markets, so more people had to crowd into those that were operating (Silverman et al., 2020).

Many Native peoples live in overcrowded homes, which made social distancing difficult. Federal funding for housing in Indian Country, part of the government's duty of care, has been blocked for decades (Jones, 2020). The Navajo tried to social distance by issuing strict curfew orders that result in arrest if violated. Other Nations set up physical roadblocks to keep away outsiders, measures taken mainly because the federal government's assistance was too limited, so more restrictive efforts were needed (CBS News, 2020). In South Dakota, Republican Governor Kristi Noem ordered the Ogala Sioux and Cheyenne River Sioux to remove those roadblocks that fall on state and federal highways and threatened a lawsuit if they did not comply. Not only did Noem's order violate tribal sovereignty, but it also violated existing agreements between the state and the Sioux governments. Harold Frazier, chairman of the Cheyenne River Sioux, responded:

> we will not apologize for being an island of safety in a sea of uncertainty and death.... You continuing to interfere in our efforts to do what science and facts dictate seriously undermine our ability to protect everyone on the reservation.

Oglala Sioux President Julian Bear Runner agreed, announcing:

> we have an inherent and sovereign right to protect our people's health, and no one, man or woman, can dispute that right. Your threats of legal action are not helpful and do not intimidate us. The only way we can get through this is to work together as a nation. (Native American tribes reject coronavirus checkpoint threat, 2020)

Outside of the United States, some very isolated groups that have little interaction with outsiders have poorly developed immunity to infectious diseases. Yet outsiders are increasingly entering these areas, such as in Brazil, where illegal logging and mining threatens not just the land but dramatically increases the risk for indigenous peoples. Some experts say "ethnocide" is likely (Marx, 2020). In the United States, the concern is that the deaths of elders will result in a loss of culture, as it is, they that teach youth the language and customs of their people. Already the smallest racial minority in the United States, as Moya-Smith (2020) put it, "when we lose an elder, we've truly been robbed of more than just a person—we've lost centuries of pre-white invasion knowledge and narrative." Nations tried to limit outsiders' access in order to curtail the spread of the disease, but that meant many people could not communicate with loved ones at all, as they lacked phones or electricity to use other means such as Facebook chats or Zoom meetings. Those that had phones were reported to be saving their battery power in case of emergency, something most white people did not have to do (Moya-Smith, 2020).

At the same time, tribal customs resulted in increased danger as well. In New Mexico, Governor Val Panteah exempted religious gatherings from stay-at-home orders. Zuni Pueblo, both the Zia and the San Felipe, contracted cases of COVID-19 at high rates in part because many participated in large group religious ceremonies. Panteah says that the state tried to test those who have done so, but limited tests made that a challenge. The virus even hit the top two officials of the Zia (Agoyo, 2020). While the choices to gather for religious services can be criticized, the history of repressing Native spiritual customs hits particularly hard for these communities. In the 1800s, the federal government adopted a Code of Indian Offenses that prohibited Native American religions and punished those practices. Punishment ran the gamut from whippings to imprisonment to withholding of rations. At the same time, Congress funded the creation of the Indian boarding school system, and Native children were ripped from their homes and forced to attend Christian church services. They were strictly punished if they were found practicing their Native religion. There have been several Supreme Court cases about Natives' rights to practice their religion. None have won, even though in 1978, the U.S. passed the American Indian Religious Freedom Restoration Act (AIRFA), which states that:

> it shall be the policy of the United States to protect and preserve for American Indians their inherent right of freedom to believe, express, and exercise the traditional religions of the American Indian, Eskimo, Aleut, and Native Hawaiians, including but not limited to access to sites, use and possession of sacred objects, and the freedom to worship through ceremonials and traditional rites. (Tatum, 2018)

On the 50th anniversary of the passage of AIRFA, Kenny Frost, Sundance Chief for the Utes, commented, "We risk losing the knowledge of traditional places as those people with traditional knowledge leaves this world. We must continue to strive to pass this knowledge on to future generations." The same is true as Native peoples cannot practice their religions due to the global pandemic (Zotigh, 2018).

Voting on Native land has always been difficult:

> The United States has a long history of suppressing the voting rights of Native Americans. Despite being indigenous to the land, they were not considered citizens for centuries and thus were not afforded the right to vote. During the Reconstruction Era, victims for civil rights and civil liberties, like the Civil Rights Act of 1866, specifically excluded Native Americans. The 14th Amendment also excluded Native Americans since they were not considered citizens at the time of its drafting.

Federal law changed in 1924 but states still tried to block Native voting; for instance, Montana passed a law requiring voters to be taxpayers, and Nations do not collect taxes (Thomas-Lundborg & Alverna, 2020). Other challenges are related to geographic isolation and limited access to postal service and transportation. Many states made it even more difficult in 2018 with strict laws about IDs and addresses. For instance, in North Dakota, a new law required a street address on the ID, but many Native Americans use P.O. boxes. Further, Native Americans are overrepresented in homeless counts, meaning they do not have street addresses (Domonoske, 2018). With a critical election in November 2020, Native people found it especially difficult to get to the polls (Jones, 2020). Nonetheless they did end up voting at record numbers and overwhelmingly supported Joe Biden.

The economic impact of lost jobs due to the pandemic has hit harder on reservations than many other places. This is partly due to high unemployment rates that preexisted the virus as well as the fact that most jobs in Indian countries are low wage. Further, those that did have decent jobs with casinos, for instance, suffered since all casinos were closed (CBS News, 2020). Joseph Kalt, codirector of the Harvard Project on American Indian Economic Development at the Kennedy School's Ash Center for Democratic Governance and Innovation, said in spring 2020:

> There is not a single Indian casino in the United States open today, and all tribal businesses are closed. Native American tribes' tax base have been cut literally to zero, and tribal governments don't have money to run the health clinic or child protection services. While state and local governments are also in trouble, at least they have a tax base, but tribes are struggling because their tax base has been wiped out.

Approximately 40% of the 574 federally recognized Nations operate casinos. The revenue generated at casinos also benefits the local, state, and federal governments. In 2019, $17.7 billion in taxes from casinos went to federal, state, and local governments. Additionally, the casinos and other tribal businesses also employ non-Natives. In 2019, tribal businesses and governments supported 1.1 million jobs, 915,000 held by non-Native Americans (Unsplash, 2020).

CONCLUSION AND RECOMMENDATIONS

> The sad truth is this is not the first time a pandemic has devastated Indian Country. Going back to the earliest days of colonization—and even as recently as the 1918 influenza pandemic, which was four times more lethal within the tribes—Native Americans have borne the worst of this country's diseases. (Jones, 2020)

But many things can be done, both now and in the future. Many organizations collected donations of funds and supplies for Native Nations. We can demand that, for once, the government comes through on its promises to Nations. Although monies were devoted to Nations in the CARES ACT, most had not received anything more than a month after it was passed. Rather than the U.S. government, a group in Ireland raised money to send to the Navajo and Hopi. This is in repayment for when the Choctaw, themselves having suffered from the Trail of Tears and despite deep poverty, sent $170 million to help with the Irish famine in 1847 (Carroll, 2020). While that is a beautiful gesture, it is beyond sad and disappointing that their generosity seems to exceed that of the U.S. Nations also supported each other; for example, the Cherokee Nation sent a large shipment of personal protective equipment to the Navajo Nation, but that does not absolve the federal government from its responsibility. Simply, much more is needed in relief for Indian Country. The government could also simplify how Nations must apply for help and equipment and unblock funding for housing (Jones, 2020). The federal government absolutely must accept Native Nations' sovereignty to take their actions to protect their people and routinely consult with tribal leaders about policy issues (Deaderick, 2020).

Additionally, the U.S. does a terrible job of educating young people about Native Americans. While changing this would do nothing in the short term, including Native American history and current challenges Native peoples face more thoroughly in school curricula in the future can help the next generation seem them not as static peoples but as living humans who have long suffered from government policy. Choctaw Keller O'Loughlin said, "Unless we educate ourselves about our history of colonization at the expense of indigenous peoples, we seem destined to continue the devastation" (Deaderick, 2020). Such education should recognize the tremendous resilience of Native people. O' Loughlin commented:

> We are still here even though we have been through the spread of disease, the removal of our ancestors from the ground, the theft of our cultural and religious objects, the theft of our children, and numerous policies throughout American history designed to dispossess us of our land and diverse cultures. (Deaderick, 2020)

Finally, Native Nations should be applauded for rolling out the COVID vaccines at far better rates than off-reservation, a fact attributed by experts to a thoughtful and centralized approach (Siegler, 2021).

REFERENCES

Agoyo, A. (2020, April 8). At this rate, the entire tribe will be extinct: Zuni Pueblo sees COVID-19 cases double as first death is confirmed. *Indianz*. https://www.indianz.com/News/2020/04/08/at-this-rate-the-entire-tribe-will-be-ex.asp?fbclid=IwAR2stSH-MgV7RuABDQoKl83p-jajNPa6k5y5gushDKqgzP7-PBERb1-8K10

Balsamo, M. (2020, April 29). Over 70 percent of tested inmates in federal prisons have COVID-19. *Associated Press*. https://apnews.com/fb43e3ebc447355a4f71e3563dbdca4f

Carroll, R. (2020, May 9). Irish support for Native American COVID-19 relief highlights historical bond. *The Guardian*. https://www.theguardian.com/us-news/2020/may/09/irish-native-american-coronavirus-historic-bond

CBS News. (2020, April 18). *Longstanding issues put Native American communities at high COVID-19 Risk*. https://www.cbsnews.com/news/coronavirus-pandemic-poverty-overcrowding-native-american-communities-navajo-shoshone-tribes/

Deaderick, L. (2020, May 10). History of inequality making COVID-19 worse for Native Americans. *San Diego Tribune*. https://www.sandiegouniontribune.com/columnists/story/2020-05-10/history-of-inequality-making-covid-19-worse-for-native-americans

Domonoske, C. (2018, October 13). Many Native ID's won't be accepted at North Dakota polling places. *NPR*. https://www.npr.org/2018/10/13/657125819/many-native-ids-wont-be-accepted-at-north-dakota-polling-places

Doshir, S., Jordan, A., Kelly, K., & Solomon, D. (2020, June 18). The COVID-19 response in Indian Country. *American Progress*. https://www.americanprogress.org/issues/green/reports/2020/06/18/486480/covid-19-response-indiancountry/#:~:text=COVID%2D19%20will%20cost%20Indian,relief%20for%20tribal%20economic%20stability.

Hilleary, C. (2020, May 9). COVID spread may put Native Americans at increased risk of violence. *VOA News*. https://www.voanews.com/covid-19-pandemic/covid-spread-may-put-native-americans-increased-risk-violence

Jones, V. (2020, May 6). 10 steps to save Native-Americans from Covid-19 catastrophe. *CNN*. https://www.cnn.com/2020/05/06/opinions/native-americans-covid-19-avoid-catastrophe-jones/index.html

Kiger, P. (2019, November 25). Did colonists give infected blankets to Native Americans as biological warfare? *History*. https://www.history.com/news/colonists-native-americans-smallpox-blankets

Marx, W. (2020, April 22). Isolated indigenous tribes risk extinction from coronavirus, experts say. *NBC News*. https://www.nbcnews.com/news/world/experts-isolated-indigenous-tribes-risk-extinction-virus-n1188586

Morales, L. (2020, April 24). Navajo nation sees high rate of COVID-19, and contact tracing is a challenge. *NPR*. https://www.npr.org/2020/04/24/842945050/navajo-nation-sees-high-rate-of-covid-19-and-contact-tracing-is-a-challenge

Moya-Smith, S. (2020, April 22). Coronavirus takes more than Native Americans' lives. Killing our elderly erases our culture. *NBC News*. https://www.nbcnews.com/think/opinion/coronavirus-takes-more-native-americans-lives-killing-our-elderly-erases-ncna1189761

National Congress of American Indians. (2018, February). Research policy update. *National Congress of American Indians*. http://www.ncai.org/policy-research-center/research-data/prc-publications/VAWA_Data_Brief__FINAL_2_1_2018.pdf

Native American tribes reject coronavirus checkpoint threat. (2020, May 11). *DW*. https://www.dw.com/en/native-american-tribes-reject-coronavirus-checkpoint-threat/a-53393465

Ortiz, E. (2020, May 6). Native American health center asked for COVID-19 supplies. It got body bags instead. *NBC News*. https://www.nbcnews.com/news/us-news/native-american-health-center-asked-covid-19-supplies-they-got-n1200246

PBS. (2005). *Guns, germs & steel*. https://www.pbs.org/gunsgermssteel/index.html

Sepkowitz, K. (2020, April 7). The risk to Native Americans from COVID-19. *CNN*. https://www.cnn.com/2020/04/07/opinions/native-american-nations-risk-from-covid-19-sepkowitz/index.html

Siegler, K. (2021, February 19). Why Native Americans are getting COVID-19 vaccines faster. *NPR*. https://www.npr.org/2021/02/19/969046248/why-native-americans-are-getting-the-covid-19-vaccines-faster

Strickland, P. (2016, November 2). Life on the Pine Ridge Native American reservation. *Al Jazeera*. https://www.aljazeera.com/indepth/features/2016/10/life-pine-ridge-native-american-reservation-161031113119935.html

Tatum, M. (2018, February 20). *No religious freedom for traditional Native religions.* Berkley Center for Religion, Peace and World Affairs. https://berkleycenter.georgetown.edu/responses/no-religious-freedom-for-traditional-native-religions

The Sentencing Project. (2016, March 20). *Race and justice news: Native Americans in the justice system.* https://www.sentencingproject.org/news/race-justice-news-native-americans-in-the-justice-system/

Silverman, H., Toropin, K., Sidner, S., & Perrot, L. (2020, May 18). Navajo nation surpasses New York state for the highest COVID-19 infection rate in the U.S. *CNN*. https://www.cnn.com/2020/05/18/us/navajo-nation-infection-rate-trnd/index.html

Thomas-Lundberg, A., & Alvernaz. 2020, L. (2020, March 12). This law makes voting nearly impossible for Native Americans in Montana. *ACLU*. https://www.aclu.org/news/voting-rights/this-law-makes-voting-nearly-impossible-for-native-americans-in-montana/

United Nations. (2020, April 24). COVID-19 and indigenous peoples. https://www.un.org/development/desa/indigenouspeoples/covid-19.html

United States Census Bureau. (2017, October 6). *American Indian and Alaska Native Heritage Month: November 17.* https://www.census.gov/newsroom/facts-for-features/2017/aian-month.html

Unsplash, S. (2020, May 8). For Native Americans, COVID-19 is 'the worst of both worlds at the same time.' *Harvard Gazette*. https://news.harvard.edu/gazette/story/2020/05/the-impact-of-covid-19-on-native-american-communities/

Wright, T. (2020, May 10). Violence against indigenous women during COVID-19 sparks calls for MMIWG plan. *CBC Canada*. https://www.cbc.ca/news/canada/manitoba/violence-against-indigenous-women-action-plan-covid-19-mmiwg-1.5563528

Zotigh, D. (2018, November 30). Native perspectives on the 40th anniversary of the American Indian Religious Freedom Act. *Smithsonian*. https://www.smithsonianmag.com/blogs/national-museum-american-indian/2018/11/30/native-perspectives-american-indian-religious-freedom-act/

CHAPTER 14

THE ASSOCIATION OF BLACK PSYCHOLOGISTS-SOUTH FLORIDA CHAPTER AND COVID-ID

Pamela D. Hall, Conswello Davis, and Jordan M. Pate-Garrett

Studies have shown that the intergenerational transmission of resources is a significant factor explaining wealth differences across racial and ethnic groups (Chiteji & Hamilton, 2002). These wealth disparities contribute to physical and mental health disparities for African Americans. The Association of Black Psychologists was formed in 1968 to nurture African Americans' mental health needs by training young scholars of African descent to facilitate healing in the African American community.

African American psychologists and healers are needed more than ever. COVID-ID (COVID-Identification), as we call it, "identified" and shed light on the fact that African Americans have been diagnosed and died from the virus at disproportionately higher rates in the United States. Systemic racism has left most African Americans overly stressed and anxious about the virus in addition to the daily problems of violence in the home and community, food insecurity, social justice, and housing concerns. African

Coronavirus and Vulnerable People: Addressing the Divide in Harm and Responses and Exploring Implications for a More Peaceful World, pp. 231–242

Americans working on the front lines in grocery stores, hospitals, or food packaging plants are considered essential but are treated as disposable.

To heed this call to address the African American community's needs during this pandemic, The Association of Black Psychologists South Florida (ABPsiSFL) chapter reached out to the local and national community, hosting a series of webinar discussions. These discussions took place primarily during the month of May in 2020. May is Mental Health Awareness Month. This chapter will discuss the purpose of the webinars, the panelists who were involved and the knowledge they brought to the discussions, and the topics covered. Due to social distancing, ABPsiSFL decided to meet our extended family virtually. Mbiti's (1991) quote, "*I am because WE are and, since we are, therefore I am,*" rang true for us during this time of social distancing, as our hearts and souls were hurt witnessing our extended family being impacted by this pandemic. The chapter will discuss the takeaways from the webinars by focusing on the participants' questions and comments posed in the chat room. These questions addressed the African American community's needs during the pandemic and ABPsiSFL's efficacy to provide support, hope, and healing during these challenging times.

The Association of Black Psychologists (ABPsi) was founded in 1968 and is an international organization with chapters throughout the country and members in numerous countries, including the United Kingdom, West Indies, and Ghana, West Africa. ABPsi's mission is the liberation of the African Mind, empowerment of the African character, and enlivenment and illumination of the African Spirit (ABPsi, 2020a). Further, ABPsi promotes African/Black psychology to heal our communities. The purpose of the members is to assist, aid, guide, and facilitate that healing. ABPsi's Call to Action for many of us is something we do, unselfishly, without regrets. In the spirit of *Ujima* (collective work and responsibility), ABPsi, along with its partners, offers various resources (e.g., podcasts, statements, webinars, etc.) to help our communities cope with the pandemic from a culturally affirming standpoint (ABPsi, 2016). ABPSi emphasizes the importance of collectivism and community. We are mothers, brothers, sisters, daughters, fathers, grandmothers, grandfathers, and aunts and uncles. We are concerned about the health and wellness of our community. Empathy is an integral component of our work, and we seek to provide a safe space in order to facilitate healing and growth.

In keeping with the organization's mission, ABPsiSFL connected with communities, built rapport and relationships, and promoted resources for individuals, families, and communities during COVID-ID. We provided a safe space to process and understand, acknowledge, and invest in the freedom of expression. ABPsiSFL sought to positively influence mental health and reduce stigmas as well as share coping and wellness strategies for the

Black community during the pandemic. It was perfect timing to address the people's needs and make an impactful connection with many individuals, as shelter at home orders began in late March and April 2020. By mid-April, the chapter recognized that pandemic was negatively impacting the lives of individuals, families, and communities of African descent. We also knew that May is Mental Health Awareness Month. Developing a series of webinars allowed us to address and discuss how the pandemic was impacting mental health for people in the community. The purpose of the webinars was to engage the community and encourage open discussions around COVID-19 as well as George Floyd. Floyd's tragic death, which happened the first week a webinar was scheduled.

What pushed the organizers of our chapter to develop this webinar series was the pain we saw among our extended family. This pain was obvious when we looked at the news or social media and when we listened to our friends and family members share the stories about police brutality and vigilantism as well as COVID. The tipping point came when the organizers saw a video on social media about a 6-year-old Black girl in the park with her mom. When a police officer approached her to say hi, the little girl began to freak out and hold her hands in the air. The little girl stood behind her mother and began to cry as if she thought she would be attacked or killed by the police officer. Small children should not be living in fear; they should be playing and living in a peaceful, not fearful, society. We watched as Black news reporters were crying on the air and had difficulty reporting other news stories. One of the organizers stated, "I have Black men calling me and asking me what I can do to help them with their fear and anger? Black men rarely ask for such support. We, Black people, are in a state of emergency and quickly becoming numb." ABPsiSFL's Mental Health Awareness Month allowed us to enact the national chapter's mission of empowerment, enlightenment, and addressing our communities' mental health.

The Association of Black Psychologists South Florida Chapter launched a four-week initiative during Mental Health Awareness month entitled "This is For Us" to address issues plaguing our community during the COVID pandemic. COVID-19 has been noted as an allegory for the Black experience in America—a respiratory disease that primarily attacks one's ability to breathe by crippling the lungs and exacerbating health and mental health disparities, resulting in high mortality death rates. In this series, four dynamic topics were addressed (1) Trauma and Social Distance, (2) Wellness in the Time of Social Distance, (3) Helping Our Youth, (4) What Have You Birthed During the Pandemic of 2020? Next Steps. An African-centered perspective was used each week, especially the concept of *Sankofa*—"go back and fetch it"—which stresses the importance of reaching back to knowledge gained in the past and bringing it into the present for positive collective progress.

MENTAL HEALTH AWARENESS MONTH SERIES

The webinars, which were held virtually because of social distancing and sheltering in place orders, were two hours long. Each week there was a panel of psychologists who were members of ABPsiSFL chapters. The panelists shared their perspective on the topic for the week and then had an open dialogue with the participants. Often the participants put their questions into the chatbox. The participants came from all parts of the country and the world. We had participants from North and South America, the Caribbean, Brazil, and Africa by the culminating event.

Week 1—Trauma and Social Distance

During the first week's webinar, professionals and participants discussed the challenges associated with sheltering in place. The panelists all shared the impact this strange new situation was having on their lives and how they found effective coping methods. The participants discussed how being at home forced them to confront and deal with thoughts and emotions they were typically distracted from because their lives were busier. Domestic violence, adverse childhood experiences and community violence were all discussed, and local resources were shared within the course of the discussion.

As the COVID-19 pandemic began, Americans were required to stay home to protect themselves and their communities. The panelists noted that the home might not be safe for many families experiencing domestic violence, including intimate partners and children. Serrata (2019) found that the social factors that put people more at risk for violence have also reduced access to resources, increased stress due to job loss or strained finances, and created disconnection from social support systems. COVID-19 has caused major economic devastation, disconnected many community resources and support systems, and created widespread uncertainty and panic, all factors that affect marginalized communities first. Data within the United States has suggested significant increases in reports of domestic violence cases, particularly among marginalized populations (Bettinger-Lopez & Bro, 2020). Violence in the home results in a cost to society, leading to potentially adverse physical and mental health outcomes, including a higher risk of chronic disease, substance use, depression, post-traumatic stress disorder, and risky sexual behaviors (Breiding et al., 2014).

Takeaways

This first webinar shed light on the rising number of sick people from the pandemic, growing unemployment, increased anxiety around financial stress, and the scarcity of community resources. Many minorities have been isolated in violent homes, without access to resources or friend and family networks. National relation boards have described an "invisible pandemic" of domestic violence during the COVID-19 crisis as a "ticking time bomb" or a "perfect storm" (Bettinger-Lopez & Bro, 2020). This "invisible pandemic" coupled with "invisible" or marginalized people became less of a worry for the macrolevel and more a charge for those working at the microlevel.

ABPsi's South Florida Chapter panelists recognized that the demand for social services and other forms of assistance had increased, especially from people in vulnerable conditions. This led to creating a point of contact for competent and appropriate clinicians of color to engage with the community. The e-mail address of ABPsiSFL was put in the chat box, and the name and number of therapists was provided if any participants felt the need for additional mental health support via teletherapy. Resources were provided for social, health, and legal services such as shelters, food banks, legal aid offices, childcare centers, healthcare facilities, and rape crisis centers. The panelists told the participants to feel free to share the information with any family and friends they felt may need it. In all, the stress of COVID was real and was compounded by the impact that preexisting trauma has on African Americans.

Week 2—Wellness in the Time of Social Distance

In an attempt to cultivate the sense of community, week two acknowledged the importance of wellness during social distance. For Black, Indigenous, and People of Color (BIPOC), health and wellness choices are essential, a matter of life and death. Long-standing health disparities have been on glaring display during the COVID-19 pandemic, a symbol of America's Black experience. The social determinants of health many Black people face, including where we live and work, and the quality of healthcare to which we have access has been unveiled. Recent data showed the rate of death for Black Americans from COVID-19 is 2.4 times higher than White people, and 2.2 times the death rate of Asians and Latinxs (American Psychological Association, 2020). Wellness, what it looked like, and how it can be executed was discussed by panelists and participants. Important concepts included meditation, natural herbs, religion and spirituality, and other related coping strategies for stress.

The infamous phrase "Black don't crack" acknowledges that externally more Melanated individuals tend to age well. But what about internally? Geronimus (1992) proposed the "weathering" hypothesis, positing that Blacks experience early health deterioration because of the cumulative impact of repeated experience with social or economic adversity and other factors contributing to marginalization. There has been substantial evidence of early health deterioration among Blacks, and racial differences in health are evident on all socioeconomic levels.

Takeaways

Both the panelists and the participants shared ideas regarding ways to reduce stress and natural remedies to protect the immune system, such as sunlight for vitamin D, herbology, the use of affirmations, prayer, and meditation. The session ended with a short meditation exercise. We spoke about the word "disease" and how having dis-ease contributes to disease, which can break down the immune system (e.g., dis-ease leads to disease). We stressed how important it was to do all we could to protect our immune systems since we were the ones with higher cases of COVID. In addition to practicing social distance, wearing masks, and sanitizing, we knew that protecting our immune system was vital. One of the affirmations put in the chat for virtual participants to practice was, "I am powerful, I am loving, I am powerful, I am loved, I am powerful, and I love it." A few comments from the participants demonstrated that the weekly webinars were indeed beneficial.

> "This was SO AMAZING!!!!!!!!!:
>
> "We needed this!"
>
> "This was such a powerful meeting. Thank you to the panelists!"
>
> "Awesome vibe/energy..."
>
> "Thank you so much, panelists! This was an excellent discussion."

Week 3—Helping Our Youth

Our youth often have specific outlets and support networks within the Black community, ranging from family members, friends and teammates, coaches, mentors, and occasionally teachers. Week three focused on reaching out to our children and youth in the middle of a pandemic.

We recognized that they might be struggling more because of the loss of social contact with their friends and peer group. We also understood that their coping strategies shifted from face-to-face to virtual. Some would believe that this was the best thing to happen to Generation Z. However, the deprivation of in-person contact within Black communities reduces the amount of support they can receive from their extended network. We had to pay close attention to our young people's needs and discuss ways to ensure that their mental health was not impacted. The panelists explained that national trends showed that rates of youth being diagnosed with anxiety and depression were rising. Thus, it was imperative to make sure our parents were armed with information to help their children or direct them to youth specialists who could help them if they struggled with the sheltering in place order.

Week three discussed grief, absence of imagination, lack of access to quality mental health, and emotional wellness services in predominantly Black areas. During this segment, professionals provided support to both the parent and child, discussing ways to connect and meet each individual where they were in the COVID-19 experience. There was no right or wrong way to experience COVID. What was important was to understand and validate the feelings of young people and to communicate. Communication often just involved listening and not judging them. Families talking to their children about other-race-related issues were now required to add yet another layer of stress to what they must now consider their everyday lives.

This session highlighted how grief could be addressed with Black youth living in higher-risk communities and the benefits of music and art therapy. Parents inquired about how to engage their children now that technology was no longer sufficient, and their children's emotions were becoming unpredictable and complicated. Everyone reacts differently to stressful situations, and people can become more distressed if they see repeated images or hear repeated reports about the pandemic in the media, especially adolescents.

Continuing with the concept of *Sankofa*, parental advice included re-engaging imagination and cultural education, empowering youth through African-centered perspectives, and cultivating the spirit of Ubuntu—believing the common bonds within a group are more important than any other individual arguments and divisions within it.

Takeaways

The panelists and the virtual participants focused on what we could do to save our youth and children. We discussed the importance of reading to our children and reading them stories with Black characters. Book titles were put in the chatbox, and an excellent documentary on colorism called *Dark Girls* (Berry & Duke, 2011) was suggested, which led to a conversation about internalized self-hatred. The webinar also focused on helping our most vulnerable youth, such as those in the criminal justice system and the foster care system. One interesting point made by a panelist who works with youth in the criminal justice system was that youth may be suffering from COVID fatigue. They had attended Zoom meetings for teletherapy and began to ask to speak via the phone because they were tired of the virtual world. This is the exact opposite of what we often think about our youth. Perhaps COVID will allow younger people to begin to appreciate talking and not just texting or even taking a break from social media. Perhaps!

Week 4—What Have You Birthed During the Pandemic of 2020? Next Steps

Birth can be defined as the act or process of bearing or bringing forth. During times of high stress and anxiety, this process may seem unfathomable; however, during the COVID-ID pandemic of 2020, participants and professionals closed out the "This Is for Us" webinar series by introducing new ideas and ventures that are being prepared to launch. Week four's final session allowed individuals to be met with love and support from a community of resources and from people who they did not know at the beginning of this journey. Marginalized people often do not have the luxury of identifying different opportunities that can be cultivated during stressful times due to more pressing survival factors. The pandemic, though exceptionally harmful, allowed for moments of stillness, meditation, and birth.

Takeaways

The last webinar ended with many participants wanting more virtual interactions because a sense of community was formed. Many of the participants attended multiple sessions. There was more interaction and sharing of ideas regarding Black empowerment and the lack of trust regarding the medical profession. Interestingly, the media did not seem to have a pulse on how Blacks feel about doctors and going to the hospital. The media seems to think presents it as though only those on the political right are anti-vaxxers. Yet, they are not the only individuals who do not trust a vaccine. Many Blacks do not believe that scientists or doctors will tell them the truth about the vaccine. There is a great deal of distrust that stemmed from experiences like the Tuskegee experiment and negative encounters with doctors. A discussion ensued around not trusting a vaccine and not wanting to be guinea pigs.

We also talked more about how the Black community needed to start supporting one another and not just focusing on the injustices that were happening, such as the murders of George Floyd, Ahmaud Arbery, and Breanna Taylor. We spent a great deal of time discussing police brutality, but we also noted that we had to begin to empower ourselves, our families, and our communities. That starts with education and empowerment, which is at the heart of ABPsi's national mission. Another surprising takeaway was the development of a book reading list authored by Africans in the diaspora. Panelists and participants put the titles in the chat box, and it was compiled and emailed to all the participants.

Juneteenth as a Culminating Event

At the end of the four-week series, many of the participants asked if we would be doing other webinars in the future. Upon reflection, we knew that Juneteenth was approaching, and it would be a great time to reconvene with the individuals who had attended ABPsiSFL's mental health awareness month webinar series. Since we had participants register via Eventbrite, we had their addresses. As such, we decided to host a Juneteenth event and invited them. For the Juneteenth event, ABPsiSFL had the opportunity to collaborate with another Black cultural organization, the Haitian Mental Health Think Tank. We engaged the communities to discuss the history of Juneteenth, its importance in America, and how it is an African American/Black celebration of freedom from slavery. The collaboration offered individuals from the African diaspora a chance to learn and understand African American culture and history and also to discuss the impact of COVID-19 and racial inequities. The Juneteenth celebration centered on "Blackness" and how we are collectively affected by America's oppression and systemic racism. The most poignant question of asked all the participants was, "when did you realize you were Black?" We used the hashtag #WDYRYWB. We then initiated virtual healing circles with the participants.

The Juneteenth event was compelling and empowering. More than 80 individuals tuned in virtually to celebrate the last state that received freedom from slavery, Texas. Juneteenth is celebrated on June 18 and is considered an African American celebration. There are Blacks from the diaspora living outside the United States, however, who not only were impacted by COVID at higher rates but were experiencing the same trauma and disenfranchisement as African Americas. They expressed feeling a connection with African Americas regarding "Blackness." Participants discussed their experiences being from America and always feeling like they had a knee on their neck. At the same time, Africans from the diaspora such as AfroLatinx participants, Africans, Brazilians, and Blacks from London and Canada shared the differences with being "Black" in their home country versus being "Black" in the United States. We also discussed the division that is often felt with regards to African Americans and Blacks from the diaspora and how we need to heal that divide. After we opened up and shared our thoughts and feelings, we ended the event with a vintage ABPsi effort called a virtual healing circle. The virtual healing circles were used as a method to connect and empower individuals to see one another and come together as a collective.

A resource and tool ABPsi established to promote Africans' healing in America is EECs. ABPsi's campaigns and initiatives encouraged members to integrate EECs into their professional identities upon completing a specific training. EECs is an evidence-informed, psychologically sound, culturally grounded process to help Black people heal from trauma (Community Healing Network, n.d.).

The newest trauma Blacks were experiencing was COVID, along with blatant social and racial injustice. EECs can be utilized in various ways with groups of people via therapy, seminars, and workshops. EECs are safe, flexible gatherings in which we as Black people can share our stories, deepen our understanding of the impact of historical forces and racial trauma on our emotional lives, and learn essential emotional wellness skills to help us be at our best (Community Healing Network, 2014).

ABPsi and made the necessary adjustments due to COVID's limitations on physical meeting, with the EECs becoming virtual healing circles. Sawubona is a term used when we facilitate virtual healing circles. Sawubona means "I/We See You" (ABPsi, 2020b, p. 13). It became a greeting for ABPsi members. These words weigh heavily on many African Americans as they acknowledge, affirm, and confirm their presence and humanity. These words are effective and thought provoking for many individuals. Again, this resource and tool aligned with healing racial trauma along with addressing COVID-ID.

We had two individuals facilitate the virtual healing circles at the end of the Juneteenth event. The healing circles lasted for about 15 minutes and required all the virtual participants to look in another person's eyes and recite empowering mantras. We looked in the eyes of six people as we recited different mantras. When we decided to do this virtually, we were unsure whether it would be as impactful as it is when done in person. However, based on the tears and the emotional reactions of the participants, it worked. We saw and felt one another. And after having such an in-depth discussion around "Blackness," it was great that we could affirm one another through the virtual healing circles.

The "This is for Us" initiative presented Black individuals with space to find community and wellness through a virtual experience: Black and well. According to the American Psychological Association's 2019 Stress in America Report, 63% of people of color say that discrimination has hindered them from having a full and productive life. The South Florida Chapter emphasizes the need for safe spaces for Black people. For most Black people in America, feeling safe, seen, and supported on our wellness journeys is far from the norm. During Mental Health Awareness Month, the Association of Black Psychologists South Florida Chapter asserted that Black people are investing in the practice of wellness on all levels not just because we want to, but because it is necessary. Ending the series with the Juneteenth event left us all feeling empowered. We know that COVID and trauma have not ended. The work of ABPsiSFL has not ended either.

Though several vaccines have been created and administered to the country, many descendants of Africans enslaved in America have not taken them for many reasons that will be discussed in the book's epilogue. So, the work of ABPsiSFL continues. Recently the ABPsi of South Florida Chapter expanded the This is For Us series to focus on Black men of the diaspora. The virtual discussion series specifically focused on Black men during Mental Health Awareness month, May 2021. Due to recent police brutality and COVID-19, we knew our Black men were being retraumatized. ABPsiSFl wanted to ensure we allowed Black men a safe and affirming space where they could freely discuss the toll being Black men in America is having on their lives and family. The goal was also to allow our expert male members of ABPsiSFl to share their feelings and provide strategies to promote wellness while living in a system of oppression. The panelists consisted of a moderator and three male panelists. The topics of discussion were Vulnerability and Masculinity and Coping While Under Scrutiny. This is who we are, and this is the work that the professional Black therapists, counselors, educators, and researchers who are members of the organization see as part of their mission. We believe that we have made headway with the Black community and have seen an upsurge in Blacks contacting us for mental health support.

REFERENCES

American Psychological Association. (2019). *Stress in America, 2019.* https://www.apa.org/news/press/releases/stress/2019/stress-america-2019.pdf

Association of Black Psychologists. (2020a). *About Us.* https://www.abpsi.org/about_mission.html

Association of Black Psychologists. (2020b). *Healing circles leader guidebook.*

Association of Black Psychologists. (2016, July). *Family-care, community-care and selfcare tool kit: Healing in the face of cultural trauma*. https://www.abpsi.org/pdf/FamilyCommunitySelfCareToolKit.pdf

Association of Black Psychologists and Community Healing Network. (2014). *Emotional emancipation initiative*. https://www.abpsi.org/pdf/EmotionalEmancipationInitiative2014.pdf

Berry, D., & Duke, B. (Directors). *Dark girls* [Film]. OWN.

Bettinger-Lopez, C., & Bro, A. (2020, May 13). *A double pandemic: Domestic violence in the age of COVID-19*. Council on Foreign Relations. https://www.cfr.org/in-brief/double-pandemic-domestic-violence-age-covid-19

Breiding, M. J., Chen J., & Black, M. C. (2014). *Intimate partner violence in the United States—2010*. National Center for Injury Prevention and Control, Centers for Disease Control and Prevention.

Chiteji, N., & Hamilton, D. (2002). Family connections and the black-white wealth gap among middle class families. *Review of Black Political Economy*, *30*(1), 9–27.

Community Healing Network. (2014). *Emotional emancipation circles*. https://communityhealingnet.org/emotional-emancipation-circle/

Geronimus, A. T. (1992). The weathering hypothesis and the health of African American women and infants: Evidence and speculations. *Ethnicity & Disease*, *2*(3), 207–221.

Mbiti, J. (1991). *Introduction to African religion*. Gaborone: Heineman.

CHAPTER 15

MIAMI-DADE ECONOMIC ADVISORY TRUST (MDEAT) YOUTH DEVELOPMENT DIVISION

Teen Court and COVID-19

Jordan M. Pate-Garrett

Youth in Miami-Dade County have begun to voice their discontent with the COVID-19 experience. They are understanding that the stay-at-home orders are about more than just social distancing, becoming the new normal. In this chapter, Teen Court participants who have been referred for mental health services share their disgruntlement and discuss how they must now genuinely sit with their emotions and identify root causes. These Teen Court participants are largely minority youth from low socioeconomic conditions. In Miami-Dade County, this includes youth from Miami Gardens, North Miami, Little Haiti, East Cutler Bay, Florida City, and Liberty City. These are areas categorized by dramatic disparities in education, unemployment, market strength and stability, business composition, and more when compared to more affluent areas of the county.

Coronavirus and Vulnerable People: Addressing the Divide in Harm and Responses and Exploring Implications for a More Peaceful World, pp. 243–248

TEEN COURT IN MIAMI-DADE COUNTY

Teen Court is an alternative sanctioning program for first-time misdemeanor youth offenders who agree to allow their peers to determine their sentencing instead of being adjudicated by the juvenile justice system. The program helps decrease juvenile delinquency by interrupting the beginning stages of criminal behavior. In 1980, riots erupted in Miami-Dade County after police officers were acquitted of beating a Black salesperson and former U.S. Marine, Arthur McDuffie. In response to community outrage and protest, the local government took responsibility for the unstable race relations, attributing them to the disparity of socioeconomic conditions affecting Black communities. In 1983, they acknowledged a need to reduce this disparity, and as a result, the Metro Miami Action Plan (MMAP) was designed to address the prosperity imbalance. It was later named the Miami-Dade Economic Advocacy Trust (MDEAT). MDEAT was charged with addressing socioeconomic disparity, home ownership, and juvenile justice within Miami-Dade County in order to ensure Blacks' equitable participation in Miami Dade County's economic growth.

Miami-Dade County Teen Court (MDCTC) was established under MDEAT as a diversion program in which peers sentence youth for minor crimes, offenses, and/or community and school behavior violations. The diversion program is a second-chance initiative intended to offer an alternative to the traditional juvenile justice system and school disciplinary proceedings. Typically, MDCTC offenders are first-time offenders under 18 who have been charged with misdemeanor or status offenses, including theft, vandalism, disorderly conduct, assault, and marijuana possession, and school-related offenses.

As cited by the American Civil Liberties Union (ACLU, n.d.), the school-to-prison pipeline is a disturbing national trend wherein children are funneled out of public schools and into the juvenile and criminal justice systems. Youth from disadvantaged backgrounds are disproportionately incarcerated through this pipeline because of increasingly harsh school policies. Zero-tolerance policies criminalize minor infractions in schools, and students of color tend to be especially vulnerable to discriminatory discipline. MDCTC addresses the imbalance of disciplinary action on minority and at-risk youth, advocating for diversion and community resources. For most students, the pipeline begins with inadequate resources in public schools; overcrowded classrooms, a lack of qualified teachers, and insufficient funding for "extras" such as counselors, special education services, and even textbooks. This locks students into second-rate educational environments (ACLU, n.d.). The ACLU further notes that while many students are propelled down the pipeline from school to jail, it is difficult for them to make the journey in reverse. Students who enter the juvenile justice system typically face barriers when attempting reentry into traditional schools, thus most of these students to never graduate from high school. MDCTC focuses on ensuring that youth offenders successfully complete sanctions resulting in no legal record for the offense and a more optimistic outlook on life. Youth learn to accept responsibility for their actions, learn good citizenship, and receive assistance through community resource referrals. Long-term behavioral changes are promoted, which leads to enhanced public safety. Negative labeling and the risk of recidivism is reduced.

MDCTC offers an avenue for engaging the community in a partnership with the juvenile justice system to respond to the problem of juvenile crime by (1) increasing awareness of the delinquency issues within the local community, (2) mobilizing community members, including youth, to take an active role in addressing the problem of juvenile crime within the community, and (3) creating youth empowerment through job readiness training and job placement opportunities to reduce delinquency and provide crime prevention measures. MDCTC is a problem-solving court within the juvenile justice system where a jury of same-aged peers can sentence teens charged with certain types of offenses. Their purpose is to provide an alternative disposition for juveniles who have committed a delinquent act, have committed a minor offense, have been charged with a misdemeanor, and are otherwise eligible for diversion. Depending on their training, community support, and agreements with traditional court systems, teen courts are recognized as valid legal venues for the process of hearing cases, sentencing, and sentence fulfillment.

COVID-19, YOUTH, AND TRAUMA

Since the inception of COVID-19, the veil has further been lifted on factors affecting minority and at-risk communities and populations, revealing dramatic disparities. The mental health team associated with MDCTC has reported treating individuals experiencing traumatic stress due to complex trauma from adverse childhood experiences and adverse community environments, referred to as a "Pair of ACES" (Ellis & Dietz 2017). With a reported crime rate of 126 per one thousand residents, Florida City has one of America's highest crime rates compared to all communities of all sizes, from the smallest towns to the very largest cities. The National Child Traumatic Stress Network (n.d.) describes complex trauma as both children's exposure to multiple traumatic events—often of an invasive, interpersonal nature—and the wide-ranging, long-term effects of this exposure. The "Pair of ACEs [ACEs] provides context to the aforementioned type of trauma; ACEs include psychological, physical, and sexual forms of abuse as well as household dysfunction such as substance abuse, mental illness, violence, and incarceration" (Campbell et al., 2016). A National Survey of

Children's Health noted that nearly 50% of American children had experienced at least one ACE, with children of color at the highest risk. With the current stay at home orders and other precautions in place, youth are now confined in homes and communities in which these factors are more present and largely unavoidable. The COVID-19 experience has prompted these youth to begin sharing grief and loss experiences, including continued community violence, home and family dynamics, and anxiety that has never been and cannot be adequately expressed with words.

It has been noted that complex trauma can have lasting effects on a child's functioning, emotions, ability to think, learn, and concentrate, impulse control, self-image, and relationships with others. This specific type of trauma is linked to a wide range of problems, including addiction, chronic illness, depression and anxiety, self-harming behaviors, and reactive aggression. Children and families are coping with trauma along with the effects of COVID-19. In and out of Miami-Dade County, youth living in adverse environments are among the most likely citizens to be exposed to trauma and the least likely to receive the services that could prevent the progression of trauma-related emotional and behavioral difficulties. Due to this present and persistent disparity, the MDEAT Youth Development Division offers free mental health services through their Teen Court program.

MENTAL HEALTH AND INTERVENTION

All too often, rather than understanding the behavior of minorities as developmental adaptations to traumatic stressors and circumstances, systems pathologize or criminalize their behavior, labeling them as mentally ill or having a conduct disorder. Common misdiagnoses of trauma-related struggles include attention deficit hyperactivity disorder—a mental health disorder that can cause above-normal levels of hyperactive and impulsive behaviors—or oppositional defiant disorder—a childhood mental health disorder that includes frequent and persistent anger, irritability, arguing, defiance or vindictiveness toward authority figures. As a result of this mislabeling, minority youth are receiving an ineffective intervention or no intervention at all.

Daily diversions of school, extracurricular activities, and alternative support systems previously took the place of intervention; however, they are non-existent with social distancing and stay-at-home orders in place. Providing interventions and appropriate coping strategies has required innovation and nontraditional techniques, especially now through telehealth. During the COVID-19 experience, Teen Court youth have responded to music-feeling associations and individual physical challenges. The utilization of current music influencers has been the most effective when asking youth to identify their feelings during the pandemic—exploring the themes presented in the songs and relating them to adolescent emotions and experience has allowed youth an escape and validation. During the therapeutic process, youth seem to acknowledge better what they are experiencing and express their feelings utilizing lyrics applicable to their lifestyle.

Some rap music highlights specific mental health themes, including depression, anxiety, and post-traumatic stress disorder, Youth with complex trauma and who have experienced adverse events can relate. While some research has been conducted on rap music as a tool to work through mental illness, there is still a gap in the literature. Rap music influences many people and has been used as a story-telling device in popular culture. According to Adam Bradley (2009), while other music genres tell stories as well, rap distinguishes itself by the sheer number of stories it conveys. This story-telling process is an important component of working through mental health issues. Like visiting a therapist, in the process of telling a story one experiences a cathartic sensation that enables the letting go of negative emotions.

Several authors have published about the use of rap and hip-hop in therapy. African American individuals listen to rap music through a cultural lens that allows them to moderate the effects of such lyrics' consumption (Allen, 1993). Elligan (2004) described how he, as a verbal psychotherapist, used rap lyrics to help young clients scrutinize their problematic behavior. According to Elligan, comparing the lyrics of rap to their own lives enabled clients to understand their own pain, provided them with hope for a better future, or made them realize they could alter their behavior. This technique has been effective when working with Teen Court participants referred for services during this pandemic.

In conclusion, this pandemic has created angst, sadness, and many changes. However, I have witnessed a common theme in working with youth. The virtual generation has grown detached from the digital world, complaining about virtual learning, virtual interactions, and virtual media. The lasting change COVID-19 may create for youth could lead to genuine interactions, intentional experiences, and the evolution of the "plugged-in teen."

REFERENCES

American Civil Liberties Union. (n.d). *School-to-prison pipeline.* https://www.aclu.org/issues/juvenile-justice/school-prison-pipeline

Allen, R. L. (1993). Conceptual models of an African American belief system: A program of research. In G. L. Berry & J. K. Asamen (Eds.), *Children & television: Images in a sociocultural world* (pp. 155–176). SAGE.

Bradley, A. (2009). *Book of rhymes: The poetics of hip hop*. Basic Civitas

Campbell, J. A., Walker, R. J., & Egede, L. E. (2016). Associations between adverse childhood experiences, high-risk behaviors, and morbidity in adulthood. *American journal of preventive medicine, 50*(3), 344–352.

Elligan, D. (2004). *Rap therapy: A practical guide for communicating with youth and young adults through rap music*. Kingston.

Ellis, W. R., & Dietz, W. H. (2017). A new framework for addressing adverse childhood and community experiences: The building community resilience model. *Academic Pediatrics, 17*(7), S86–S93.

National Child Traumatic Stress Network. (n.d.). *About child trauma*. https://www.nctsn.org/what-is-child-trauma/about-child-trauma

CHAPTER 16

RECONCEPTUALIZING THE AMERICAN DREAM FOR RACIAL/ETHNIC MINORITIES DURING COVID-19

The Intersection of Health and Mental Health Disparities

Elizabeth F. Louis

INTRODUCTION

O say can you see by the dawn's early light. What so proudly we hailed at the twilight's last gleaming
Whose broad stripes and bright stars through the perilous fight
O'er the ramparts we watched, were so gallantly streaming?
And the rocket's red glare, the bombs bursting in air. Gave proof through the night that our flag was still there
O say does that star-spangled banner yet wave. O'er the land of the free and the home of the brave

—The Star-Spangled Banner
(National Anthem for the United States of America)

Coronavirus and Vulnerable People: Addressing the Divide in Harm and Responses and Exploring Implications for a More Peaceful World, pp. 249–261

Lift ev'ry voice and sing
'Til earth and heaven ring
Ring with the harmonies of Liberty
Let our rejoicing rise. High as the list'ning skies
Let it resound loud as the rolling sea
Sing a song full of the faith that the dark past has taught us
Sing a song full of the hope that the present has brought us
Facing the rising sun of our new day begun
Let us march on 'til victory is won

—Lift Every Voice and Sing
(National Anthem for African Americans)

Suppose one were to ask about the meaning of the national anthem of the United States. In that case, you might get different responses depending on the lived experiences and historical background of each person's descendants. Although it is sung in English, Spanish, and Native American languages such as Lakota and Apache, the national anthem does not capture the essence of the native, enslaved, and immigrated peoples that compose the American population. While the "Star-Spangled Banner" proudly professes the land of the free and the home of the brave, the "Lift Every Voice and Sing" version recounts the historical sacrifices, the intentional marches for freedom, and the continuous pursuit of victory not only for African Americans but also for other racial and ethnic minorities. Below you will find the beginning verses of "America" (My Country, 'Tis of Thee), where freedom is assumed to be an inherent right of Americans, yet this freedom is reserved for those who did not inherit the land of pilgrims' ancestry and who are of Eurocentric lineage.

My country, ' tis of thee,
Sweet land of liberty, of thee I sing;
Land where my fathers died,
Land of the pilgrims' pride,
From every mountainside, let freedom ring!

—America (My Country, 'Tis of Thee)
—Patriotic Song for Americans

The American Dream is one of the pillars of the U.S that has been sought after for generations by diverse groups of people (Musick & Wilson, 1998). Many have voiced their opinions on what exactly is meant by the American Dream. DeSantis provides a critical analysis inclusive of different disciplines, including philosophy, communication, sociology, folklore, and anthropology, to identify eight themes regarding the ideal of the American Dream (DeSantis, 1998). These are the themes of equality, freedom, wealth, democracy, puritan work ethic, religious independence, new beginnings, and consumption and leisure. According to DeSantis (1998), the American Dream is a myth that "posits that with effort, hard work, optimism, and egalitarian cooperation, anyone in America can morally achieve material success and enjoy the freedom, leisure, and religious and social independence that attend wealthy economic status." Yet, this framework assumes that every person has been provided with an even playing field, where hard work is the key variable to elevate oneself socially and economically. The American Dream is the idea that any achievement is possible with hard work and sacrifice, and that anyone is the overseer of their life and directs their path to success. The American Dream has been more attainable for white Americans given their history regarding the genocide of the native people. slavery, and inherited wealth, this country's norms. Generally, this country's history aligns with Eurocentric values. Yet, the pursuit of the American Dream has not stopped the descendants of slavery from believing in Dr. Martin Luther King Jr.'s *I Have a Dream* speech (Illuzi, 2014). Some immigrants crossed borders and seas for a chance at life-changing opportunities. This was seen throughout Barack Obama's campaign strategy in 2008. He strived to share his message of a "more perfect union," acknowledging that the American Dream could only be achieved when race is confronted and addressed (Rowland & Jones, 2018). For the American Dream to be a reality all Americans need to have this type of hope and vision.

THE PURSUIT: AMERICAN DREAM

The sacrifices and victories of racial and ethnic minority communities to attain their version of this dream can be illustrated through changes om policies and laws. Demographic shifts involving minorities serving in various positions of power and other immeasurable contributions to this nation are imprinted in our minds. For example, the Great Migration of 1915–1919 found African Americans leaving the south to find employment and be better able to meet their basic needs. They were fleeing from social and political oppression and wanted to be closer to loved ones who had already migrated north. African Americans embraced their agency to search for dreams this nation had only postulated through broken promises. They decided to leave their families, farms, and towns to get a chance at fulfilling their aspirations in northern cities. Opportunities were portrayed as more attainable and feasible in the north, which shifted the African Americans demographic population for generations. However, this relocation did not prevent African Americans from experiencing discrimination. Further, it illustrated the barriers that exist for Blacks to achieve their dreams.

The U.S. is comprised of different groups that have settled here for a variety of reasons. Crises from Central America have created a humanitarian emergency that has produced unaccompanied minority crossing the borders and caregivers migrating to the U.S for a chance at better life conditions. Presently, policies such as the Development, Relief, and Education for Alien Minors (DREAM) Act and Deferred Action for Childhood Arrivals (DACA) have posed questions about the country's approach to vulnerable populations who are fleeing unsafe environments. The DREAM Act is a "proposed a path that would have granted citizenship to immigrants that illegally crossed the border with their families when they were children," DACA "grants them the possibility to receive renewable two-year work permits to avoid being deported" (Tinoco, 2018). The migratory stories of Latinos and other Caribbean and African immigrants are sacrificial ones where a safe passage to the United States is not guaranteed. Many risks and hardships are encountered along the way. Although that is true, this form of migration violates federal laws. Still, pursing the American Dream fosters hope for migrants and their families who reside within and outside the U.S. and can help break a generation of poverty, reduce the risk of violence, ameliorate unfavorable living conditions, and provide better access to jobs, education, health, and security.

Immigrants to the U.S. come from myriad backgrounds, including Africa. Some Africans come from economically successful premigration status, while some have limited resources and seek asylum (Knight et al., 2015). There was an increase in African immigrants with the introduction of the 1965 Immigration Act, and this group is known to have the highest educational attainment among all other immigrant groups in the United States (U.S. Census Bureau, 2019). For some African immigrants, the American Dream involves economic and educational success, reinforcing the belief in meritocracy, or the "agency of the individual to 'work hard.'" With the American Dream, more opportunities are available; one can exercise freedom of choice and have a fulfilled life that was not afforded to them in their home countries. The strong familial expectations and emphasis on excelling in school are common themes that motivate African immigrants to work harder than their counterparts.

As of July 2019, the U.S. population is over 328,239,523 million people with 60% white, 18.5% Hispanic or Latino, 13.4% Black or African American 5.9% Asian, 2.8% two or more races, 1.3% American Indian and Alaska Native and 0.2% Native Hawaiian and other Pacific Islander. Schaeffer published a study where it was found that the most common age among white Americans was 58, while racial and ethnic groups were much younger, with an average age of 27 (Schaeffer, 2019). For example, the most common age for Hispanics was 11, 27 for Black, 29 for Asians, and for those who identified with two or more races, it was three. This demographic shift is a depiction of the changing representations that exists in the United States. These age differences and the increase in racial and ethnic minorities will inevitably influence the American Dream.

CONTRIBUTIONS TO AMERICA

Historically, the essence of the U.S. is a compilation of contributions and the positionality of Native Americans, immigrants, migrants, and enslaved descendants. These diverse groups have helped make America one of the world's most powerful countries. The innovations, education, sacrifices, spirit, sweat, blood, and tears of those who came before us have shaped America today. For instance, the White House was built by slaves as were other institutions such as Georgetown University. Blacks and African Americans have contributed to agriculture, bringing our cultural and ancestral mechanisms that have supported the farming industry as well as to science, such as African slave Onesimus, who shared his knowledge of the African practice of inoculation that was used with American soldiers during the Revolutionary War. The march from Selma to Montgomery, Alabama that was led by Martin Luther King Jr. was the catalyst for the passing of the Voting Rights Act. America has also been gifted by civil rights activists, writers and poets including Maya Angelou, James Baldwin, Ruby Bridges, Sojourner Truth, and Langston Hughes. They critiqued and challenged the status quo. and were rebellious in speaking their truths to cultivate spaces for racial and ethnic minorities (Guillaume, 2020). With the increase of Black immigrants, making more than 1.3% of the American population, there are more than 2.3 million eligible Black immigrant voters and many hold positions in the healthcare industry like nurses, nursing assistants, and personal care aides, which helps diversify these fields (New American Economy, 2020). Also, Black immigrants contribute to the economy; for instance, in 2018, "Black immigrant households earned $133.6 billion, paid $36.0 billion in taxes ($22.8 billion in federal income tax and $13.2 billion in state and local taxes), and had a spending power of $97.6 billion."

When considering Native Americans, the first people to call the America their home, it is obvious that they provided the foundation for the way of life and natural resources we use today. This includes the fine art of turquoise jewelry, woodcarvings and beadwork, foods we consume such as corn, beans, tomatoes, peppers, melons, their farming methods which helped the European colonizers to survive, their invention of the canoe for transportation and their form of government system that adopted by the American federal system that Benjamin Franklin wanted to form. The usage of language that is widely part of the American culture, such as hurricanes, barbecues, and the naming of cities such as Seattle, Miami,

Milwaukee is all part of U.S heritage; they even developed a form of sign language to communicate between tribes and to facilitate trading. And, as the bearers of their native lands, they helped preexisting navigation of America and informed the colonizers who brazenly stole their land (U.S. Department of Agriculture, n.d.). Similarly, Hispanics have demonstrated their cultural values and traditions in the United States. Whether is it through food that ranges from Mexican and other Latin American cultures, they have influenced the music we listen to and inspired labor leaders and civil rights activists such as Cesar Chavez, who raised national consciousness around labor considerations and advocating for humane work conditions (Liherald, 2018). According to the New American Economy (2020), "almost 12 percent of all Hispanic immigrant workers worked for their own business in 2017, making them 24.5 percent more likely to have their own business than the overall U.S. population" and reinforces their influence in the economy and further exposure to their innovation, ideas, and culture. Also, Hispanic households earn and consume a tremendous amount that includes paying more than $252.2 billion in taxes and spending more than $780.7 billion, which strengthens the U.S. economy.

Furthermore, Asian Americans have been pivotal in the development of America. When it came to birthright citizenship, the 1898 decision by the U.S. Supreme Court was that children born in the U.S. to foreigners were indeed American citizens. This ruling came after Wong Kim Ark's legal battle. He was born to Chinese immigrants in San Francisco and paved the way for others. Similarly, Dr. Tuan Vo-Dinh has helped care. Amanda Nguyen's advocacy as a rape survivor ensured that sexual assault survivors received help. The innovation of e-mail, online portals, and video-sharing has forever changed the internet and digital platforms that are readily used and function in many aspects of American society, such as in business, education, and other sectors (Chan, 2020).

HEALTH AND MENTAL HEALTH DISPARITIES AND COVID-19

Despite the insurmountable contributions these diverse groups have made and continue to make to this nation, they have endured many health scandals, including the unethical Tuskegee syphilis study and the inappropriate use of Henrietta Lacks's DNA. In 1932, the rights of Tuskegee African American sharecroppers were violated by doctors from a U.S. government entity that knowingly withheld information and treatment and allowed their biases and prejudices to be carried out a study on syphilis (Nix, 2019). Years later, the cells of Ms. Lacks, who was being treated for cervical cancer, were part of the first human cells grown in a lab, all without her consent. Ms. Lacks's cells pioneered breakthroughs for vaccines and cancer treatments.

Still, it all came at a cost that violated delivery principles of fundamental medical care and her family was kept out of these healthcare developments (Ritter, 2013). Times have changed to improve ethical practices, but these circumstances illustrate the challenges racial and ethnic minorities face in accessing and receiving quality healthcare. Among them is a lack of trust, given that minorities have been lied to or not fully informed about medical procedures and tests, as these examples illustrate.

With the coronavirus (COVID-19) pandemic, "deep-seated inequities in health care for communities of color" has amplified "social and economic factors that contribute to poor health outcomes" (Substance Abuse and Mental Health Services Administration [SAMHSA], 2020). Longstanding racial disparities have resulted in disproportionate healthcare access and treatment for racial and ethnic minorities. For example, according to the Centers for Disease Control and Prevention (2020), although Blacks make up about 13% of the population in America, they accounted for 30% of COVID-19 cases, and Latinos comprised 17% of COVID-19 cases given their 20% makeup of the U.S. population. According to SAMHSA (2020), People of Color (POC) face increased risk for COVID-19 since they have higher rates of "underlying health conditions, such as diabetes, asthma, hypertension, and obesity compared to Whites. POC are more likely to be "uninsured and to lack a usual source of care, which impedes accessing COVID-19 testing and treatment services." The population of POC is also more likely to work in settings where they do not have the luxury to work from home. They disproportionately work in service-oriented industries such as hospitality, retail, and restaurants, which puts them at risk for their health and their economic stability. Given the context that POC live in, they are more prone to have multigenerational housing structures and home settings where it is difficult to engage in physical distancing or isolation. They are more likely to use public transportation, which furthers their exposure to COVID-19.

The social determinants that are governed by systemic oppression, stereotypes, and racial inequities position POC to be even more vulnerable to contracting COVID-19. Studies have demonstrated how discrimination, which includes racism, can lead to chronic and toxic stress and shapes social and economic factors that put some people from racial and ethnic minority groups at increased risk for COVID-19. These forms of discrimination exist in multiple levels in our society, from the micro to macro layers, including education, housing, healthcare, finance, and the criminal justice system. During this pandemic, there have been futile attempts to improve access and utilization of services to support POC. There are circumstances that place them at a disadvantage when it comes to mode of transportation, the privilege to take time off work, childcare, language, and communication barriers, the gaps in representations of providers who culturally resemble patients, and continuous biases that exist in care systems that are not designed for serving POC with their best interests in mind (American Psychological Association, 2020).

Racial and ethnic minorities have faced insensitive approaches to address their mental health needs before and during the pandemic (Schwartz et al., 2014). The APA estimates that about 18% of U.S. adults are diagnosed with a mental disorder every year, with 43% of people receiving some form of mental health treatment. However, racial and ethnic minorities have a "higher burden of disability resulting from mental disorders." For example, the rates of depression are Whites (34.7%), Blacks (24.6%), and Hispanics (19.6%), In addition to being overrepresented, racial and ethnic groups experience more persistent mental health problems. One may ask why mental health issues are more persistent for racial and ethnic groups. There are myriad reasons, including access and utilization of services. Also, cultural perceptions and stigma, environmental, financial, and social stressors, and the influence of religion and spirituality. In addition, engrained self and communal concepts of wellness, such as the stereotype of being exceedingly strong to buffer underlying pain and suffering, contribute to these problems. Native Americans reportedly have the highest rates of post-traumatic stress disorder and alcohol dependence among all racial and ethnic groups, even though they consist of a small percentage of the American population. Their narratives, historical forms of oppression and being survivors of genocide and other injustices have contributed to their scarred emotional wellness and maladaptive coping techniques. The consequences of past atrocities still leave imprints on the youth and generations to come. Further, although racial and ethnic minority youth may engage in similar misbehavior patterns, they are more likely than White youth to be placed in the "juvenile system than to specialty primary care than White youth" (Underwood & Washington, 2016).

The COVID-19 pandemic has further revealed and exacerbated existing mental health disparities (Yancy, 2020). There already existed a cultural divide in how providers misdiagnosed and underdiagnosed racial and ethnic minorities due to bias, misunderstanding of cultural differences, and lack of sensitivity to recognize culturally based symptoms expressed outside the Western, White conceptions of mental health disorders. Before COVID-19, professionals were already aware of the challenges to access and the mental health burden on ethnic and racial minorities. Yet, during this pandemic, the slow response and sometimes ineffective strategies implemented in mental health services that POC usually utilize, such as outpatient, prescription, and inpatient, were not adapted to consider these existing structures. According to SAMHSA (2020), Asian Americans are less likely to use mental health services than all other racial and ethnic groups. During the pandemic, this group experienced discriminatory slurs (e.g.,

Chinese virus) and prejudices. This could have been an opportune time to learn how to connect more with this community. While Native Americans and people who identify with two or more races are more likely to use outpatient services, including prescriptions, more steps could have been taken to make sure these services remained available, especially with physical distancing and telehealth challenges. Also, when accounting for gender, women in all racial and ethnic groups (except for Native Americans) are more likely to utilize mental health services, given this information, as pillars of many cultures and communities. Specialized and considerate services inclusive of gender could also be garnered to alleviate stress and foster wellness. Additionally, Blacks and Latinos with mental health and substance use disorders are more likely to experience incarceration and homelessness, which increases their risk for COVID-19 due to the limited ability to follow health guidelines in prison or on the streets.

RESILIENCE

One common and interwoven thread among racial and ethnic minorities is their cultural forms of resilience. Despite the challenges that racial and ethnic minorities have faced, their resilience and cultural responses have signified a collective bond to overcome adversity. Racial and ethnic minorities have demanded that the U.S. revisit their risk and protective factors before and during COVID-19 (Villarosa, 2020). America can learn from these diverse groups. Despite all they have overcome and continue to struggle with, their hope in transcending through the American Dream is an enduring spirit.

Studies that have focused on Hispanics/Latinos have found factors that can contribute to resilience, including religious involvement, community networks, and significant relationships with family and friends (Consoli et al., 2013). When facing adversities, some Latinos have implemented a "getting through" mentality to reassure themselves that they will be "better off" after the adversities. Consoli et al. (2013) identified internal mechanisms that supported Latinos in maintaining their resilience, including "positive thinking and internal strength." These strategies reaffirm the body of literature on "cognitive framing affecting behavior and outcomes." Within the context of Asian Americans, Murjani (2014) argues that Yosso's six forms of "non-dominant cultural capital" can represent how resilience is manifested for this diverse group. The six types include aspirational capital, which is defined as holding steadfast to hope regardless of structural forms of inequity; linguistic capital, evidenced by communicating via interpersonal, and intellectual skills gained through bi/multilingualism; familial capital, which refers to knowledge of heritage that provides a meaningful sense of "community history, memory, and cultural intuition"; social capital, which is composed of support networks and resources within the community; navigational capital, which "refers to skills of maneuvering through social institutions not created with Communities of Color in mind"; and resistant capital, or the "knowledge and skills fostered through oppositional behavior that challenges inequality." These culture-specific forms of resilience help racial and ethnic minorities survive and even thrive to pursue their American Dreams.

For the African American/Black American community, protective factors such as strong racial socialization and social support contribute to their resilience. In the Brown (2018) study, "messages emphasizing cultural pride and having knowledge of African heritage were significantly related to the resiliency of participants." Social support is also not limited to the family context but can be through mentors, role models, or significant others who play a vital role in people's lives. Support within the community can come in the form of church or religious places of worship, spaces that alleviate emotional distress. Cultural factors that help to build and sustain the Black self-concept are very salient to developing resilience. Within the Native American context, Goodluck specified strengths-based forms of resilience that are commonly used (Goodluck, 2002). For example, the themes included the "power of the group or communal interdependency and support, spirituality and related ceremonial participation, humor, cultural identity, political relationships and factors (i.e., political involvement, activism, and affiliation), language and stories, tribal values, children, education, and the land or environment" (Belcourt-Ditloff, 2007). Belcourt-Dittloff (2007) explored how humor, community, spiritual orientation, and historical resilience are buffers for positive coping mechanisms and help to alleviate psychological distress.

Within the era of COVID-19, health and mental health systems in America can implement these cultural forms of resilience paramount to the wellness of diverse racial and ethnic groups. We recognize that COVID-19 has changed our lives, yet we must not forget what has worked before to help minority groups defeat challenges. The disruptions of community and familial forms of support, interruptions of routine faith practices, economic instability, and tested pre-existing forms of coping and resiliency have created a compounded and complicated situation for many. This critical period calls for collective action not only among members of racial and ethnic minority groups but also community and faith-based groups, governments, and systems-level approaches to sensitivity that encourage the implementation of culturally appropriate services and resources.

THE RECONCEPTUALIZATION OF THE AMERICAN DREAM

With this call for action and response, a new paradigm of hope and reconceptualizing the essence, reality, and attainment of the American Dream for diverse racial and ethnic groups given the health and mental health disparities that exist, can hopefully provoke community, institutional, and systemic change. The voices of racial and ethnic minorities are present and significant and are urging strategies and solutions to be enacted in order for our fellow brothers and sisters to thrive during and beyond COVID-19. The American Dream can be that guiding light that helps instill hope in people during this pandemic. We cannot afford to pursue this dream the same way we did before COVID-19. Still, we must evoke our cultural strengths and resilience to redefine the dream we hope will become realized and not let a global crisis take us off track, as so many previous historical and present-day oppressions have attempted. To re-conceptualize the American Dream, the collective movement of racial and ethnic minorities who are positioned to soon be the majority of America can demonstrate to Americans and the world during the pandemic how to thrive. We can and must rewrite history through the lens of our diverse narratives, histories. This will promote unity.

REFERENCES

American Psychological Association. (2020). *Mental health disparities: Diverse populations.* https://www.psychiatry.org/psychiatrists/cultural-competency/education/mental-health-facts

Belcourt-Dittloff, A. (2007). Resiliency and risk in Native American communities: A culturally informed investigation. *ScholarWorks at University of Montana*, 1–169.

Brown, D. (2008). African American resiliency: Examining racial socialization and social support as protective factors. *Journal of Black Psychology, 34*, 32–48.

Centers for Disease Control. (2020). *COVID-19 in racial and ethnic minority groups.* https://www.cdc.gov/coronavirus/2019-ncov/need-extra-precautions/racial-ethnic-minorities.html

Chan, J. (2020, May 13). 10 Asian American contributions that need more recognition. *IntheKnow.* https://www.intheknow.com/2020/05/13/10-asian-american-contributions-that-need-more-recognition/

Consoli, M., Ayala, M., López, S., Gonzales, N., Cabrera, A., Llamas, J., & Ortega, S. (2013). Resilience and thriving in the Latino/A population: Intersections and discrepancies. *Revista Interamericana De Psicología/Interamerican Journal of Psychology, 45*(3).

DeSantis, A. (2009). Selling the American Dream myth to Black southerners: The Chicago defender and the great migration of 1915–1919. *Western Journal of Communication, 62*(4), 474–511.

Goodluck, C. (2002). *Native American children and youth well-being indicators: A strengths-based perspective*. Casey Family Programs.

Guillaume, M. (2020, February 2). 29 notable African Americans who helped change the world. *6ABC*. https://6abc.com/black-history-month-notable-african-americans-most-influential-famous-people/5888312/

Illuzi, M. (2014). Lincoln's "race of life" is not the American dream of equal opportunity. *American Political Thought: A Journal of Ideas, Institutions, and Culture* 3, 228–253.

Knight, M., Roegman,, R., & Edstrom, L. (2015). My American Dream: The Interplay between structure and agency in West African immigrants' educational experiences in the United States. *Education and Urban Society, 48*(9). 827–851.

LiHerald. (2018, September 17). *Celebrating Hispanic contributions to America*. https://www.liherald.com/stories/celebrating-hispanic-contributions-to-america,96054

Murjani, M. (2014). Breaking apart the model minority and perpetual foreigner stereotypes: Asian Americans and cultural capital. *Recreating New Domains: The Future of Higher Education, 35*(10), 79–90.

Musick, M., & Wilson, J. (1998). Work, race and the American dream. *Sociological Focus, 31*(1), 17–30.

New American Economy. (2020, March 19). *Power of the purse: The contributions of Black immigrants in the United States*. https://research.newamericaneconomy.org/report/black-immigrants-2020/

Nix, E. (2019, July 29). Tuskegee experiment: The infamous syphilis study. *History*. https://www.history.com/news/the-infamous-40-year-tuskegee-study

Ritter, M. (2013, August 7). NIH, family of Henrietta Lacks reach deal on access to DNA code. *Washington Post*. https://www.washingtonpost.com/national/health-science/nih-family-of-henrietta-lacks-reach-deal-on-access-to-dna-code/2013/08/07/68f3da04-ff8b-11e2-96a8-d3b921c0924a_story.html

Rowland, R., & Jones, J. (2018). One dream: Barack Obama, race, and the American Dream. *Rhetoric and Public Affairs–Michigan State University Press, 14*(1), 125–154.

Substance Abuse and Mental Health Services Administration. (2020). *Double jeopardy: COVID-19 and behavioral health disparities for Black and Latino communities in the U.S.* https://www.samhsa.gov/sites/default/files/covid19-behavioral-health-disparities-black-latino-communities.pdf

Schaeffer, K. (2019, July 30). The most common age among Whites in U.S. is 58—More than double that of racial and ethnic minorities. *Pew Research Center*. https://www. research.org/fact-tank/2019/07/30/most-common-age-among-us-racial-ethnic-groups/

Schwartz, B., Bernal, D., Smith, L., & Nicolas, G. (2014). Pathways to understand help-seeking behaviors among Haitians. *Journal of Immigrant and Minority Health, 16*(2), 239—243.

Tinoco, S. (2018). Reconceptualizing "The American Dream" for undocumented immigrants: The yearning for a lost sense of family, identity, and belonging. *Pacific Coast Philology, 53*(2), 289–307.

Underwood, L., & Washington, A. (2016). Mental illness and juvenile offenders. *International Journal of Environmental Research and Public Health, 13*(2), 228.

U.S. Census Bureau. (2019). *Quick facts*. https://www.census.gov/quickfacts/fact/table/US/PST045219#PST045219

United States Department of Agriculture. (n.d.). *Native American contributions*. https://www.nrcs.usda.gov/Internet/FSE_DOCUMENTS/nrcs141p2_024206.pdf

Villarosa, L. (2020, April 29). A terrible price: The deadly racial disparities of COVID-19 in America. *The New York Times*. https://www.nytimes.com/2020/04/29/magazine/racial-disparities-covid-19.html

Yancy, C. (2020). COVID-19 and African Americans. *JAMA, 323*(19), 1891–1892.

CHAPTER 17

SOUFRANS AYISYEN

An Emerging Theoretical Construct of Haitian Suffering and Resilience

Guy C. Jeanty

COVID-19, a virus that is now ubiquitous globally, is the light at the dawn of the 21st century that lays bare the putrid maladies that we have known and felt for a very long time lurking deep inside our collective consciousness. We have resisted. Still, the ferocity and scope of the coronavirus is no match for our denials and the desperate need to pretend that all is well in a diseased body. COVID-19 is a triple pandemic revealing blatant racism, the unrelenting and disproportionate impact of the virus itself, and the unique suffering of Haitians. This chapter will address a conceptual framing of suffering that emerged during the COVID-19 pandemic specific to the Haitian people's historical and multigeneration suffering. In Haitian parlance, the suffering which will be addressed is called *Soufrans Ayisyen.* Suffering holds a dubious distinction in Haitian life. In a sense, it is ubiquitous; it's so common that it seems to fill the air. We have learned to coexist with it like an unfriendly neighbor. Molefi Kete Asante's foreword in former president Jean Bertrand Aristide's *Haïti-Haiti? Philosophical Reflections for Mental Health Decolonization* captures Haitians' coexistence with suffering. Asante says of Aristide's goals during his first presidency of Haiti, "Indeed,

Coronavirus and Vulnerable People: Addressing the Divide in Harm and Responses and Exploring Implications for a More Peaceful World, pp. 263–291

he [also] balanced the federal budget for the first time that anyone could remember. In his [Aristide] words, his goal was to move the country from misery to poverty with dignity" (Aristide, 2016, p. 2).

The word "misery" holds a unique place in the Haitian vocabulary; it is a reference point of a kind of imminent hell that lurks around every corner that one seeks to evade. Thus, this kind of suffering, *Soufrans Ayisyen*, is embedded in our very being. What then is the definition of *Soufrans Ayisyen*? *Soufrans* in Haitian Creole means suffering. *Soufrans Ayisyen* is the Haitian's collective and individual, historical, psychological, emotional, social, economic, and spiritual trauma caused by enslavement and maintained by Euro-American's continued exploitation and global domination. This chapter is a preliminary articulation of *Soufrans Ayisyen* and will cover the following topics: (1) the linguistic challenges in formulating *Soufrans Ayisyen*; (2) a discussion on the origin of *Soufrans Ayisyen*; (3) the premise of *Soufrans Ayisyen*; (4) the philosophical underpinnings of *Soufrans Ayisyen*, and (5) recommendations for clinical application.

LINGUISTIC QUAGMIRE

We often boast as humans that language is the sine qua non of our superiority over all other life forms. But in reality, we are often prisoners of our linguistic conventions. We all too often are chagrined by the myriad ways in which language fails. Language limitation frequently stymies our attempts to get at the true essence of our deepest thoughts and feelings. This failure of language exists even in one's native tongue. The frustration is even greater when another's language is imposed upon us. The social and psychological conventions of colonial languages corral us and limit our ability to fully express ourselves because the oppressor's very language is also our enemy. It disenfranchises our very sense of being. In my opinion, no one speaks about the limitations of language more poignantly and with as much eloquence accessible to the familiar person as James Baldwin.

Having joined the ancestors' rank, Baldwin, is someone I humbly consider a "spirit" mentor. As such, his ideas are deeply personal to me, and I strive diligently to use those ideas as a compass with which to navigate turbulent moments. In the opening statement of his speech at the University of California, Berkley in 1979, Baldwin (published in 2019) stated in his distinct cadence and rhythmic oratorical style like that of a Baptist preacher:

> I am going to improvise like a writer on some assumptions. And though I feel a little uneasy in saying this, nevertheless, what a writer is obliged, at some point, is to realize that he's involved in a ***language*** which he has to

> change. For example, for a ***black writer***, especially in this country, to be born into the English language, realize that the assumptions of the ***language***, the premises of which the ***language*** operates ***are*** his enemy. [Emphasis added]

Baldwin's astute observation is that another's language strictures dictate and restrict one's ability to use that other individual's language to appropriately articulate the true essence of one's own experience. For example, Africa's European descendants (or so-called "white" people) have perfected language as a weapon of warfare. They have imbued an arbitrary word like "white" with false meanings and assumptions to their benefit and others' detriment and destruction. Parenthetically, this fact is not only true of the English language; French, Spanish, and Portuguese are just as lethal. Also, the English language is rife with self-serving and fork-tongued proclamations such as:

> **We hold these truths to be** [Emphasis added] self-evident: that all men are created equal; that their Creator endows them with certain unalienable rights; that among these are life, liberty, and the pursuit of happiness.
>
> —Thomas Jefferson

The same language, as Baldwin (2019) would say, "is a trap bag." The language, or words, say one thing but mean something entirely different, deceiving the writer and reader (or nonreaders). Such vile use of language, in my view, renders a language duplicitous, untrustworthy, and dangerous for all. For example, the mere thought and struggle in this chapter about whether or not to use the word "white" either as an adjective or a noun demonstrates both the word's absurdity and the fact that the word/language is my enemy, as Baldwin suggested. This conundrum is so pervasive that even "white" writers cannot escape it.

Jacqueline Battalora (2013), in the prescient text *Birth of a White Nation*, argued that:

> Academic discourse on race is further complicated by terminology that asserts a "natural" status. By this, I mean that use of common race terminology such as "whites" to talk about people of European ancestry works to give a "truth" status to the social meanings that have been attached to it … I have found no reasonably useful way out of the conundrum that using terminology for so-called racial categories presents. (p. xix)

Similarly, Robin Diangelo (2018), in her book, *White Fragility*, lamented.

> Throughout this book, I argue that racism is profoundly complex and nuanced, and given this, we can never consider our learning to be complete

> or finished. One example of this complexity is in the very use of the racial categories "white" and "people of color." I use the terms white and people of color to indicate the two macro-level, socially recognized racial hierarchy divisions. Yet using the terms, I am collapsing a great deal of variation. And though I believe (for reasons explained in chapter 1) that temporarily suspending individuality to focus on group identity is healthy for white people, doing so has very different impacts on people of color.

An alternative to this linguistic quagmire is a factual and historical approach. Richard King (1990, pp. 22– 23), in his formidable work, *African Origin of Biological Psychiatry*, said:

> Today's human forms: African, Asian, European, Latino, and Oceanic are very recent children of their black African parents, the Annu, Twa people. All humanity started in Africa and then migrated to the different corners of the globe, changing in superficial aspects due to climactic-sunlight exposure conditions. All humanity has a vast black origin, Black Dot, in Black North-East Africa. European-Africans must not forget Europe's first historian, Herodotus, who said that "the Egyptians, Colchians, Nubians, and Ethiopians have thick lips, broad nose, wooly hair and are burnt of skin (Jochannan, 1971)"... In this way, we can account for the evolution of the blond northerner (white-European-African).

King's (1990) historical and anthropological description of "white" people as "European-Africans" is scientifically corroborated; however, neither historical or scientific facts are any match for the brazen allegiance to lies, particularly in an era where these melani- deprived Africans unashamedly assert a notion of "alternative facts." As such, rather than getting too bogged down into the social constructionist quagmire, similar to King and Vernon Dixon (1971), before him, who used the term "Euro-American," I am opting for the designation European to refer to the de-pigmented Africans who as a consequence of the ice age became deficient in melanin. The burden (or lack of precision) and responsibility of this designation belongs to those who have manipulated language.

SOUFRANS AYISYEN: ORIGIN OF THE CONCEPT

The concept emerged from a confluence of events and experiences, including my own (i.e., my family of birth), the Haitian collective, and the writings of African American scholars. Three key factors account for the conceptual creation of *Soufrans Ayisyen*. First, my lived experience as a Haitian/Haitian American. Second, my reading of African American social scientists, which has been and remains critical. Third, a serendipitous conversation with a colleague who encouraged me to articulate the concept in writing.

I was conceived when my father made several attempts to flee Haiti, specifically the *ton-ton macoutes*, who wielded tremendous power to spare or take life at will during Francois Duvalier's presidency. That turbulent experience, which nearly resulted in my father's death and possibly the demise of our family, is central to our family narrative. True to our culture's oral tradition, even the third generation born in the United States knows about great grandpa's fortuitous escape from Haiti disguised as a woman in order to board a ship bound for the Bahamas. My father settled in Nassau and then eventually migrated to Miami, Florida. The retelling of that story, one that I never heard my father talk about, became a portal for my mother and older siblings to look back at our family's precarious existence in Haiti, our familial "*soufrans*." *Soufrans*, it seems in Haiti, readily crosses the invisible barriers of class, race, and religion within changes in political regimes. It is a part of the Haitian narrative, more catastrophic for some than others. The plight of the Haitian collective, the common man and woman, mainly those considered *nèg mòn* (i.e., mountain people, people assumed to be a lower class), is one of historical and perpetual struggle. This constant and pervasive struggle seems to exist at every level of Haitian society and is a kind of struggle that seems passed from one generation to the next much like a hereditary disease that cannot be cured. So much so that in day-to-day conversation, the fact of actual or future *soufrans* permeates the minds and language of the Haitian collective; *soufrans*, it seems, shapes our mental maps and creates a collective consciousness of suffering. *Soufrans* is woven seamlessly into the Creole vernacular.

As a consequence, a common retort among practically all Haitians, regardless of class, race, or religion, is the statement: *Pa fè m' soufri* (i.e., Don't make me struggle), or to put it differently, "Don't put me through misery." That statement is so emotionally and psychologically loaded for Haitians that it conveys a willful act of barbarism, the ultimate fate to that can befall someone.

My passion for bibliotherapy is such that very often when I read, the experience between me and the author I am reading often morphs into a passionate dialogue, similar to the call-and-response experience of a Black church where a fiery Black preacher is preaching and I, as a congregation of one, respond enthusiastically to the authors. It is the seminal works and voices of African American scholars in the best tradition of Pan Africanism combined with my own lived experience and thoughts that have given rise to *Soufrans Ayisyen*. These scholars include individuals such as Professor James Smalls, Professor Kaba Hiawatha, Kamene, Dr. Leonard Jeffries, James Baldwin, Dr. Edwin Nichols, Dr. Wade W. Nobles, Dr. Bobby E. Wright, Dr. Asa Hilliard, Dr. Frances Cress Welsing, Dr. Amos Wilson, Dr.

Joy Degruy, and many others. Dr. Wade Nobles' seminal work, *The Island of Memes: Haiti's Unfinished Revolution*, is pivotal in the birthing of *Soufrans Ayisyen* as a theoretical construct.

During the early months of the COVID-19 pandemic, a serendipitous conversation occurred with Dr. Charlene Désir. I discussed my clinical impressions of Haitian clients with her using the term *Soufrans Ayisyen* to describe a phenomenon that I had observed. Dr. Desir was intrigued by the idea and suggested that the view be developed. I agreed and began the process of articulating the framework of *Soufrans Ayisyen*. I am confident that had that conversation not occurred, *Soufrans Ayisyen* would have remained locked in my mind.

As a construct, *Soufrans Ayisyen* is a complex, multilayered trauma experience that affects the consciousness and identity of Haitians. Such a phenomenon makes life grueling and creates a state of despair for Haitians. Misery and misfortune are expected, and Haitian life is marked by a perpetual and transgenerational struggle experienced by Haitians globally regardless of social-economic status. Enslavement is but one critical aspect of *Soufrans Aysyen*. Enslavement is the genesis of Haitians' suffering and Haitians' distinction as the only Black nation to gain independence from it by overthrowing white domination in armed conflicts. These complex realities are the root causes of *Soufrans Ayisyen*, thus contributing to and perpetuating Haitians' continued trauma.

THE PREMISE OF *SOUFRANS*

There are five key assumptions in conceptualizing *Soufrans Ayisyen*,. First, the acts, conditions, and mentality that caused *Soufrans Ayisyen* were purposeful and meant to destroy us or keep us in a perpetual state of oppression. Second, the goal for those who perpetrated those acts of exploitation, and their attempts to eradicate us, was to have their descendants carry out the same oppressive and barbaric behavior. Stephanie E. Jones-Rogers (2019, pp. 1–2) courageously chronicles this fact after combing through voluminous historical documents of female slave owners. Jones-Rogers revealed the precarious existence of the enslaved being subjected to the whims of the children of enslavers. She cited a specific case:

> Lizzie Anna Burwell was like many other white girls growing up in slaveholding households in the Linesville, North Carolina area in 1847. She loved flowers and often strolled through her parents' garden with Fanny, the enslaved woman charged with her care. After spending so much time with Fanny, Lizzie Anna developed an intense bond with her [Fanny], but one day Lizzie Anna became "vexed" with Fanny, so she went to her father and demanded that he "cut Fanny's ears off" and get her, Lizzie Anna,

> "a new maid from Clarksville." Lizzie Anna was three years old.... White southern girls like Lizzie Anna learned how to be mistresses and slave owners through an instructional process that spanned their childhood and adolescence. (Jones-Rogers, 2019)

If after Haiti's independence in 1804, and if after the Emancipation Proclamation in 1862, Africans in the Caribbean and the United States continue to suffocate, it is not accidental. It is because the descendants of oppressors remain just as committed to their privilege and our collective demise. It is necessary to speak clearly and accept the hard truth about how systems of oppression get passed on, to name them. We must say precisely how these oppressive systems are perpetuated through the teaching and indoctrination of children with their predecessors' pathology. Iyanla Vanzant is known for her remark: "You've got to know what your 'thing' is, and you've got to call it a 'thing,' whether it's meanness, nastiness, un-forgiveness, arrogance, ego, resistance, rebelliousness, or defiance." We must face this fact and call it by name. Children are born innocent into situations that they did not create but are often socialized consciously to think and behave according to their social group's normative behaviors. We cannot escape the brutal truth that people who commit atrocious acts were once children, deliberately taught and indoctrinated with false beliefs of superiority and entitlement. They also are poisoned with the false teachings of the inherent inferiority of people of African descent. Over time, many such children evolve into callous, destructive, and all too often murderous human beings. In contrast, this matter is further complicated because Europeans often perceive African descent children as much older than their age and see them as threatening—a phenomenon that, in Europeans' minds, turns our children into dangerous perpetrators.

Third, the ideologies and systems from which *Soufrans Ayisyen* was created, maintained, and passed on to subsequent generations of oppressors cannot be used to liberate African descent people who suffered due to these very ideological social structures. Put differently, the system that created the problem cannot be used to solve the problem. Fourth, *Soufrans Ayisyen* is a multidimensional trauma experience. Put differently; it is collective trauma, individual trauma, and transgenerational trauma. Joy Degruy (2005) stated, "Recent research in the field of epigenetics ... has revealed that trauma can actually impact an individual's DNA, and the manifestation of the traumas experienced by prior generations can be passed along genetically to future offspring" (p. 9). Lastly, personal or amicable experiences with individual Europeans or single institutions are irrelevant because the oppressive behaviors that are detrimental to African people persist unabated despite the occasional encounters with some Europeans who may not be overtly hostile or may even be allies of African descent people. Because of

Europeans' group behavior and their control systems, they always override single Europeans and individual acts. Therefore, individual encounters or actions of civility with specific Europeans is irrelevant in the face of systemic structural oppression.

To eradicating these domination systems, many scholars and advocates of African people's full citizenship have identified at least three critical areas. Those areas are culture, economics, and politics (See Leonard Jeffries, Claude Anderson, Edwin Nichols). For *Soufrans Ayisyen*, the culture will be the focus. Edwin Nichols' philosophical argument about the role and relationship of culture to human behavior and thought process is vital in advancing this argument. Nichols proposed that cultural differences are best understood by interrogating a groups' axiology (i.e., values), epistemology, and logic system.

THE AXIOLOGY OF *SOUFRANS*

Central to the discussion of *Soufrans Ayisyen* is the belief systems embedded in the behaviors that caused and sustained Haitian suffering. Edwin Nichols's (1986) research on the philosophical aspects of cultural difference provided a lens to understand the values, behaviors, and rationale of those who caused this specific experience, *Soufrans Ayisyen*. Vernon Dixon, a Pan Africanist economist, is acknowledged by Nichols as a critical influence in developing the Nichols' model. In an interview, Nichols lamented that Dixon did not receive as much credit as he should have for his contribution in delineating Europeans and Africans' worldviews and the harmful impact of Europeans' system of logic.

Nichols's (1986) ideas provided a point of departure to begin to construct a theory of *Soufrans Ayisyen*. Nichol's model delineates three key components, axiology, epistemology, and logic, which he argues relate to cultural differences and group behavior. Nichols's central thesis is that one's cultural conditioning affects the way that events encountered by an individual are interpreted and acted upon. Nichols identified four large social groups to demonstrate and substantiate the theory of cultural difference. Those groups include European (Euro/American), African (African American, Caribbean, and Hispanic), Asian (Asian/American and Native American), and Mediterranean (Middle Eastern). Each group possesses a discrete value system, a method of knowing and logic. In this work, the focus will be on two cultural groups, Europeans and Africans.

In his schema, Nichols (1986) argued that the climate that shaped Europeans' ecology significantly impacted their value system, which was necessary to survive and thrive in their ecology after coming out of the ice age. Philosophically, he argues, "The European focus of Man-Object dictates that the highest value lies in the object or the in the acquisition of the Object" (p. 11). Nichols argues that such a value system comes from what was necessary for Europeans to survive and thrive as an ethnic entity starting in Europe. Because of the harsh climatic environment, the object itself–food, clothing, shelter, and safety—was the most important thing because those things were not omnipresent. Nichols illustrates this point in an interview wherein he explained the tremendous difficulties associated with European's growing and harvesting crops and the absolute necessity for precise planting and harvesting. He stated:

> So if they [Europeans] didn't plant at the right time in which to harvest and to store and learn how to preserve and be very careful in their measurement of time, even in the measurement of how much food they could eat per month because they could run out if they overate in one month (E, Nichols, personal communication).

As such, Nichols argued that European society is very much into counting and measuring, which became their epistemology. This value system was necessary for their survival and to thrive. This axiology is not inherently immoral; it was necessary for their survival. Hence, the highest value for Europeans lies in the object and the acquisition of the object. Some of the things that could be classified as "objects" would be land, work, time, etc. However, when this value system is placed in a broader, global context, exploitation is the logical extension.

To extend this argument further, it can be said that the European tends to become obsessed with the "object" and the impulse to possess the "object" at all costs. Put differently; Europeans are blinded by the physical object and the drive to conquer what is seen. As a consequence, the European becomes blind to the metaphysical aspects of what is unseen. Thus, he sees the land, earth, as something to be possessed and exploited without any inherent sense of an interdependent relationship between himself and the land. So, everything which can be seen is to be possessed and thereby objectified, human beings included.

In contrast, Nichols stated, "In the African axiology, the focus is on Man-Man. Here, the highest value lies in the interpersonal relationship between persons" (p. 11). Vernon Dixon (1971) originally described these two paradigms as follows: "The dominant value-orientations in the Euro-American world view is what I term the Man-to-Object relationship; while for homeland and overseas Africans, it is what I term the Man-to-Person relationship" (p. 22). This view is widely held among Pan Africanist scholars such as Linda James Myers, Kobi Kambon, John Henrik Clarke, Naim Akbar, Molefi Kete Asante, Wade Nobles, Karanja Keita Carroll, and others.

Nichols further stated that differences in basic survival needs shaped the value differences between Europeans and Africans:

> Ecologically, food for Africans was omnipresent; their environment provided an abundance of food and other resources. The challenge was more about storing and preserving food supplies than desperately trying to cultivate and produce crops. Hence, the most important thing for people in that ecology was establishing and maintaining relationships. (E. Nichols, personal communication)

Nichols suggested, appropriately so, that "If Man-Object were the axiology of Black people, we would all be dead" (E. Nichols, personal communication). Because it is interpersonal relationships, particularly for African Americans, that enabled them to survive the great tragedy of enslavement, Jim Crow, and systemic discrimination and death at Europeans' hands. The same is true for Haitians and other Africans in the Caribbean and the Americas; the highest value is the person-to-person relationship. That personal bond was intended to be broken so the enslaved would comply with those conditions, infecting the minds. Wade Nobles (2015), in his work *The Island of Memes: Haiti's Unfinished Revolution*, makes a similar point about African axiology:

> People of African ancestry share specific orientations that are based on a common spiritual essence and similar cultural beliefs and practices as well as concrete historical experiences.... Relying on the principles of harmony within the universe as a natural order of existence, African-centered psychology recognizes that (1) spirit permeates everything; (2) everything in the universe is interconnected; (3) the collective is the most salient element of existence; and (4) communal self-knowledge is the key to mental health.

Both Nobles and Nichols advance the same argument about the value system of people of African descent. The person-to-person (or the relationship) axiology of Africans is central to our survival wherever we are on the planet. And acting contrary to that has been and remains detrimental.

The dilemma concerning *Soufrans Ayisyen* then, it seems, is that axiologically, we are adrift, caught between the Europeans' craven objectification/acquisition worldview and the African's interpersonal, inter-dependent value system of "I am because you are." This creates an axiological conflict for Haitians, which contributes to and perpetuates *Soufrans Ayisyen* both individually and collectively. The European mentality of objectification and domination has infected Haiti's minds, leading to an individualistic mindset and rampant materialism, which are counter-productive to the wellbeing of Haiti and to Haitians' well-being. European values and African values have collided, and the European values have saturated the minds of Haitians. Nobles (2015, p. 53) aptly described the root of this phenomenon root as a "memetic" infection, a virus that has infected Haiti. He stated that:

> Critical to understanding the clash of culture and consciousness is the idea of memes and memetic ideation and their role in Europe's psychological domination of Africa's mind....The meme itself is defined as a unit of information residing in the brain.... Words, skills, behaviors, etc., are the outward and visible manifestations of the memes within the brain, which are transmitted between individuals via the sense organs. Memes use their possessor's communication and imitation skills to replicate themselves and influence the world in which their possessor dwells.

Therefore, *Soufrans Ayisyen*, in part, is perpetuated by Haitians' adopting European axiology of "man-object" rather than "person-to-person." Karanja Keita Carrol argued that African's worldview "is grounded in cooperation and collective responsibility; incorporates interdependence, spiritualism and circularity" (Carroll, 2008, p. 10). This is the opposite of European axiology, which is founded on competition, individualism, and materialism. The European value system has seeped deeply into the Haitian psyche, aggravating the systemic suffering. Radical changes are necessary to shift the Haitian mindset and adopt a value system that will reduce suffering and enable Haitians to thrive. This will include adopting a holistic value system based on what is best for the collective rather than the individual.

THE EPISTEMOLOGY OF *SOUFRANS*

Epistemology refers to the nature of knowledge. It raises two fundamental questions. How do you know what you know? What are the processes that are used to know something? There is a distinct difference between European and African epistemology. Jimoh (2017) stated that "There is a distinctive African way of perceiving and reacting to the world.... This consists of how African see or talks about reality" (p. 4). Dixon (1971) identified a similar distinction between the Euro-American view, which he refers to as "Object-Measure Cognition," and the African view, which he refers to as "Affect-Symbolic Imagery Cognition" (p. 131). The epistemological difference between the two worldviews is found in what Dixon referred to as "empty perceptual space." Put differently, the "empty perceptual space" is a perceived gap on the part of Euro-Americans which suggests a separation of the self from the phenomenal world. This "empty perceptual space" within the Euro-American epistemology is distinguished from an African epistemology.

Dixon (1971) argued that this positivistic mentality born out of the Enlightenment era cemented European's proclivity to view themselves as separate and apart from everything around them. It leads them to believe that they can somehow hold an "objective" stance to everything around them and that whatever cannot be "verified" empirically does not exist. An alternative epistemology conceptualized by Dixon is "diunital" (p. 131), which suggests a "Both-And" perspective or the "In-Between" as elucidated by Nichols (1986). Diunital logic will be discussed in more detail in the logic section of this work.

An epistemology of *Soufrans Ayisyen* must take into consideration the fact that Haitians are first and foremost sons and daughters of Africa who, before enslavement, shared the same epistemology. Remnants of Haitians method of knowing are evident in the traditions of Haiti, particularly in the cultural traditions, the spiritual systems, the remnants of our oral traditions, indigenous songs and dance and our relationship to nature. Etta and Offiong (2019), in *The Reality of African Epistemology,* stated that "African epistemology is deeply rooted in African tradition; it is metaphysically and spiritually inclined" (p. 280). Additionally, the epistemology of Africans is highly experiential and rooted in the experience of the collective. As such, it operates from the premise of "I feel, therefore, I am." Thus, African epistemology is deeply rooted both in thought and sensory experiences.

Additionally, epistemology for the African starts with the premise, "We are therefore I am." It is an epistemology that is focuses on being one with nature and emphasizes spirituality and an understanding of the world through a spiritual source. African epistemology regards the experiential world and the non-experiential world as causally related.

In contrast, Western culture's fundamental teaching is that knowledge consists of the mind's ability to represent reality accurately, whereas, argued Jimoh (2017), "the African theory of knowledge postulates a cultural and situated notion of knowledge" (p. 1). This postulation rests on the African ontological notion of reality as a continuum in which human beings are interdependent with the physical and the metaphysical.

In the field of psychology, Nichols (1986) expanded Dixon's (1971) idea, stating that, "Africans know through symbolic imagery and rhythm, while Europeans know through counting and measuring." This epistemology connotes a separation of the self from nature. Because axiology and epistemology are interdependent, it follows that axiology informs epistemology. Nichols stated that European epistemology follows their axiology, wherein the object and acquisition of the object are the highest value. Hence, Europeans' reliance on the senses as a means of cataloging, measuring, weighing, and adding to acquire objects is consistent with their value system. In contrast, African axiology in which the highest value is in the interpersonal relationship (Man-Man) follows their epistemology of knowing through symbolic imagery and rhythm.

There are different ways of knowing. Africans, in particular, have modes of knowing that are uniquely their own. According to Etta and Offiong (2019), those are "oral tradition [which] is the method in which history, stories, folktales, and religious beliefs are passed on from generation to generation" (p. 293). Additionally, intuition is also an accepted form of knowing. Etta and Offiong described intuition as "a truth by which the knowledge comes to an individual; it is accepted as a kind of certainty that could suddenly come upon somebody as a flash of light" (p. 296).

The epistemology of the African then is most often gained by feeling or intuiting what lies behind appearances and superimposing this information onto what can be ascertained by the senses. Bynum (2012, p. 297). in *The African Unconscious: Roots of Ancient Mysticism and Modern Psychology*, made a similar point in stating that:

> The traditional African religious intuition believes in and observes an energy and information field around all things, especially human beings (Somé, 1994). The paradigm accepts that all things are, in some sense, alive and remain alive despite their apparent, manifest transformation in the energetic field of space and time.

Africans' ways of knowing are extensive and also include mystical knowledge, rational knowledge, ancestral knowledge, communal knowledge, and ontological knowledge, by which is meant the very "being" or the essence of being human and being able to recognize the interdependent relationship between humans and the universe. This is a profound way of knowing the self and everything else outside of the self. The epistemology of Africans is very experiential.

Hence given this context, I would argue that the epistemology of *Soufrans Ayisyen* is also highly experiential. The collective and individual experiences that gave rise to *Soufrans* are the lived experiences that occurred or were imprinted in our bodies, minds, and spirits. The *Soufrans* (trauma) are embedded in our very consciousness. We know what we know experientially, and epistemology is sometimes reflected elegantly in our various art forms and spiritual traditions but at other times manifested in our unhealed traumas where we end up also traumatizing each other. In Haiti's case, from the very beginning, the numerous coups d'etat against the government and the endemic distrust, disrespect, and impatience towards one another are also ways in which *Soufrans* is perpetuated. The epistemology of *Soufrans* then is a continuous loop of cycling and recycling of the experience of physical enslavement, isolation, and hypervigilance. These forms of knowing must be utilized to enable us to move beyond survival and towards thriving as a collective.

THE LOGIC OF *SOUFRANS*

There is a symbiotic relationship between axiology and epistemology from which logic derives. According to Nichols (1986), logic quite simply is how one reasons to answer and justify conclusions. The axiology of a social group primarily determines logical outcomes. For Europeans, the highest value is in the object or acquisition of the object. Given that axiology, what is their logic system? Nichols states that "The European logic system has its basis in dichotomy, by which reality is expressed as either/or" (p. 14). The logic system of Europeans is dichotomous logic wherein choices are binary, "either-or."

This form of logic is neither inferior nor superior to any other method of logic. However, the problem arises when a binary system of logic is applied to human beings. People are complex; thus, an algorithmic form of logic can cause significant problems when the wrong people are in power positions. For instance, in Euro-American society, much of the public discourse is scattered with binary memes such as being "pro-life" versus "pro-choice," championing "law and order" versus "civil liberty," or "capitalism" versus "socialism." These binary formulations towards public policy inevitably result in winners or losers, which leads to an adversarial environment. More subtle and pernicious effects of dichotomous logic can be seen in the following group of words identified by Nichols (1986, p. 14):

Assertive	Submissive
Aggressive	Passive
Powerful	Powerless
Strong	Weak
Intelligent	Ignorant
Independent	Dependent

This list of traits organized as opposites is inconsequential until conscious or unconscious cultural bias is superimposed. For example, if maleness in society is superimposed on the positive side, males then are socialized to think of themselves as assertive, aggressive, powerful, strong, intelligent, and independent. If femaleness is superimposed on the negative side, women are then trained to be submissive, passive, powerless, weak, ignorant, and dependent.

Dichotomous logic is similarly problematic for perceived "minorities." A Black male who is surrounded by predominantly white males and who attempts to follow the assertive-independent paradigm in the left column is perceived as dangerous. For the Black male to neutralize the danger, as perceived by Europeans, he is often physically or psychologically forced into the dichotomy's negative side (the right column). These binaries often create stereotypes, which are then used to justify oppressive behavior and conditions. People often find themselves locked into one paradigm or the other. Adult Black males, forced to vacillate between being assertive at home and submissive in public, internalize a great deal of anger, resulting in hypertension, relationship breakdowns, and a higher mortality rate for Black men, perpetuating stress and trauma.

The effects of dichotomous logic and its symbiotic relationship to *Soufrans Ayisyen* can be illustrated in these groups of words:

European	African
Educated	Ignorant
Sophisticated	Backward
Rich	Poor
Upper-Class	Lower Class
Mulatto	Black
French	Creole
Christian	Vodoun

In Haiti, the left column is frequently used to describe social class and race differences, real or perceived. These binaries persist and continue to divide Haitians in Haiti and in the diaspora. Wade Nobles correctly ascertained that the lingering effects of enslavement in Haiti has resulted in "the shattering of consciousness and fracturing of identity" (Nobles, 2015, p. 129). These binaries shape the consciousness and distort the identity of Haitians, making *Soufrans Ayisyen* ubiquitous and widespread.

In contrast to the European's dichotomous logic system, Nichols (1986), influenced by the economist, Vernon Dixon (1971) stated that the African logic system is diunital (a term Dixon coined), or characterized by the union of opposites. Nichols (2015) illustrated dichotomous logic and diunital logic by employing the narrative of Adam and Eve. God says to Adam, "Who ate the apple?" Adam replied, "The **woman** whom you gave me gave me the apple to eat." Adam's dichotomous logic blames Eve. In the African diunital logic, the story goes as follows. God says to Adam, "Who ate the apple?" Adam replied, "**We** ate the apple [Emphasis added]." Adam does not blame Eve because the highest value is in the relationship. Kobi Kambon, as cited by Carroll (2008), argues that the African's axiology is "grounded in cooperation and collective responsibility; corporateness and interdependence; and spiritualism and circularity. This is contradistinction to the European axiology founded on competition and individual rights; separateness and independence; and materialism and ordinality" (p. 10). Nichols is correct in stating:

> [If] the highest value lies in the relationship, as Africans we can't use that logic system [dichotomous logic], the reason is it won't keep the [African] value system in place because in that logic system [dichotomous logic] if I'm right, you to have been wrong. If you're right, I have to be wrong. How long then can we keep a relationship as the highest value? We cannot. (E. Nichols, personal communication)

Within the context of *Soufrans Ayisyen*, Haitians, like Esau, have unknowingly traded their birthright, diunital logic, for the poison pill of dichotomous logic, which perpetuates the Willie Lynch syndrome of division; mitigate real progress and still worse, epigenetically transmit the virus of "shattered consciousness and fractured identity." Therefore, we must employ a logic system that can support or complement a value system that benefits the collective.

It is essential to reiterate that there is nothing inherently bad about dichotomous logic; it works well in industry and computer science, which are particularly based on either-or logic. It is, instead, the misuse of dichotomous logic that is detrimental in social systems. The misuse of dichotomous logic forms schisms among groups by utilizing cultural biases to privilege some people (e.g., Europeans). The word privilege is worth a closer look. By definition, privilege is "a right or advantage held as a prerogative of status or rank and exercise to others' exclusion or detriment." When the "white" male is privileged, it is to the exclusion or detriment of others. The logical extension is that the "white" male has the right and privilege to exclude others to the detriment of those so excluded.

Whether based on race or class, privilege is socially constructed and very often shaped by cultural bias. Cultural biases are made real via socialization, which begins early in life, shaping people's beliefs about privilege or about those supposedly not deserving of benefits granted to others. Socialization imprints racism, sexism, and oppressive behavior, granting those prejudices a true status by repeating and reinforcing the biases. Cultural biases are particularly damaging when enshrined into law as real, for instance, chattel slavery in the United States, anti-miscegenation laws, or the Code Noir, which governed Haitians' lives before the war for Haitian independence and the effects of which continue to be felt at this present time (Nobles, 2015).

SOUFRANS AYISYEN: DISORDER OR SYNDROME

As a construct, *Soufrans Ayisyen* reflects a complex, multilayered trauma experience that affects Haitians' consciousness and identity. This phenomenon is pervasive and infects every Haitian regardless of class, religion, gender, economic status, or location in the world. It is a traumatic experience that resulted from actual events, both historical and contemporary. However, given that psychological wounds are not visible to the eyes, the vast majority of Haitians are not necessarily aware of this injury and attempt to function normally, unaware of the spreading infection. As Bessel Van Der Kolk (2014, p. 1) rightly pointed out:

> Traumatic experiences leave traces, whether on a large scale (on our histories and cultures) or close to home, on our families, with dark secrets being imperceptibly passed down through generations. They also leave traces of our minds and emotions, our capacity for joy and intimacy, and even our biology and immune systems.

As Phillipe Shock Matthews often declared about African descent, "Nothing is *wrong* with us; something *happened* to us" (personal communication). And that "thing" which happened to Haitians is being kidnapping from their homes and separated from their families, enslavement, rape, torture, murder, attempted genocide, war, continued threats of war, economic embargos, deprivation, created/sustained political unrest, social disruption, sowing of the seeds of division, orchestrated/systematic coups, and the formation of alliances to punish and keep Haitians in a state of constant unrest.

Soufrans Ayisyen can be and should be considered from the perspective of actual physical and psychological violence perpetrated against real victims. Thus, *Soufrans Ayisyen* can be viewed as a disorder, or a syndrome caused by violence. Definitions of the terms disorder and syndrome is important. A disorder is defined as "A disturbance of function, structure, or both, resulting from a genetic or embryonic failure in development or exogenous factors such as poison, trauma, or disease." In Haiti, the disruption of function and structure is self-evident in every stratum of Haitian society. In her formidable work, Joy Degruy (2005) in *Post Traumatic Slave Syndrome*, courageously stated, "significant life-threatening experiences alter genetic coding and is heritable in subsequent generations" (p. 102). Consequently, children conceived with "post trauma" acquire the adaptive genetic traits, thereby inheriting a legacy of trauma.

In the case of Haitians—during enslavement, after independence and the U.S. occupation, and still after—the acts of violence and sustained threats of violence designed to terrorize compromise Haitian well-being in every conceivable manner. Considering just the physical impact, our immunity to illness is compromised, and morbidity and mortality are exacerbated. Also, constant economic embargos against Haiti, exorbitant interest on loans, and being driven out of desperation to flee Haiti only to suffer human rights abuses in the United States and the Dominican Republic results in additional trauma and compounds the effects of existing trauma. The current data on trauma is incontrovertible; trauma negatively affects biology. Additionally, the factors that caused the damage to Haitians were exogenous. As Phillipe Matthews said, "something ***happened*** to us [Emphasis original]" (personal communication).

A syndrome is defined as "The aggregate of symptoms and symptoms associated with any morbid process, together constituting the disease's picture." *Soufrans Ayisyen* is a composite of historical and current symptoms of oppression (i.e., "white" supremacy or sustained impact of colonization), resulting in the Haitian society's systemic malfunctioning, both for the Haitian collective and individuals. *Soufrans Ayisyen,* in effect, is a manifestation of a constellation of trauma-induced symptoms. Thus, it is a disease caused by history and maintained by current oppression. As stated earlier, epigenetics research has revealed that the environment influences the functioning of genes, and trauma can be transmitted over generations (Dugruy, 2005).

Two significant studies prove this phenomenon. From an epistemological perspective, this is, in fact, part of the bind that African people confront. African people's experience and knowledge base on our epistemology does not exist or matter until European "research" says it does, and only when the subjects are "white." Perhaps the most famous of the two studies is the Dutch Hunger Winter, which lasted for two years, 1944–1945. The study found that "Women pregnant during the period gave birth to babies who were affected by health problems throughout their lives" (Zimmer, 2020). When they became adults, those children suffered higher rates of obesity, diabetes, and schizophrenia; all these health conditions were traced back to their mothers' food deprivation.

A more recent study analyzed data of Union soldiers who were captured and held as prisoners of war by the Confederate army. The researchers found that the sons of ex-POWs in the worst camp environments were 1.11 times more likely to die at any given age after 45 years old than the sons of non-POWs and 1.09 times more likely to die at any given age than the sons of POWs where camp conditions were better (Costa et al., 2018). The impact of these hardships did not stop with those who suffered them; those adversities also affected the prisoners' children and grandchildren. Epigenetics is a fact about how one's environment influences genes. Joy Degruy (2005) describes this phenomenon as "genetic memory."

> Behavior can be affected by events in previous generations that have been passed on through a form of genetic memory.... A body of research shows that your DNA may contain a biological memory of the stress your grandparents endured. Can trauma, stress, and even nightmares be passed down from generation to generation? Scientists say yes. (p. 101)

Given the scientific data, I argue that *Soufrans Ayisyen* is a unique syndrome that affects Haitians in Haiti and those in the diaspora. Former President Jean Bertrand Aristide (2011, p. 27) in his impassioned work, *Haïti-Haiti? Philosophical Reflections for Mental Decolonization*, states in his poem, Operation Kidnapping, the brutal reality that confronted Africans, resulting in *Soufrans Ayisyen Syndrome*:

> Notwithstanding the trauma, pain, and unimaginable suffering already endured by [the enslaved] after the unleashing of operation kidnapping, the end of the hellish voyage at sea meant a greater hell on another land. The whips and cudgels of the colonists were to become more powerful than ever. For the victims, the message was crystal clear.

In contrast to the Dutch Hunger Winter and the imprisonment of ex-POWs of the U.S. civil war, *Soufrans Ayisyen* lasted far longer, and the enslavement, dehumanization, brutality, destruction of our culture, destruction of families, creation of a false racial construct, torture, and murder were all weapons used against us and codified into laws. In effect, the "laws" are weapons of mass destruction, a poison completely infecting the Haitian mind. As a weapon of warfare, this insidious use of laws by governments or religious institutions continues to this day through policies that maintain Haitians' trauma. The false construct of race was created by law and through those laws that have been eradicated in Haiti and the infection persists.

Concerning the racial construct created by the Europeans and imposed on Haitians, Wade Nobles (2015) states, "To understand the contemporary problems of color and class in Haiti, one has first to understand the Haitian mind as infected by Spain and France and their European 'memetic' ideation" (p. 63). In 1452, Pope Nicholas V issued the papal bull, Dum Diversas, which authorized and formally launched the West African slave trade. The document stated:

> We grant you [Kings of Spain and Portugal] by these present documents, with our Apostolic Authority, full and free permission to invade, search out, capture, and subjugate the Saracens and pagans and any other unbelievers and enemies of Christ wherever they may be, as well as their kingdoms, duchies, counties, principalities, and other property ... to reduce their persons into perpetual slavery. (Dupuy, 2019)

In 1501, the Spaniards began the systematic kidnapping of Africans, believing them to perform physical labor to enrich themselves. French invaders, pirates, and criminals followed the Spanish. Later, King Louis XIV (1638–1715) of France authorized the kidnapping and transport of Africans to Saint Domingue. Louis XIV sought to increase his power by instituting Code Noir (the Black Codes). The Black Codes contained a set of regulations that governed the enslaved Africans' lives and the masters who held them captively (Nobles, 2015). President Jean Bertrand Aristide says of The Black Code that it was "A black cord to hang blacks." According to Article 2 of the code, "All the slaves who will be on our island will be baptized and educated in the Catholic, Apostolic and Roman Church." President Aristide appropriately said of the code, "religion came to resemble a weapon of war. In addition to other deadly weapons, the colonists carefully selected the Catholic religion as an evil weapon with which to wage war" (Aristide, 2011, pp. 27–29). It is essential to understand the word "war" not as hyperbole or metaphor but as an actual and ongoing assault of Haitian culture and the Haitian mind. It is a real war.

Nobles (2015) is correct in concluding that "The *Code Noir* can be reread as memetic ideations" (p. 69). Fouchard, as cited by Dupuy (2019), stated, "Haiti's elite, in their attachment to their Christian, European, and bourgeois values, considered Vodou repugnant and condemn it as a gross superstition or some inherited defect that is best forgotten" (p. 46). This weaponization of religion was meant, at the very least, to undermine but at worst to destroy the axiology, epistemology, and logic system of enslaved Africans. However, the resiliency of the African ancestors was formidable. President Aristide's (2016) statement brilliantly captures the resilience and resistance of our ancestors.

> The Africans cultural root and reality were so firm that the only riches that the [enslaved] were able to bring with them from Africa were precisely the roots of their beliefs, traditions, religion, culture, history, languages and all the other toots of remembrances buried deep in their memories anchored firmly, like an umbilical cord, to the entrails of Mother Africa, always alive in their spirit.

The African consciousness bent but never broke despite the vilest and barbaric acts that the Europeans could imagine and inflict on Africans, Africans in the bleakest hour called on Mother Africa. That same spirit would later be summoned at Bois Caïman in 1791.

It is through the creation and amending of laws that Europeans empower themselves but oppress Africans. As stated earlier, the declaration of independence is a prime example that even when a law appears noble and just, such laws in practice do not apply to much less benefit African people. Jacqueline Battalora's (2013) analysis of Virginia and Maryland's anti-miscegenation laws in the 1600s reveal two critical things. In the United States and the colonies, European' laws were designed to expressly disenfranchise African people. The laws were painstakingly created and underwent several iterations until the right combination of laws could be enacted to guarantee the total and complete subjugation of Africans as property and free labor. While the colonists in Haiti were enacting The Black Code, the Euro-Americans simultaneously were finetuning anti-miscegenation laws to gain maximum control economically, politically, and socially. These laws in the United States, whether independent of the French in Haiti, also created the label "white" as a means to confer benefits for those who were designated "white." European men in particular were granted rights and benefits which previously did not exist.

These laws constructed "realities," which existed not only on paper but, through socialization and punishment, poisoned the minds of "white" people in the United States. The Black Code in Haiti had the same nefarious result. Jacqueline Battalora (2013) and Nobles (2015) made the same point about the codification of racism, misogyny, and bigotry into law. Nobles (2015. p. 70) correctly stated:

> The memetic ideation of the *Code Noir* essentially codified the European memetic cluster and created laws, which resulted in a symbiotic infection of human consciousness to support behaviors that reinforced and propagated "whiteness." Frenchness, as sensate sensoria, had the attributes of sacred, superior, authoritative, accountable, deserving to be obedient to, omnipotent, having the power over life and death.

As Dupuy (2019) argued, Haiti's elite has rejected Haitian culture's essence in their attachment to European axiology, thus their African heritage. Similarly, Aristide opined that "Slavery by itself was infused and infected with prejudice. Any scheme to further infect the minds of [the enslaved] with the virus of an inferiority complex yielded significant benefit to the colonists." Haiti's elite also became Europeans in "blackface." This virus not only infected the mind but, as Nobles (2015) suggested, caused a tremendous rupture in the psyche of Haitians, resulting in a "shattered consciousness and fractured identity." This memetic infection has caused Haitians to disassociate from their fundamental axiology, epistemology, and logic system.

Given the systemic and sustained multigenerational trauma that Haitians have experienced and continue to live with, I have identified this phenomenon as *Soufrans Ayisyen Syndrome* (SAS). What are the characteristics of *Soufrans Ayisyen Syndrome*? The features of SAS include but are not limited to the following:

- A historical and pervasive contemporary trauma affecting the Haitian collective and individual
- A trauma previously codified in law with present and future effects.
- Multigenerational

- Epigenetic experience
- An impulse or desire to disassociate from Haiti, Haitians, Black, or anything pertaining to Africa
- Self-defeating behaviors
- Vacant esteem (seeking identification with Frenchness, European, Spaniards, or "whiteness")
- Shame and low self-esteem associated with being Haitian or of Haitian descent
- They are viewed as carriers of diseases such as HIV/AIDS, malaria, etc.
- Shattered consciousness and distorted identity
- Distorted view of race/class
- Confusion, hate, and embarrassment of Vodou
- Preference for European culture and religion but contempt for indigenous Haitian culture and spiritual system
- The experience is global
- Reflexive distrust of other Haitians
- Disregard of fellow Haitians
- Believing the worse and expecting the worse of fellow Haitians
- Believing that Haitians are inherently incapable of working together
- Suicidal ideation and or suicide

Soufrans Ayisyen Syndrome is a complex, multilayered experience of trauma that affects Haitians' consciousness and identity. This phenomenon makes life grueling and creates a state of despair for Haitians. Misery and misfortune are expected, and Haitian life is marked by a perpetual and transgenerational struggle experienced by Haitians globally regardless of social-economic status. Enslavement is but one critical aspect of *Soufrans Ayisyen Syndrome*. Enslavement is the genesis of Haitians' suffering, along with Haitians' distinction as the only Black nation to gain independence by overthrowing white domination in armed conflicts s. These complex realities are the root causes of *Soufrans Ayisyen Syndrome*, thus contributing to and perpetuating Haitians' continued trauma.

THE THREE PILLARS OF *SOUFRANS AYISYEN*

Soufrans Ayisyen, as presented, is a multilayered phenomenon. Several root causes have been presented. Nobles (2015) identified two critical consequences from the Haitian struggle for freedom: shattered consciousness and fractured identity. The preconditions of shattered consciousness and fractured identity, he argued, is "the concept of 'meme,' sensoria-information structure or contagious information patterns that replicate by symbiotically infecting human minds and altering behavior causing them to propagate the pattern" (p. 62). It is a fact that Europeans, by invading native lands (inadvertently in some cases), brought with them diseases that later infected native peoples. However, the more virulent disease that the Europeans carried and infected indigenous people with was their objectification mentality and the insatiable greed to acquire everything with value or perceived value. In addition to shattered consciousness and fractured identity, I believe another element is necessary: ancestral fragmentation. I would respectfully add this as a third consequence which is just as real but more metaphysical, ancestral fragmentation. In my view, a rupture has occurred between Haitians and the spirit of our ancestors. The fragmentation between us, Haitians in Haiti and the diaspora, and our ancestors' metaphysical reality needs to be restored.

Shattered Consciousness

It seems to me that the matter of consciousness is a constellation and extension of axiology, epistemology, and logic. As presented above in Edwin Nichols and Vernon Dixon's works, axiology, epistemology, and a groups' logic system are, in effect, that groups' conscious ways of living and behaving among themselves and with different people. The distinct consciousness bequeathed to Haitians, Nobles suggested, is an "African heritage replete with an elegant, elaborate, and extraordinary conceptualizations of human knowing and awareness, ergo consciousness" (Nobles, 2015, p. 103). This heritage is a composite of the material and immaterial fact of existence and the African as an expression of both the physical and metaphysical reality. This reality is deeply rooted in spirit, the unseen realities of the universe where the African is a visible manifestation. Furthermore, Nobles (2015) stated:

> At the most fundamental level, consciousness is found in the 'pulse' that gives us life. In contestation to a European worldview and consciousness, consciousness relative to African people should be thought of as a construct representing human beings' ability to know, perceive, understand, and be aware of self in relation to self and all else. (p. 163)

An epistemology grounded in the notion that the self is an extension of a collective that knows and sees itself as part of a Divine and cosmic order would create a human being in harmony with self, the collective, nature, and the universe. Before European enslavement and attempted genocide, the African consciousness is one of infinite possibilities of cooperation with the divine order. Enslavement, however, shattered that consciousness by the barbarism of Europeans. It is not surprising that for enslaved Africans in Haiti to organize themselves to wage war for independence against European domination, they had to reconstitute themselves first by appealing to the Divine forces (i.e., Vodou Lwas: Ogou, Legba, Damballah, and others).

In effect, *Soufrans Ayisyen* is a manifestation of the shattered consciousness of Haitians. It is imperative that this crime perpetrated against us is brought to our conscious awareness, including how thoroughly it is in infecting our entire being. Every part of us has been infected by European barbarism, and the lingering effects permeate every single area of life.

Fractured Identity

Consciousness and identity are inextricably connected. However, consciousness is fundamentally metaphysical, in the sense that consciousness has to do with the awareness of the self and experience in relationship to a cosmic reality far greater than the self. On the other hand, identity connotes an immediacy of the self's experience in space and time. The African proverb speaks to that ontological reality. Vernon Dixon (1971), in talking about the African ethos of communalism, stated, "I am because we are; and since we are, therefore I am" (p. 129). Nobles (2015) further substantiated this idea of identity by stating that:

> Included in the African notion of identity is the belief that the complexity of being "a person" (immaterial and material) gives one an intrinsic human value and that the "person" is a "process" characterized by the divinely governed laws of essence, appearance, perfection, and compassion. (p. 104)

Taken together, Dixon and Noble's arguments were that African identity, fundamentally, was a metaphysical phenomenon and always a collective experience that passes from one generation to the next. This is a fact that Edward Bruce Bynum (2012), elegantly and through painstaking research, articulates in his book *The African Unconscious*. He stated,

> The primary matrices or reflections of the African unconscious can be found in the emphasis on group or tribal, or community consciousness as opposed to egoic or individualized or autonomous consciousness...This wider environment includes not only the somatic expression of the body but also the health of the family, the community, and a person's relationship to the gods. (p. 97)

Therefore, this fundamental rupture of the African's identity in Haiti is both profound and transgenerational. As such *Soufrans Ayisyen* is a grave and potentially fatal disease that continues to metastasize in Haitian life. How then did this fractured identity occur? By introducing rogue cells in the Haitian consciousness, the group's cohesive nature was compromised and eventually undermined. Through intimidation, division, fear, deprivation, rape, torture, separation of families, denial of practicing indigenous faiths, race, class, and murder, Haitians were systematically assaulted. The traumas, despite the hard-fought victory of independence, epigenetically have taken root in the form of "memes" in the consciousness and identities of Haitians, perpetuating *Soufrans Ayisyen*.

Ancestral Fragmentation

The idea of ancestral fragmentation is based on my belief that a disconnection exists between a current-generation (or individual) and their ancestors due to trauma. Understanding and treating ancestral fragmentation is a process in need of development. The process is akin to a psychological autopsy.

The theory of ancestral fragmentation is based on the principle of conducting a psychological autopsy of the ancestors, reconstructing the fundamental factors of their experience of being kidnapped, becoming disoriented by violence—the destruction of homes, murder of men, women, and children—and shackled, physically and mentally, as objects. The process is to identify critical elements of the ancestors' experience and how those experiences began to alter their mental maps, while they attempted to maintain some semblance of equilibrium psychologically and spiritually. The onslaught of trauma, I believe, would have caused immediate physiological and psychological effects, such as hypervigilance and distrust of other enslaved Africans. They became so traumatized that those fearful Africans began to form an emotional and psychological alliance with the perpetrators.

This is based on the idea that the trauma experienced by those who fought and died for freedom was at a high cost to themselves and those that they loved. This is also based on the idea that some of our ancestors, to do the most good for the most people, had to kill "weaker" Africans due to brainwashing by the enslavers. Perhaps such fragmentation has been transferred epigenetically, and we, Haitians, continue to suffer the effects of it and must recognize and heal ourselves from our actual trauma and ancestral trauma.

RECOMMENDATIONS

This work is the initial theoretical and clinical foray in dealing with *Soufrans Ayisyen Syndrome,* a problem caused by and maintained by systemic European oppression. The responsibility for solving the issues associated with *Soufrans Ayisyen Syndrome* rest with Haitians and other African descendants. The philosophy underpinning *Soufrans Ayisyen Syndrome* needs to be developed further from an African perspective. Similarly, clinical applications also need to be developed and researched by Haitians and people of African descent.

Proposed clinical applications of *Soufrans Ayisyen Syndrome* may include ancestral mourning, ancestral healing, ancestral reverence, identity pre-enslavement, ancestral reconnection, transforming the collective/individual, and resiliency then and now.

Ancestral Mourning

The total number of our ancestors killed and died because of enslavement can only be approximated. The inhumane conditions in which they suffered and died must be acknowledged and mourned. Untold numbers died, some valiantly, staring the oppressors and death in the face. Others died in fear, traumatized by an experience that they could not make sense of. Many died alone, and many voluntarily chose while some begrudgingly chose death for their children rather than subjecting them to enslavement. We need to mourn them, to pay respect to their life, death, and life in the afterlife.

Ancestral Healing

Many of the ancestors suffered tremendous damage to their soul, and I believe that some of the ancestors are not entirely well in soul or spirit. As such, we have a responsibility to mourn them, convey our love and express gratitude that their lives and deaths were not in vain. We must find and create ways to encourage and participate in their healing and rest.

Ancestral Reverence

We Africans are fundamentally spiritual people. We are soulful people. The spirit which influences our art, music, our creations, our literature is vibrant energy. That energy connects us to our ancestors; it is our ancestors. As such, we must consciously recognize and pay homage to that spirit that connects us to each other and connects us to them because without them, there is no us. We must revere the ancestors.

Identity Pre-enslavement

Treating and recovering from *Soufrans Ayisyen Syndrome* necessitates restructuring and realizing our reality and identity before enslavement. This process entails an immersive experience of our identity, the knowledge of self, so that we can become conscious of who we indeed are.

Ancestral Reconnection

To reconnect with our ancestors, we have to know who they were, including our African ancestors and our Haitian ancestors. Before we were Haitians infected by European ethos, we were Africans: Dahomians, Igbo, Nago, Hausa, Aja, Ewe, and Fon from West Africa (currently, Benin, Togo, and Nigeria) and BaKongo and Mandigo from Central Africa (currently, Angola and Kongo). We became Haitians and are today the sons and daughters of Africa. Part of reconnecting with our ancestors means knowing our African origins and our story before enslavement. Knowing which tribal groups, we are a part of would go a long way towards reconnecting with our ancestors and our current tribes, which would be a significant part of the collective healing.

Transforming the Collective/Individual

The Europeans' divide and conquer strategy continues to plague Haitians, along with class, race, and religion. This has created tremendous division among Haitians and has spawned an individualistic mentality and rampant materialism. This European axiology must be systematically dismantled to help bring us back to our true selves, our connection with the collective first. From that springs our individuality. Individually "successful" Haitians mean little if the Haitian collective is suffering from *Soufrans Ayisyen Syndrome*. If the Haitian collective is suffering, it reflects on individual Haitians. All of the negative stereotypes ascribed to being Haitians will continue to be imposed on individual Haitians and be their burden to carry regardless of personal success. Transforming Haitians as a collective necessitates planning and collaboration with Haitians who have the group's interest as their chief focus and collaborating with Haitians in Haiti and the diaspora.

Resiliency Then and Now

This content area essentially is about the fundamental question: Who were we? How did we cope with and overcome adversity? We were in harmony with nature and everything around us, both the seen and the unseen. We were stargazers, builders, architects, scientists, mathematicians, philosophers, priests, spirit beings, organizers, entrepreneurs, lovers of humanity, and family. We were profoundly conscious and present and fascinated students with stories about the universe and the seen and unseen realities of which we were a part. We were undaunted by the mysteries of the universe and thus created all manner of things that still astound the best European minds to this very day. Resiliency is in our genes; survival of enslavement and systemic disenfranchisement is evidence of our resiliency. Imagine who we would be and where we would be if European domination was0 lifted and our minds truly set free, decolonized. We are resilient.

CONCLUSION

The experience and concept of *Soufrans Ayisyen* arise out of a deliberate strategy and ruthless implementation of social, cultural, political, and economic practices designed to dominate Haitians completely. The results are the insertion of European values, epistemology, and logic systems into Haitian consciousness, causing a shattered consciousness, fractured identity, and alienation from the Haitian self/African ancestral spirit. The COVID-19 pandemic has further exacerbated *Soufrans Ayisyen* with dire physical consequences, social isolation, and economic hardship. An equal or greater determination—socially, culturally, politically, and economically—is necessary to decolonize the Haitian mind and practice appropriate behavior. The heightened awareness of racial injustice is an opportunity to hone this theory, create specific clinical applications, and heal *Soufrans Ayisyen* in solidarity with Pan African people and their allies.

REFERENCES

Aristide, J. (2016). *Haïti-Haitii? Philosophical reflections for mental health decolonization*. Routledge.

Baldwin, J. (2019, October 2). *Speech at the University of California, Berkley, 1979* [Video file]. YouTube. https://www.youtube.com/watch?v=cnh0pxOTvh8&ab_channel=NarrativeAfricaTV

Battalora, J. (2013). *Birth of a White nation: The invention of White people and its relevance totoday*. Strategic.

Bynum, E. (2012). *The African unconscious: Roots of ancient mysticism and modern psychology*. Cosimo Books.

Carroll, K. (2008). Africana studies and research methodology: Revisiting the centralityof the Afrikan worldview. *The Journal of Pan African Studies, 2*(2), 4–27.

Costa, D., Yetterb, N., & DeSomer, H. (2018). Intergenerational transmission of paternal trauma among US Civil War ex-POWs. *Proceedings of the National Academy of Sciences, 115*(44), 11215–11220.

Degruy. J. (2005). *Post traumatic slave syndrome*. Uptone Press.

Diangelo, R. (2018). *White fragility: Why it's so hard for White people to talk about racism.* Beacon Press.

Van Der Kolk, B. (2014). *The body keeps the score: Brain, mind, and body in the healing of trauma*. Penguin Books.

Dixon, V. (1971). African-oriented and Euro-American-oriented worldviews: Research methodologies and economics. *Review of Black Political Economy*, 7(2),119–156.

Dupuy, A. (2019). *Rethinking the Haitian revolution: Slavery, independence, and the struggle for recognition*. Rowman & Littlefield.

Etta E., & Offiong, A. (2019). The reality of African epistemology. *International Journal of Innovative Science, Engineering & Technology, 6*(10), 279–305.

Jimoh, A. (2017). An African theory of knowledge. In I. E. Ukpokolo (Ed.), *Themes, issues, and problems in African philosophy* (pp. 121–136). Palgrave Macmillan.

Jones-Rogers, S. (2019). *They were her property*. Yale University Press.

King, R. (1990). *African origin of biological psychiatry*. Afrikan World Books.

Nichols, E. (1986). Cultural foundations for teaching Black children. In *Teaching mathematics: Culture, motivation, history, and classroom management* (Vol 1, pp. 10–16. Institute for Independent Education.

Nobles, W. (2015). *The island of memes: Haiti's unfinished revolution*. Black Classic Press.

Zimmer, C. (2020, August 5). The famine ended 70 years ago, but Dutch genes still bear scars. *The New York Times*. https://www.nytimes.com/2018/01/31/science/dutch-famine-genes.html

CHAPTER 18

REIMAGINING *SOUFRANS AYISYEN* (HAITIAN SUFFERING)

Cultural and Clinical Narratives During the COVID-19 Pandemic

Pascale Denis, Elizabeth Louis, and Charlene Désir

Fèy, o! Sove lavi mwen. Nan mizè mwen ye, o!
(Oh leaves, save my life. I'm in misery. Oh!)

—Traditional Haïtian song

As Haitians, we narrate life through extraordinary songs, dances, and wisdom-filled proverbs so colorful that they also sing. Songs and proverbs about suffering abound including the traditional song above. These expressions of struggles are intertwined and point to ways of living and not just surviving. There is in Haiti an orally transmitted knowledge of plants, leaves, and their healing power and uses. Traditional medicine is used for everything, from headaches and lack of sleep to fertility issues, and now to address the ravages of COVID-19. Whether in Haiti or in the diasporic communities around the world, Haitian people share with each other their knowledge of this or that plant, and the many ways they can be

Coronavirus and Vulnerable People: Addressing the Divide in Harm and Responses and Exploring Implications for a More Peaceful World, pp. 293–310

used to cure their ailments. Psychologically, in a world filled with fear and uncertainties, Haitians and Haitian Americans, can turn to the familiar, to soothe themselves and regain some sense of agency. We connect with each other, remind ourselves of past recipes and in so doing recreate an internal landscape made up of memories, smells, sounds, and transmitted wisdom that can help us weather this frightening time. Akhtar (2011) speaks of the destabilizing effect for human beings when they experience what he calls the trauma of geographical dislocation. For Haitians and Haitian Americans in the United States, there is creative energy and repair in mobilizing ideas from the motherland, which then have a stabilizing effect. These can then help us regain a sense of competence, a gathering of our personal and communal strengths needed to face this new threat.

Hardships and how we overcome them play an important part in the way we build our identities; in the ways we understand ourselves and interact with the world. We are spoon fed, resist against, and/or resign ourselves to hardships. They seep through constantly, shaping and coloring our attempts at making sense of our lives. Speaking at the Haiti pavilion during the Chicago exposition in 1893, Frederick Douglas expressed admiration about the fact that Haiti still existed despite being boycotted by the entire Christian world. We have been, and continue to experience tremendous situations of sufferings, at home and in the United States, as recent immigrants, and as U.S. born citizens. Yet, we sing, we laugh, and fight, demanding a better life, a better future, for us and our families.

How are we to make sense of this *Soufrans Syisyen*? (Haitian Suffering) this seemingly "patat cho" or hot potato that we pass from generations to generations, from Haiti to all our diasporic homes? How does it inform this particular moment we are in? The purpose of this chapter is to explore the cultural and clinical narratives that inform the ways we live in the world, in Haiti and in our diasporic dwellings. We want to better understand that suffering, the space it takes in our lived experiences, and how it has and still informs who we are, hoping to free ourselves, to embody and intentionally cultivate our liberating stories and songs.

COVID-19- FEAR, ISOLATION, AND OPPORTUNITIES

The United States started addressing and enforcing measures to contain the COVID-19 pandemic later than other countries. Messages from elected officials, guidelines and recommendations were often confusing and erratic. The Black community in the United States is among those hit the hardest by the COVID-19 pandemic, in which they are three times more likely to die from the coronavirus than White Americans and have five times higher rates of hospitalization than non-Hispanic White people (Centers for Disease Control and Prevention, 2020; Pilkington, 2020). These morbid statistics are a consequence of the deep legacies of racism, systemic health disparities, and the broader social repercussions of pervasive racial injustice. One area that these injustices are evident is in the sharp disparities in health care. Early on, the disproportionate impact of the virus on minorities became clear creating even more fear and a sense of being left alone without a social safety net or a larger community of care. According to the Migration Policy Institute (2017), the Haitian diaspora in the United States comprises approximately 1.1 million individuals who were either born in Haiti or report Haitian ancestry. Haitians, as a subset of those minority groups, are heavily comprised of those called "essential workers," thus more exposed and witness to the devastating effects of the pandemic.

Psychosocial Effects of Stay Home Orders

The aloneness that one might feel as an immigrant and is constantly being negotiated to maintain a sense of identity, is now compounded with the forced isolation of COVID-19. Instead of being able to rely on the network they have built over time, they are now told that they need to socially distance, isolate from the very people that could help them weather this frightening moment. Families, especially the older members, if living alone, are cut off from their loved ones, their daily routines upended. Economic pressures, health and preexisting conditions and the risks they carry are now part of the everyday conversations, creating added anxiety and fear. In cases of death, people who could no longer rely on cultural rituals of mourning have been feeling guilty about their inability to fulfill their duties. In spite of that retreat into social distancing which came with the pandemic, and is now becoming the norm, people have found ways to meet virtually, reflect, and creatively address this moment. Haitian therapists are also providing therapeutic supports and engaged in conversations to support the growing mental health needs in the Haitian community.

Haitian Mental Health Think Tank

The Haitian Mental Health Think Tank was created during the COVID-19 pandemic. At the end of March 2020, in response to the growing mental health needs of Haitian clients due to loss, social isolation and fear, a group of Haitian and Haitian American mental health professionals from different disciplines including school, counseling, clinical psychology, mental health, social work, behavior analysis and conflict resolution met to develop a think tank to delve deeper and exam historical and cultural influences on

Haitian mental health. The context of shifting ways to approach therapy and mental health support during COVID-19 propelled us to go deeper into our practice and to use this opportunity to provide support to each other as therapists of Haitian descent and, more importantly, create a research lens to coconstruct knowledge about the cultural understandings of mental health within our community.

Our goal is to shift the narratives and ways of understanding as we work with trauma in the Haitian community. For example, as witnessed in past catastrophes in Haiti and in the United States (i.e., earthquake, Hurricanes Mathew and Katrina, school shootings, and other hate and gender-based violence, etc.), there is a mobilization of a service industry to address trauma, that works and makes money out of the consequences of trauma, and the suffering of others, while not addressing the root causes of those issues. The trauma is real but there is not an in-depth cultural lens to address and prevent additional traumas. Mental health intervention from abroad and created out of cultural and historical context of clients can be counterproductive for ethnic populations such as Haitians. There is money in global mental health interventionalists; often experts do not include local and cultural knowledge, and further, and then they often exclude root causes or local/cultural understandings of mental health and healing, particularly in the Haitian context.

The purpose of the Haitian Mental Health Think Tank is to ultimately integrate relevant clinical and behavioral interventions that are culturally based while integrating historical influences of generational trauma toward recovery and sustained mental wellness. It is imperative to create clinical healing models that highlight and promote resiliency and thriving communities of Black wellness. The Haitian Mental Health Think Tank is a space for therapists of Haitian descent to share, research, and develop successful practices and resources.

As the Haitian Mental Health Think Tank met, we began to foster the emergence of a different concept of suffering that was particular to a Haitian experience of being in the world and with each other. At the same time, we quickly became wary of not developing a concept that would be reductive. We wanted to remain aware of all-encompassing experiences or different expressions of what that suffering would and could mean to different subgroups, in age, in location, and both inter and intra generations. Thus, the concept of *Soufrans Ayisyen*—Haitian suffering emerged as relevant conceptual Haitian mental health framework.

CULTURAL NARRATIVES—MAKING SENSE OF *SOUFRANS AYISYEN*

For Haitians, in Haiti and in the diaspora, one of the lenses that we internally carry and through which we understand the everyday events of our lives is the concept of *Soufrans Ayisyen*.

Whether it be historically, as a consequence of the dehumanizing displacement of millions of enslaved Africans, or currently, due to their struggles in modern Haiti and in their diasporic homes, there are multiple layers and avenues of understanding *Soufrans Ayisyen* and the ways it has been resisted against. This section will first explore the ongoing presence in music and proverbs of *Soufrans Ayisyen* and its cultural narrative expression in its colonized context. It will then focus on its manifestation in stereotypes and the resulting distancing of people from each other. *Soufrans Ayisyen* will be also related to the continued societal violence of our present, in Haiti and in its diaspora. By highlighting their resilience and creative imagining of themselves as complex human beings, this section will argue throughout that Haitians and Haitian Americans have never stop resisting this idiosyncratic suffering.

Soufrans Ayisyen, a colonization of the mind, a foreign or secondary identity and the name Ayiti

Mwen malad m kouche m pa ka leve/ Palmannan o, m pa moun isit o.........

O Sàn o lamizè pa dous o, ago e / Lamizè pa dous o, ago e / M pwal chache lavi yon lòt kote o.

(I'm sick, I'm resting, I can't get up / Palmannan, I'm not of here.......

Oh spirits, misery is not sweet / I'm going to find life in another place)

In the song *Lamizè pa dous*, a traditional Haitian song, the singer voices *"m pa moun isit o,"* a reminder that we are not of here, a statement that resonates with the experiences of the Haitian people. It is a lyric that encapsulates the experience of displacement, that is, having been forcibly taken away from one's home and family, put as merchandise goods in ships where they were subjected to gruesome and murderous weeks of voyage through the middle passage, brought to, and bought for slave work in another land, one in which they would be subjected to the most cruel and demeaning life. The statement speaks to an ongoing, centuries long experience of suffering, one in which the enslaved experience of self was constantly confronted with a reality that wanted to force her/him into a perception of being subhuman. It also speaks to a refusal of what was the norm then, serving as a reminder of, and a longing for a "before" life. In singing it now, it also talks to a similar refusal of a life of misery. It points to a will for a better life, a better place, a better option, it points to a will to continue fighting. That experience of suffering mixed with a longing for, and internal knowing of a life elsewhere, the words and music that carry and transmit those experiences are just one of the specific ways that *Soufrans Ayisyen* colors how we know ourselves. This suffering and its accompanying resistance are expressed and used to make sense of our hardships, past and present. That resistance was enacted once in the uprising that resulted in our independence, and it continues to this day in the homeland and in the diasporic communities, in which pride of our traditions and cultures is still cultivated. Churches, Ounfò, vodou temples are such places, where this cultivation happens. Because of COVID-19, they had to close their doors, resulting in an added sense of loss for many, one that might reignite a deeper, underlying sense of suffering.

Another way of thinking of *Soufrans Ayisyen* is also in not owning the term, but writing it in its French version, *Souffrance*, as something that has to do with our circumstances, as people brought to Haiti, captured and enslaved, making Haiti the site of suffering, and not its inhabitants. One is reminded of Fanon's realization of his own "blackness" when faced with racism: "Look, a Negro." That experience felt alien to how he knew himself, an imposed gaze, whose understanding would then shape many of his experiences, his interactions, and his thinking. *Soufrans Ayisyen*, when experienced as imposed by the other/s, but not essential to one's identity, can be explored, held, questioned, in ways that can free spaces for the other experiences of selves that we carry. Yet, it remains, often forefront, reinforced by the ongoing difficulties, the obstacles of the making of a nation, of finding a common voice, a common project. There is work to be done in searching for another narrative, in developing awareness of all the ones we carry, while listening to, acknowledging, and making sense of that *Soufrans Ayisyen*. There is a need to reconnect with the different facets of who we are, while integrating the many ways our centuries long interactions and interdependence with that land, its language, sounds, its nature, have also shaped who we've become. One can wonder if the reappropriation of the Taïnos's name of the land, Ayiti, was not a first attempt at that, a reminder of a young nation's task of imagining itself as more than a gathering of suffering people, a reclaiming of the other "before" of the land, of its culture, creativity, models of being with its surroundings.

Is there then a place, alongside that particular suffering, for expansion and inclusion of those former experiences of selves, a space for reinhabiting, intentionally, a lived memory of our beings in Africa, the traditions and countries we have come from, their knowledge and wisdom? How do we appropriate/reappropriate a sense of self that was ours before arriving in Haiti, and is also made of our encounter with this land?

Internalized and Embodiment of *Soufrans Ayisyen*—Resilience, Liability, or Survival?

Is *Soufrans Ayisyen*, because of its pervasiveness, a perpetual, historic state, so embodied in us that it is showing up in all our experiences of life? Has it become so much part of our identity that we seem now to have become the image of it? In the news, and in stories, we continue to be described as the poorest country in the western hemisphere, the unmanageable country that cannot maintain political stability, one in constant need of international aid. Is our survival of this constant state of affairs a form of resilience? Or a forced identity that is maintained by the constant precarious state that we live with? Is our experiencing of *Soufrans Ayisyen* one that has been projected upon us and that we have internalized along the way?

The experiences of Black people have been and continue to be viewed in stereotypes, used as a way to dehumanize them. Even when some of those stereotypes are presented as positive qualities: The strong Black woman (*Fanm Djamn*) who can endure anything is an example of one which can serve as a way to distance, alienate, and not empathize with what is praised. "Black women, and black people don't experience pain as acutely, they can take it." There is a normalization of that suffering that is profoundly racist, and that allows for a continued viewing Black women as a spectacle, but not a situation that bothers or disrupts. This dehumanization functions psychologically as a way to constantly maintain the other in that sociopolitical space, one in which human rights do not apply the same way and allows for continued racist attacks whether overtly and/or subtly. There is then an experience of each other, of the other, that is informed by those views, which through time, have become part of our vocabulary.

Reductive single stories are created. Though some seem empowering, such as the resilience of Black women, the Haitian *Fanm Djanm*, they also carry hidden messages, like double edged swords that render that same woman, her pain, and her struggles, invisible. We praise and in doing so, we distance ourselves and we do not necessarily feel a commonality with what is narrated as extraordinary and extra human, disengaging us from feeling compassion and empathy, and taking action in our joint responsibility of participating and lightening the burden of that person who is seen as so strong.

Precarities, ongoing societal violence, that happen when conditions for basic needs are constantly not provided, result in physical and psychological suffering, only leaving space for surviving. People are in survival mode (fight, flight, or freeze). They hold on tightly to their idiosyncrasies, more than they do to their larger commonalities, because they need reassurance quickly in the face of danger, threat, and abandonment. In situations of threat, both physical and emotional, they reach for ways to regain homeostasis and soothe themselves. Familiarity is a great way to do so, and bonding against a singular enemy, more manageable than the overpowering systemic one, gives back agency. We are no longer thinking, just reacting, wanting to feel better. Because those conditions are ongoing, there is no longer space for an evolving story of ourselves, of a learning of new adaptive ways of being in the times we live in. We are, as Christina Sharpe (2016) says, "encountering a past that is not past" (p. 13). The story of the "Men anpil chay pa lou, many hands make the burden light" gets lost in that context. Connecting, netting all our stories together, creating a complex narrative is a task of every moment, if we are to move away from just surviving.

Human beings exist in community and through community. Ubuntu is an African philosophical concept that expresses our interconnection and interdependence, in an essential way, that a person is a person through other people. "I am, because you are." We build our identities and sense of selves in community, and more so in communities of care, ones that let us know that we matter. We are, in those communities of care, seen as complex persons, whose experiences take place inside a body of knowledge, of skills, and of beliefs that inform what we know about life, and inform the ways we know to survive and thrive in this life. But we also carry pain and trauma that have been transmitted intergenerationally and that inform who we are in non-verbal ways. We often act our lives and interact with others without a conscious awareness of what is being played out in our relationships, or in our expectations of ourselves and/or our communities.

Those communities are also made of our governments, laws, and societal arrangements. In societies that do not create the conditions for the institution and implementation of care for their citizens, there is precarity, an absence of a holding and an absence of an acknowledgement of all as equal contributors to a common goal and purpose. There is divisiveness and othering, a disdain and plain abandonment; the usage of the majority by a minority, leaving very few spaces for breathing, belonging, let alone expansion. Distrust is now the norm; stereotypes, fixed views of self and others abound, all becoming sources of suffering, of *Soufrans Ayisyen*. Those views get shared over and across time, from one generation to the next. Overtime, and even when removed from some of those situations of trauma and nonrecognition, we know ourselves, understand and transmit stories of our identity, with past data, are more often than not in a "frozen Present"

(Browne, 2017).[1] Though some of these narratives have been sources of resilience, survivorship, and resistance, they are also sources of rigidity.

A major form of resistance to slavery, in Haiti and elsewhere, known as *marronage*, developed as an applied practice born from a profound need for freedom. It has also become the way that we shield ourselves away from real and perceived sources of subjugation, of exploitation, and it informs how we view others. It requires vigilance that can result into a lessened experience of relating to, and counting on, one another. *Marronage* demands and nurtures an intelligent understanding of one's physical and social environment, and of one's ability to survive in it. This understanding is a strength but also entertains and reinforces. In a larger community in which there is such lack of care, a suspicion of the other, before solidifies a certain way of being in life. Though a creative, lifesaving way to escape an experience of suffering and its resulting psychological impact, it lingers in people's psyche as a mode of surviving the present, one in which the endangerment of the citizens is very real.

"Depi nan Ginen, nèg rayi nèg—Since Guinea, since time immemorial, man has hated man" is another one of those truths that are transmitted intergenerationally to explain the mistrust and animosity that can show up in between subgroups of Haitian people. Differences are pointed to, focused on, as a displacement and a way to make sense of the precarity and the violence of the environment. Others' differences are used to alleviate powerlessness. Those "truths," those sayings, are used to move anxiety and threat away from the structural societal violence that continues its attack on the body and mind of the majority, restoring an illusory sense of agency, even if for a short period of time. From those shared, ongoing experiences of lacking, narratives emerge that provide meaning making views, albeit maladaptive ones, of life.

As Haitians and Haitian Americans, we have survived, and continue to survive tremendous hardships. *Soufrans Ayisyen* is one of the ways we know ourselves, experience our lives. It is nonetheless not the only way we exist. In the midst of precarity, there is constant bustling, a communal life celebrated with laughter, music, storytelling, and a presence to loved ones, all in the absence of societal care. Joy is present, close, and never excluded of our everyday lives. Precarity, and the ongoing experience of life as suffering, seem to have accentuated the preciousness of every moment. People have learned to live with suffering and death. Yet, they narrate an existence in which joy is cultivated, one in which every moment counts. Numerous stories of individual successes are shared, sources of pride and perseverance that are partly rooted in the rallying of forces and strengths of families and smaller groups. However, our larger communities are disjointed, unable to reach across for a greater goal, a common dream, one in which we can see and bear witness for each other. "Men anpil chay pa lou" one of our most famous proverbs, a testament of our wisdom, and an indication of a way forward, has started to sound empty. We need a new dream, one that pays homage to our struggles, our strengths, and that also acknowledges and faces the causes.

Volkan's (1997) concepts of chosen glory and chosen trauma are tools that can help us acknowledge and work with our internalized, fundamental, basic assumptions. Chosen glories (e.g., the first Black republic of the world, the only successful slave revolt in history…) are sources of self-esteem, cultural and psychological sources of pride about a common past history. The group feels pride when narrating their chosen glory. Chosen glories do not burden the next generation with unfinished, unresolved psychological tasks, as do chosen traumas. Chosen traumas are narratives about massive traumas that continue to be experienced as sources of helplessness and humiliation. They inform the identity of groups, enhancing their sense of belonging, and are often experienced as an us-them feeling that gets easily exploited in the absence of spaces of healing in which the trauma can be addressed. When those traumas are not addressed and processed, they are passed to the next generation, becoming transgenerational unresolved tasks.

Immigrant people of color live a precarious life. Although Haitians in their homeland live a difficult life, they are nested in their social surroundings and network. Though their bodies suffer from diseases and economic hardships, their souls are not always experiencing precarity. They still have access internally, and in community, to a larger repertoire of stories, of ways of being. They construct meanings that are colored by this *Soufrans Ayisyen*, told through the songs, the lessons, and expectations that they share with their family and loved ones, but they do so with and as part of their communities, ones that also offer solace and support, spaces to embed those meanings into a larger understanding of life. Haitian Americans' social networks no longer exist in the same way, whether in their adoptive country, or back home, once they have left for a fantasized dream of a better world. Dr. Annie Lee Jones writes, in an essay published in 2016, that for some Black immigrants, the encounter with "the plague of American racism based on skin color" is particularly traumatic and leaves them with little hope. Once confronted with a different, often hostile reality, they must mobilize all sorts of resources to make a dignified life for themselves and their families, while mourning their losses. Their unresolved legacy of trauma, of *Soufrans Ayisyen*, continues to color theirs and their children's experiences in a context in which their community of care is not as strong, is less accessible.

Transgenerational Differences, Racism, and *Soufrans Ayisyen*

Haitian Americans live with ambivalent messages; with parents, caregiver or families who are not entirely here, longing and finding purpose in an absent, longed for homeland that they cannot experience as viscerally (Bibb & Casimir 1996). Haiti, its history, myths (Chosen Glory) can be both that source of pride while also the site of resentment for what can never be enough in their own places of birth. There remains a silent space between them and their loved ones, memories that they will never share, can only join in vicariously, and can never really know. They cannot console, soothe the sadness of what they have not caused. They also carry a sense of suffering that, if not explored, talked about, remains an unknown part of themselves, that can be triggered, an inherited frozen present. Their developmental task of individuation and separation is more difficult, complicated by both verbal and nonverbal clues that they keep misreading, is not significantly attended to. Kirkland C. Vaughans (2017) reminds us that according to Volkan (1997) "children can become the reservoir for unresolved mental representations of the trauma of previous generations who have been unable to come to terms with issues of humiliation and loss."

Young and U.S.-born Haitian Americans grow up in a different culture than that of their parents, caregivers, and family members, often relating more to the one they live, and can be made to feel that they are no longer Haitian. This ambivalence of identity can at times feel disjointed given the ethnic and racial identity development first- and second-generation Haitian Americans wrestle with. Historically, the notions of identity in the form of race and ethnicity have theorized by African American psychologists such as Cross (1995), Helms (1990), Berry et al. (2006), and Phinney et al. (2006). Perspectives on models of racial identity have attempted to compass this trajectory within different internal phases that one has to confront directly or indirectly. These models of identity usually have a sphere of preferred attainment to achieve some form of internal equilibrium or wholeness. It is difficult to pinpoint which model best represents the lived experiences of first- and second-generation Haitians, yet these frameworks along with ones that address ethnicity and culture can assist Haitian Americans in their pursuit of affirming and reimagining what their identity is within the American context and beyond. For example, according to Berry et al., the ethnic minority identity development model includes assimilation, separation, marginalization, and integration. Each of these categories may or may not be stagnant but fluid depending on the awareness, knowledge, understanding and meaning making that Haitian Americans are brought into while residing in the United States. While

Berry et al. argues that the last stage is integration, which encompass valuing and integrating one's culture and the majority culture, they may not resonate with many Haitian Americans. Given the ongoing pandemics of racism and COVID-19, the shift in positionality and reckoning with how Haitians and Haitian Americans fit into this current wave of antiracism and anti-Blackness, integration may not be as balanced as one may pursue.

The shifting of self-awareness emerges at different periods in one's life. Whether it is from the major sacred settings of home, religious/spiritual space, and school for Haitian culture or from other environments within and outside of the United States, Haitian Americans are constantly faced with choices to prove or disprove perceptions placed upon themselves by society or others (Sue & Sue, 2013). For many Haitian Americans attending schools, it was common to hear descriptions of your people by other Black racial/ethnic minorities with phrases such as "boat people," "Vodou," "AIDS carrier." During the formative years of development, Haitian American youth have to constantly assert their Blackness and sometimes have to choose if they will be African American or Haitian American or Black American, depending on the day and context. Reliance on parents, caregivers, and family members to assist with this journey of self-discovery, self-restoration and self-preservation was at time futile due to their own wrestles and entanglements that they were also facing.

The moment of self-realization of belonging within the Haitian narrative can be at times an oxymoronic experience in which one feels part of this group yet also feels lost or criticized due to not fully embodying what it means to be Haitian minus the hyphenation of American. Being Haitian for Haitian Americans can mean different things depending on the generation. For example, language is a significant aspect of Haitian culture and when Haitian Americans can either understand but not speak or speak but with an American or diasporic accent, they can at times be shunned, made to feel embarrassed or deemed to be not Haitian enough. Other forms of these test of Haitianess can be in the form of knowledge of Haitian traditions, visiting/living in Haiti, proper usage of proverbs, writing Haitian Creole, and knowing how to cook different Haitian cuisines. These are all some form of cultural staples or recognition that Haitians check off to assess how Haitian may be. Yet, there are some in the first and second generation who proudly and authentically represent what it means to be Haiti within their own sense of knowing, regardless of if it may not fit a particular cultural imprint.

The COVID-19 pandemic has revealed many challenges intergenerationally and first- and second-generation Haitian Americans have not been excluded from experiencing them given the pandemic of racism and growing up Black in America. These racial disparities and antiracism movements have intersected and further revealed where Haitian Americans footprints lie in this juncture of yet another uprising. We have accompanied our fellow African American sisters and brothers and support them during this collective *soufrans*. The *soufrans* of the younger generation of Haitian Americans seems to coincide more fluidly or more overtly in tangent with the experiences of other Black Americans more so than with the *soufrans* of Haitians in Haiti. There are multitude of reasons for why movements such as Black Lives Matter unconsciously engaged more Haitian Americans than movements against corruption and injustice in Haiti. Could it be that the *Soufrans Ayisyen* that is occurring in Haiti is more detached and geographically out of reach to the younger Haitian Americans and the stories of their parents, caregivers, and the media portrayal of this form of soufrans is enough to paint a picture but not engage in this collective experience? Or could it be that there are new layers and elements of *Soufrans Ayisyen* that the younger generations of Haitian Americans are schooling us and consciously living out the soufrans of the past in the present, intertwined with similar principles of soufrans. The Haitian American youth of the present day reflect the images, patterns, behaviors, consciousness, and spirit of yesterday's past *soufrans*.

> "To accept one's past—one's history—is not the same thing as drowning in it; it is learning how to use it."
>
> —James Baldwin, *The Fire Next Time* (1963)

Narratives are complex, emotional, and often contradictory. They are charged with meanings that are experienced viscerally, experienced as true, whether consistent with, or regardless of, the lived external realities. We inhabit physical spaces that have been and continue to be challenging, in Haiti, in the U.S. as immigrants, and with now the added reality of fighting a lethal virus. We also inhabit the psychological spaces that enable us to make sense of them.

Narratives are frames inside of which we construct our views of ourselves, of others and of the world in which we live. They inform our understandings of our past, influence our interpretation of our present and how we imagine our future. They are the building blocks of those meaning making structures, inherited hauntings from an unresolved past, being reworked continuously in the lives that we are making. How do we pay attention to, grow an awareness of, the hauntings we carry, those stories that shape us and the many ways we continuously rewrite and celebrate our lives?

CLINICAL NARRATIVES AND EMERGING MENTAL HEALTH CONSIDERATIONS

In working therapeutically with *Soufrans Ayisyen*, embracing its multiple facets, we can both honor our resilience, our creativity, and intentionally let go of what is no longer serving us. In therapy, we can hold the spaces in which the hauntings that we carry can be acknowledged, and relief can be provided. In discussing and validating the social realm in which their suffering is embedded, we, as therapists, can engage in conversations in which individuals can feel heard about real external hardships, while also working at recognizing narratives that they carry, ones that they might unintentionally act out, reclaim ones that can strengthen their senses of selves, free them to start imagining and better align with the lives they want (Nicolas et al., 2006).

The therapist remains curious, not jumping to conclusions or preconceived ideas. The British psychoanalyst Wilfred Bion's (1984) concept of negative capability comes to mind, a capacity to hold uncertainty, not rushing to offer interpretations, keeping an open mind even in moments when both therapist and patient feel challenged (Bion, 1984). The therapist will at times let the patient guide her/him, working at opening thinking in a manner to include what might not be immediately inscribed in a concrete reality, as opposed to only operating within a structuralist epistemology. By opening spaces of exploration, of questioning of their lived experience, both internal and external, therapist and client can work at freeing, liberating, and cocreating new versions of their identities. The following are approaches which members of the Haitian Mental Health Think Tank have or are exploring to incorporate in their clinical work with Haitian clients to recognize and explore cultural relevant practices toward healing *Soufrans Ayisyen*.

Social Dreaming Groups

Social dreaming matrices (SDM) focus on the social aspect of dreams, as those dreams can help understand the processes at play in groups and in societies at large. The dreams, not the dreamers, are the focus. The working hypothesis is that dreams shared reflect a collective cultural experience, a social unconscious made of social, political, and cultural experiences, that have been dissociated. For George Bermudez (2018) social dreaming matrix groups are spaces in which members participate in communal dream sharing. Those dreams' social meanings are made visible when shared and discussed. Themes that have been identified by all can then be processed and worked through.

Working with dreams might resonate well culturally. Dreams, as messages from the spiritual realm, the ancestors, are embedded in the traditional Haitian culture, and might also serve as a bridge to engaging those places of tension and distrust, or of nonattunement. They might allow for the unthought knowns, the emergence of what is often held in silence. Dreams are personal and intimate. Common goals or approaches might emerge, and when experienced as coming from their own minds, might feel as ones that they have ownership over, which might allow for the imagining of alternate narratives. Some of the social dreaming group assumptions are that the dreams shared can help elaborate new thoughts about systems, organizations, that the participants might be involved in reworking cultural scripts and deep-seated convictions. Other times, shared dreams might help a particular individual use the content of the dreams towards a social role that she/he might be struggling with.

Hypnosis

Hypnosis is rooted in Kemetic spiritual sciences and is merely a small aspect of the sacred sciences of Kemet (Ashby, 2002). King (2012) in *African Origin of Biological Psychiatry* argues convincingly, as do many others that there is a well-established history of physiology and psychology in African cosmology and the spiritual sciences. Breath is central in hypnosis as it represents a conscious observing and appreciating of miracle of life. Incorporating the idea with clients is a way of demonstrating how their bodies are supposed to be sustained and care for. Incorporating breathing exercises in therapy through hypnosis, assist uncovering intrusive thoughts and behavior to help bring them under control. A simple yet effective way of introducing hypnosis is to ask a client to consider the times that their mind operates independently of their conscious awareness. People instantly recognize that the mind has the capacity of functioning on multiple levels and that they can have such profound experiences and still remain in control. Hypnosis, in effect, is utilizing the senses as portals into the subconscious or accessing our intuition which functions on a metaphysical level.

Drumming

Drumming (Fleurant, 1996) is one of the few forms of music that is easily accessible to almost anyone. The resounding effect is that one is instantly connected with ancestors who have been struck by the drum in the very same way as you will experience. The expression of pain and pleasure are all there for you to explore as you play the drum. You and the drum create something like a fingerprint, the sound you create is unique to you and can never be replicated by anyone else. It is your song of the heart, the music of your soul an offering to the universe to take your grief or gratitude into the heavens. Within five minutes of engaging in drumming you access an alternative form of expression. Nonverbal expressions are fundamental existence and deeply healing. Sometimes there are no words to express *soufrans*/suffering in therapy, but one can create rhythm for it. To express an emotion is to move it along from our inner being and into the universe, it is a prayer without words. As we are able to express and release emotions, we make room for new ones. Drumming can help find creativity, healing, and transcendence for those in clinical treatment.

CONCLUSION

COVID-19 has acutely reminded us of our human fragility, made us aware that we are all in this together and has given us an opportunity to reexamine one of our most enduring narratives. We have a chance to dream together in another way to create a larger more inclusive community. One that can tackle the immense task of creating a space of care, inside and outside the boundaries of Haiti, a community in which we can all thrive and feel safe. The Haitian Mental Health Think Tank, in integrating health professionals from different perspectives and specializations, is itself an experiment of such inclusiveness toward Pan African wellness. For example, the first author of this chapter, Pascale Denis was a psychiatrist in Haiti, where she worked for more than ten years, identifies as Haitian and now works as a mental health therapist in the United States. The other two authors identify as Haitian American. Elizabeth Louis was born in the United States, is a counseling psychologist who has worked in Haiti, United States, and Rwanda. Charlene Désir was born in Haiti migrated at a young age to the U.S. and is a trained school psychologist and researcher. The Haitian Mental Health Think Tank is a container for weaving community narratives with clinical narratives and interventions to evolve both concepts utilizing emerging frameworks such as *Soufrans Ayisyen* that are relevant to the Haitian community. Fundamentally, weaving these fabrics together forms a foundation for revolution—changing the social conditions of racism and White supremacy while recognizing and centering self/group care for Haitian mental health practitioners. Based on the emerging experiences of *Soufrans Ayisyen* during COVID-19, Haitian American mental health practitioners are weaving cultural and clinical narratives to sing a new song and illuminate new spaces and ways of liberation.

REFERENCES

Akhtar, S. (2014). *Immigration and acculturation: Mourning, adaptation, and the next generation*. Rowman & Littlefield.

Ashby, M. (2002). *The African origins: Book I–Part 1. African origins of African civilization, religion, yoga mysticism and ethics and philosophy*. Cruzian Mystic Books/ Sema Institute of Yoga.

Baldwin, J. (1963). *The fire next time*. Modern Library.

Bermudez, G. (2018). The social dreaming matrix as a container for the processing of implicit racial bias and collective racial trauma. *International Journal of Group Psychotherapy, 68*(4), 538–560.

Berry, J., Phinney, J., Sam, D., & Vedder, P. (2006). Immigrant youth: Acculturation, identity, and adaptation. *Applied Psychology, 55*(3), 303–332.

Bibb, A., & Casimir, G. (1996). Haitian families. In M. McGoldrick, J. Giodano, & J. K. Pearce (Eds.), Ethnicity & family therapy (pp. 97–111). Guilford.

Bion, W. (1984). *Attention and interpretation*. Karnac Books.

Centers for Disease Control and Prevention. (2019). *COVID-19 in racial and ethnic minority groups*. https://www.cdc.gov/coronavirus/2019-ncov/need-extra-precautions/racial-ethnic-minorities.html

Cross W., Jr. (1995). The psychology of Nigrescence: Revising the Cross model. In J. Ponterotto, M. Casas, L. Suzuki, & C. Alexander (Eds.). *Handbook of multicultural counseling* (pp. 93–122). SAGE.

Helms, J. (1990). *Black and White racial identity: Theory, research, and practice*. Greenwood Press.

Ivor Browne: The Frozen Present. (2017, April 1). *Network Ireland, 100*. https://networkmagazine.ie/articles/ivor-browne-frozen-present

Fleurant, G. (1996). *Dancing spirits: Rhythms and rituals of Haitian vodun, the rada rite*. Praeger.

Jones, A. (2016). Relational dynamics of loss, grief and fear in everyday lives of African-American women. *American Psychoanalyst, 50*(3), 1.

King, R. (2012). *African origin of biological psychiatry*. Afrikan World Books.

Migration Policy Institute. (2017, August 2). *Haitian immigrants in the United States*. https://www.migrationpolicy.org/article/haitian-immigrants-united-states-2015

Nicolas, G., DeSilva, A. M., Grey, K. S., & Gonzalez-Eastep, D. (2006). Using a multicultural lens to understand illnesses among Haitians living in America. *Professional Psychology, Research, and Practice, 37*, 702–707

Phinney, J., Horenczyk, G., Liebkind, K., & Vedder, P. (2006). Ethnic identity, immigration, and well-being: An interactional perspective. *Journal of Social Issues, 57*(3), 493–510.

Pilkington, E. (2020, May 20). Black Americans dying of Covid-19 at three times the rate of White people. *The Guardian*. https://www.theguardian.com/world/2020/may/20/black-americans-death-rate-covid-19-coronavirus

Sharpe, C. (2016). *In the wake: On Blackness and being*. Duke University Press.

Sue, D., & Sue, D. (2013). *Counseling the culturally diverse: Theory and practice* (6th ed.). John Wiley & Sons.

Vaughans, K. (2017). To unchain haunting blood memories: Intergenerational trauma among African Americans. In J. Salberg & S. Grand (Eds.), *Wounds of history*. Routledge.

Volkan V. (1997). *From ethnic pride to ethnic terrorism*. Farrar, Straus & Giroux.

NOTE

1. "Once that shut down happens, then that experience is frozen. So it is not a case of a threatening memory being repressed, it is that it has never gotten in properly. Once it is frozen it is outside of time, so twenty years later this can be activated some everyday event can trigger it—and you then experience it as if it is happening now. You don't think about it and remember it—you feel it and experience it. And of course at that point you think you are going nuts because you look around and nothing traumatic is happening, yet you experience this traumatic feeling. That is why I called it 'the frozen present,' because when it comes, it comes through as the present, not as the past" ("Ivor Browne: The Frozen Present," 2017).

CHAPTER 19

VULNERABLE POPULATIONS AND COVID-19

The Challenges of Black, Brown, Indigenous People of Color and the Poor During a 100-Year Pandemic

Ruban Roberts

INTRODUCTION

Since March 2020, in the wake of the COVID-19 pandemic, the global society has adopted to—with varying degrees of acceptance—what has been referred to as "the new normal." Within a month of the first cases being diagnosed, the United States government hesitantly issued stay-at-home orders to "slow the spread." However, the unexpected consequences of these preventative orders soon revealed what many already knew and even more perhaps suspected: large swaths of Black, Brown, Indigenous, and poor populations were affected disproportionately by the virus for wildly varied reasons ranging from health to technology. What was known or suspected had previously been revealed during U.S. disasters like Hurricane Katrina in 2005, which raged through New Orleans and crippled its predominantly Black-populated 9th Ward. The aftermath of Katrina's destruction put a

Coronavirus and Vulnerable People: Addressing the Divide in Harm and Responses and Exploring Implications for a More Peaceful World, pp. 311–325

fine point on a population that can be described as "working poor." Slow government response exacerbated issues within the community that existed well before the storm. Fifteen years later, they are still felt. The storm's scars are still clearly visible, even though now many blocks show the inevitable signs of gentrification. Katrina revealed the inequities experienced by the poor, and specifically, that poor Blacks were especially vulnerable in times of disaster. Still, it appears that no real panacea was put in place to deal with future disasters. The stay-at-home orders instituted to slow the spread of COVID-19 only served to highlight how this country continues to underserve Black, brown, indigenous, and poor populations.

In the relatively short history of this country, class inequities have been commonplace though rarely honestly addressed, as the gap between the wealthy and the poor is considered a necessary ingredient of the American fable—where individuals with indefatigable pluck and perseverance can traverse the gap from poor to rich. That is the American way. Therefore, discussions about the overwhelming disparities found in poor communities are relegated to political talking points and locked in bureaucratic systems' wastelands. The spread of the U.S.'s COVID-19 virus reveals the stark reality and near-insurmountable numbers of underserved communities. When initial stay-at-home orders were issued, this country was not prepared to have the wealth gap listed as a contributing factor to the spread of the virus among communities of color. How could it? Stay-at-home orders for the middle class and wealthy Americans meant something quite different from those same orders for Black, Brown, Indigenous, poor, and working poor communities. In these communities, stay-at-home orders meant individuals sheltering in homes that housed multiple generations and extended family, living in communities where maintaining advisable "social distance" is not possible, or working in an industry or position considered "essential" where attendance is mandatory.

> There are a lot of theories why Blacks are dying at higher rates than other races during this pandemic," says Fares Qeadan, Ph.D., a U of U Health biostatistician and senior author of the study. "However, our descriptive study strongly suggests that Blacks are not dying from COVID-19 because they are genetically more susceptible, have more comorbidities, or aren't taking the necessary precautions. Instead, it is likely because they are working in jobs where they have a greater risk of coming in contact with the virus day in and day out. "The "efficiency" of the virus was discovered early in the pandemic, but the efficiency with which it affected communities of color was underestimated when stay-at-home orders were issued. (University of Utah Health Sciences, 2020)

One interesting factor regarding policymaking that is too often overlooked is that it stems from the policymakers' personal viewpoints and experiences.

It is not surprising that Black, Indigenous, and People of Color (BIPOC) and poor communities were not at the top of policymakers' minds when stay-at-home orders were enacted. This is not to say that these orders were in error but to point out that policymakers did not offer sufficient guidance for BIPOC and poor communities to navigate the pandemic safely. Considering the differences that BIPOC and poor communities navigate daily, the pandemic further highlighted disparities with regards to health, social justice, finances, and mental health.

As a country, we are now navigating the phased reopening of the economy across the country. The frontline workers widely praised have been primarily first responders: nurses, doctors, emergency medical technicians, police officers, and the like. Little recognition has been paid to those working at grocery stores, gas stations, big box stores, the post office, other delivery services, and wage workers with little choice but to be in the workplace during stay-at-home orders. These workers are made up primarily of BIPOC and the poor. Like first responders, they have been on the front lines of exposure and suffer more deeply than any other due to these myriad issues affecting their community.

The spread of the COVID-19 virus took the world by storm and required international cooperation, including instituting "social distancing" and stay-at-home measures. In the United States, the concept of social distancing is considered a draconian measure in some circles, but it is particularly foreign to many marginalized populations that reside in densely populated communities—particularly for BIPOC and poor populations with limited resources. In these communities, social connection and interaction are vitally important and provide a form of social capital and enable people to have pride and functionality. BIPOC neighborhoods tend to be densely populated. Prior to the COVID-19 outbreak, one would find groups of people gathered on the front porch or stoop or at local parks, recreational centers playing sports, or frequenting cafes, bars, restaurants, or local sporting events. The "new normal" we are all forced to adjust to is another factor that will leave scars on these communities for generations to come, le Hurricane Katrina. To understand why people in these groups have been disproportionately affected by what would appear to be a simple stay-at-home order, it is necessary to delve deeper into how they became vulnerable in the first place.

HEALTH DISPARITY AND DISPROPORTIONALITY IN VULNERABLE POPULATIONS

According to the 2010 U.S. Census, approximately 36.3% of the population consists of a racial or ethnic minority group: American Indian or Alaska

Native, Asian American, Black or African American, Hispanic/Latinx, and Native Hawaiian or other Pacific Islander (Grief & Miller, 2017). In the United States, ethnic and minority groups have markedly greater instances of chronic disease and premature death compared with their White counterparts. We find that as socioeconomic status rises, chronic disease and premature death decreases. There are several contributing factors to higher rates of disease discussed in an insightful article written for *The Annual Review of Public Health*. Authors Gary W. Evans and Elyse Kantrowitz argued that the apparent link between income and health arrive at the confluence of

> a plethora of suboptimal environmental conditions ... (and) the poor are most likely to be exposed not only to the worst air quality, the most noise, the lowest-quality housing, and schools, etc. but of particular consequence, also to lower-quality environments on a wide array of multiple dimensions. (Evans & Kantrowitz, 2002)

Before the COVID-19 pandemic, health inequities found amongst racial and ethnic lines were widespread but discussion of them was typically relegated to polarizing political debates about universal healthcare. In the end, not shockingly, little public policy addressed the dearth of adequate healthcare for populations in lower socioeconomic strata, thereby leaving millions of Americans with little defense against the eventual outbreak of COVID-19. There are few recorded instances in our country's history when socioeconomic disparities related to health have been revealed as starkly as they have since this pandemic. As mentioned earlier in this chapter, BIPOC and poor people have long suffered from ailments specifically linked to their socioeconomic position. There is well-documented demographic evidence of the higher prevalence of diabetes, high blood pressure, asthma, obesity, and other chronic diseases in BIPOC and poor communities compared to their middle-class neighbors. Figure 18.1 illustrates a survey conducted that shows higher reported asthma and diabetes rates among Black, Native American, Hispanic, and Hawaiian/Pacific Islanders. Immunocompromised individuals with chronic comorbidities find themselves at the mercy of this new threat, and with multiple contributing factors at play, there is little wonder that the novel coronavirus had a swift and devastating impact on these communities nationwide.

In examining this clear and present danger to our most vulnerable citizens, we must first address the illnesses that provide fertile ground for diseases like COVID-19 to have a devastating effect. If we are to protect the most vulnerable people from the spread of the virus, we must also address the pervasive, underlying health problems that are commonplace within their population.

Figure 18.1

Percent of Nonelderly Adults with Selected Health Conditions by Race/Ethnicity, 2018

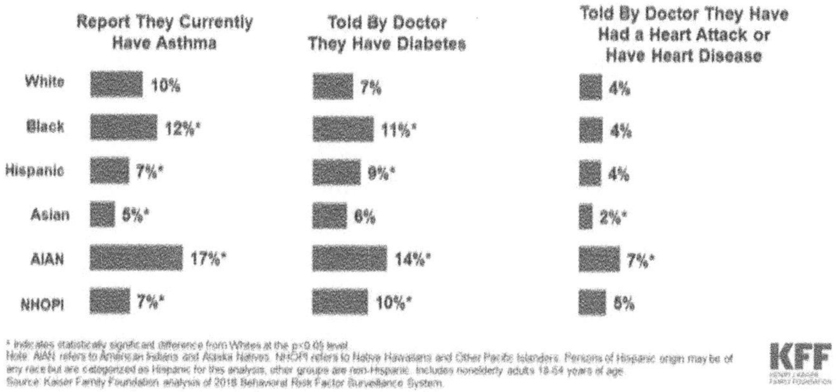

Race/Ethnicity, 2018.

Kaiser Family Foundations (2020).

As noted in the Evans and Katrowitz (2002) article, there is a correlation between crowded housing conditions, below average municipal services, access to quality food and health services, and constant exposure to high-stress environments to the chronic health issues found in underserved areas. BIPOC and poor individuals living in crowded areas and working low wage jobs that have been labeled "essential" places these people at further risk given their propensity to have underlying health issues known to increase the likelihood of COVID-19 related hospitalization, if not mortality.

The correlation between poor health and socioeconomic status is clear; however, COVID-19 did not cause the problem, the virus exploited it. Generations of BIPOC and the poor have long subsisted on easy access foods with low nutritional value, and the results have shown a predictable line drawn across racial and ethnic lines for heart disease, hypertension, diabetes, obesity, asthma, and other chronic illnesses. People living in more impoverished communities are offered few healthy options in these "food deserts," as fresh, affordable food options are few and far between and younger generations have been raised on a diet of easy access, low nutritional value foods high in artificial sweeteners, salt, and trans fats. Now, imagine being forced to shelter in place with a small budget for food. The most easily accessible, affordable foods are unhealthy, and there is a virus that preys on people with diabetes and hypertension. Over the last five months, the virus has forced many to make choices about their overall health, and many are demanding that the government do a better job to ensure food equity. Unfortunately, this is precisely the type of dilemma vulnerable populations have—feed their families what is available and affordable or invest in more expensive, healthy foods that over stretch their budgets. We must ask our government officials to take a harder look at the underlying factors contributing to increased numbers of BIPOC succumbing to the virus. It is well-known that high salt and sugar content in food consumed by vulnerable populations leads to diagnoses of comorbid illnesses, which have been painfully exploited by the COVID-19 pandemic. The fact is that poor and working poor families rely on our government to legislate and regulate funding and laws on their behalf; therefore, governing agencies like the FDA may have to reconsider policies regarding food additives and look at reallocation of government agriculture surpluses to vulnerable populations. In addition, there is a need for preventative health care and education in these communities to aid in preventing deaths from COVID-19 or the next pandemic caused by comorbid illnesses.

Adding to the stressors resulting from comorbid illnesses, "social distancing" requirements are complex for BIPOC and poor populations. These measures represent "a bridge too far" because BIPOC and poor populations tend to live in smaller homes that house multiple generations or reside in housing projects with narrow hallways or small elevators. Simply put, these folks live and breathe where finding a consistent "six feet of separation" may as well be like finding a mile. In these same living situations, many inhabitants—considered essential workers—do not have space to allocate "clean rooms" to safely disinfect before coming into contact with others in the home. At this point, we have all heard the anecdotal stories of families and friends gathering at celebrations, then reporting multiple cases of contracting the virus afterward. Suppose we can easily find cases where multiple family members contracted the virus after a Memorial Day barbecue. In that case, we must understand the complete devastation that the virus causes for individuals forced to live in close quarters over several months. In living situations where maintaining a safe distance is simply impossible, there is little wonder that the virus has affected these communities far more swiftly than others across the country. The coauthor of a University of Utah study, Charles R. Rogers, PhD, an assistant professor of public health, stated, "Black essential workers could be bringing the disease home from work and inadvertently spreading it among their family members—especially considering some Blacks live in multi-generational, high-density housing" (University of Utah Health Sciences, 2020).

In addition to the Centers for Disease Control's (CDC) main recommendations to maintain social distance, use masks, and disinfect regularly, the CDC has also recommended testing as a means of slowing the spread of the virus. Here again is another area where the recommendations have not fully considered the ramifications of systemic classism and racism. Early on in our country's lockdown, the president claimed, "Anybody that wants a test can get a test. That's what the bottom line is" (WhiteHouse.gov, 2020).

It did not take long to realize that there was an actual shortage of tests which required authorities to limit those that received them.

> Testing has hobbled the American response since the earliest days of the pandemic. As our reporting revealed, the U.S. had tested fewer than 3,000 people for the coronavirus by March 5, even though the virus's community spread had been detected more than a week earlier. In the following weeks, states and hospitals rationed access to tests, granting them only healthcare workers and the sickest patients. This meant that many people who may have had the virus, especially in the Northeast, were never tested for it. (Madrigal & Meyer, 2020)

We have seen municipalities work to allocate testing sites to underserved communities by enacting walk-up sites in addition to drive-through testing sites. At sites in these areas, a number of tests were allocated for individuals to be tested without making a prior appointment—a key accommodation needed for these communities where working parents, senior citizens, homeless, or individuals dependent on public transportation. These are changes municipalities instituted after seeing a surge in transmission and deaths among underserved populations. However, like walk-up facilities and no-appointment testing, one major barrier to testing was the cost. How were citizens in underserved communities going to pay for these tests? After a significant amount of posturing on both sides of the political aisle, federal lawmakers finally agreed that getting tested and treated for COVID-19 should not be a financial decision, but that decision too came at a cost.

Prior to the passage of the Coronavirus Aid, Relief, and Economic Security (CARES) Act, a $2.2 trillion relief bill that earmarked funding for a number of aid programs for citizens, health insurance plans did not cover COVID-19 testing or treatment—a practice which resulted in millions of uninsured or under-insured Americans without access to testing.

> Covid-19 also creates unique affordability challenges related to surprise medical billing, which can occur when a patient receives treatment from an out-of-network physician at an in-network facility. Staffing shortages and triage protocols make it more likely that patients will be sent to out-of-network facilities or be seen by out-of-network providers when they cannot check providers' network status. Furthermore, provider shortages may require providers to fill in care gaps for many conditions, not just Covid-19, expanding the potential for out-of-network care and surprise bills during this time. (King, 2020)

Weeks later, we were still at a tipping point. Testing facilities remained overwhelmed with the sheer volume of tests they received. The number of tests available to the public remains variable, even as businesses pushed to reopen and people get back to work. Our most vulnerable populations, BIPOC and the poor, danced on the head of a pin as they continued their daily struggles to make ends meet in a society where the concept of "working poor" seems hyperbolic. In short, the clarity with which the pandemic exposed systemic vulnerabilities in health care was revelatory in that the comorbidities found in BIPOC and poor populations were revealed as was the fact that they lacked appropriate avenues to quarantine and practice social distancing, lacked access to testing facilities, and encountered other barriers to treatment as well.

MENTAL HEALTH AND WELLNESS DURING COVID-19

Understanding how BIPOC and poor communities are affected physically makes up a fraction of the challenges for this group in the age of COVID-19. The "certainty of the unknown" has affected the mental health of vulnerable populations during this pandemic. Surveys administered by the CDC (2020) found that 40.9% of respondents reported at least one adverse mental or behavioral health condition, including anxiety disorders or symptoms of depressive disorders. More disturbing, in that same survey, "the percentage of respondents who reported having seriously considered suicide in the 30 days before completing the survey was significantly higher among respondents aged 18–24 years (25.5%), minority racial/ethnic groups (Hispanic respondents [18.6%], non-Hispanic Black respondents [15.1%]), self-reported unpaid caregivers for adults (30.7%), and essential workers (21.7%)" (Czeisler et al., 2020). Considering such a large swath of the population is likely suffering from mental wellness challenges during the pandemic, it would come as no surprise that BIPOC and poor communities are experiencing the compound effects of the stressors that come from their socioeconomic status and also the immediate concerns due to coping with the effect of COVID-19 on their health, finances, housing situation, and employment. The "certainty of the unknown" does not generally rest well with wealthy Americans but certainly adds even more to the agitation and anxiety of the poor. Community-level intervention and prevention efforts, including health communication strategies launched to reach these groups, could help address various mental health conditions associated with the COVID-19 pandemic. However, BIPOC and poor populations deal with economic hardships and issues related to food and shelter insecurities, access to education, childcare, and social justice in the best of times. The overall fear of the unknown has risen exponentially as people of all socioeconomic strata cope with feelings of anxiety and depression resulting from stay-at-home orders.

Scholars in the field of mental health all posit that emotional stability is largely dependent on regular routines and daily functions. These norms have been disrupted by this pandemic and have forced all of us out of our routines. The usual concerns and struggles of our most vulnerable populations have been magnified in the "age of COVID-19."

The daily concerns of BIPOC and low-income families include struggling with the realities of how to pay bills and ensuring that their families are safe and secure. As a society, our main concerns are how long will this last and when things return to normal; however, these are constant questions for this population that have been exacerbated by the widespread uncertainty this pandemic has caused. Now add to this with the concept of social distancing and the difficulties that vulnerable populations endure because of crowded living conditions, their statuses as essential workforces, comorbid illnesses, and social justice issues and it is easy to see that this is a perfect storm of stressors.

Although some of us would describe ourselves as introverts or extroverts, all human beings are social and creatures of habit by nature. Our dependence on socialization is key to how we transact our daily lives, whether going to school, going to work, or spending time with our family and peers. Prior to the initial shutdown, the U.S. celebrated one of the country's largest sporting events, the Super Bowl. Attended by tens of thousands, viewed live by billions, this event illustrates how we connect through sports, church, local restaurants, bars, and even through social activism. You see, we are social beings but with the ability to gather and bond suspended indefinitely only adds to the myriad stressors experienced in BIPOC and poor communities.

We cannot underestimate how the existing stressors affected these individuals prior to COVID-19. Heart disease, diabetes, obesity, and asthma are statistically higher in these communities versus their White, middle-class counterparts. Now, add to this premature births, heart attacks, strokes, domestic violence, gun violence—again, all pre-COVID-19—then add incarceration, substandard education, housing inequities, and substandard living conditions, and you push already vulnerable populations to the brink. Understand, given the existing stressors they already deal with regularly, it is sad that individuals and families alike in our most vulnerable populations have challenges accessing or even seeking out mental health services. The subject of mental health awareness and COVID-19 has not received the attention that it deserves for this population, nor is it deemed a priority because getting the economy back on track and getting people back to work is vitally important. The fact is COVID-19 has devastatingly impacted vulnerable populations, and it will require concerted attention to specifically address the mental health needs of BIPOC and poor populations.

Earlier in this chapter, I discussed the arrogance exhibited by our lawmakers as they developed stay-at-home guidelines. However, there is yet another area that those existing just outside the BIPOC, and poor strata take for granted but have leaned on quite heavily in light of social distancing and partial economic shutdown—the internet. When speaking of social connection, an interesting fact is that during the ups and downs of the economy and stock market, social media stocks have been one of the few stable segments during this time. Again, we find that the pandemic reveals systemic injustices. It is shocking to find that when schools first began to delve into an e-learning format, millions of students did not have access to the internet in their homes. Our reliance on the internet to interact now determines the success of our children in school. A parent's ability to provide stable, working internet access to homeschool their children adds to the stress and anxiety they already feel.

Unfortunately, there is a major drawback for BIPOC and poor communities regarding the use of technology during forced isolation. Serious technological inequities were discovered by school districts assigning work to students and unemployment offices accepting online applications. The technological resources, that is, computers and internet access, deemed ubiquitous to most, are unavailable in many communities of color; therefore, they are even more isolated during the period of lockdown. Many parents were happy to send children back to school when they began reopening, perhaps because they lacked the tools to educate them at home properly. Adults and children are looking for stability in these challenging times. The disarray caused by the shutdown, semi-shutdown, and phased reopening put everyone in situations that challenged their mental well-being. Even now, we can see no quick end to this challenge; however, as a larger community, we must deal with the systemic disparities and mental health needs our BIPOC and poor populations live with daily if we truly want to repair our economy.

VULNERABLE POPULATIONS AS ESSENTIAL WORKERS DURING COVID-19

Beyond the mundaneness of a daily routine from the social distancing orders, the shutdown's impact has been emotionally and mentally draining for everyone. However, the pressures are wildly exacerbated in BIPOC and poor populations. Over the years, researchers have written about the adverse effects of social isolation and its correlative relationship to mental illnesses and disorders such as depression and PTSD. To that end,

I strongly suggest that we shift the dialogue from the concept of social distancing and instead invoke the concept of physical distancing in its place. In essence, shifting the emphasis to maintaining a safe physical distance from others while remaining socially connected via our devices (phones, laptops, tablets, desktops). This effort affords all populations vulnerable and privileged to remain socially connected while adhering to public health mandates.

Since the beginning of the pandemic, our national news networks started to highlight how the virus affected our food chain. Stephenson (2020) stated:

> Numerous COVID-19 outbreaks in meat and poultry processing plants erupted not long after cases emerged in the United States. On May 1, a study published by the CDC said that 19 states had reported 4,913 cases and 20 deaths among approximately 130,000 workers at 115 meat and poultry processing facilities. (Stephenson, 2020)

These essential workers in the farming and meatpacking industry exhibiting symptoms admitted to not informing their employer. As shocking as this may seem, these workers may not report sicknesses because they lack personal time off, do not have insurance, or both, and they cannot afford to lose valuable work hours. For these people, sustaining their families and paying their bills far outweighs the possibility of contracting or spreading the virus. Therefore, one of the issues that we must consider for our BIPOC and poor populations are lasting protections for essential wage workers who are without medical coverage, sick or paid leave, and are unable to receive unemployment compensation.

Here again, the pandemic has exposed an issue of workforce reforms and regulations that has been politicized as a left-wing talking point. It is not a matter of left-wing versus right-wing when we consider the butterfly effect these choices have on the nation. An infected essential worker has the ability to infect, exponentially, if that worker is directly involved with our food chain. While I do not support draconian measures like arresting those that do, we need to understand the mitigating factors behind their choice while maintaining the position that the sick should have access to healthcare and allowed the time necessary to heal without fear of redress.

This potential dilemma further illustrates the responsibility that employers have to provide a safe, open, and supportive workplace for essential low-skilled workers. The irony here is that the low wage workers at chicken farms, fruit orchards, meat processing plants, the hospitality industry, in foodservice, in-home health care, and transportation workers—just to name a few—are those same people suffering from the added stressors of living with comorbid illnesses, housing inequities, and job insecurities in the age of COVID-19. Economic hardships have disproportionately affected the BIPOC and poor communities. The resulting economic shutdown forced many low to moderate-income BIPOC families to put their lives at risk and return to work prematurely or work while ill just to pay their bills. As of the July 2020 jobs report, the unemployment rate stood at 10.2%, a reduction compared with previous months but still its highest level in over a decade (U.S. Bureau of Labor Statistics, 2020). Businesses have been forced to close or drastically reduce their staff to adjust to the pandemic. Still, our essential workers—many of which are part of our vulnerable population—manage the day-to-day challenges of working in the "new normal" while keeping their families together.

SOCIAL JUSTICE PROTEST AMONG VULNERABLE POPULATIONS IN COVID-19

While still firmly under stay-at-home orders, the world witnessed the senseless murder of George Floyd at the hands of officers sworn to protect and serve the people. Unfortunately, police shootings and the murders of Black people occurred long before the pandemic; however, something was starkly different this time. Perhaps, one would posit that the stress of stay-at-home orders and the media bombardment of death tolls from the pandemic struck a social nerve already pulled taut. The outrage expressed over the murder of George Floyd murder transcended race, age, and ethnicity. In my lifetime, I have never seen so many people from such diverse backgrounds and walks of life rally in solidarity to condemn the murder of a Black man by a police officer. Through the protests that followed, it was clear that the confluence of events that the stark reality of racism and systemic injustice—highlighted in the senseless killings of George Floyd and Breonna Taylor—existed also in healthcare, technology, and housing, as well as our criminal justice system. The rise of social justice protests opened the eyes of many to the shortfalls that have plagued BIPOC and poor communities for decades. COVID-19 has forced the issues of racial hatred and systemic injustice to the front and center. These two pandemics seem to have caused a rebirth of our nation. Conversations about race and racial attitudes are happening on topics such as dismantling systemic and structural racism, police reform, and economic inclusion in all society sectors. By and large, this country is finally beginning to accept and acknowledge that there have been two Americas—one for the privileged and another for those who struggle each day to "just get by."

THE AFTERMATH: IS THERE A POST-COVID-19?

We are truly in an unprecedented time when we have, as a nation, been confronted with our strengths and our weaknesses. Right now, we absolutely find ourselves at a crossroads and must decide how we move forward with no real end of COVID-19 in sight. Over the last several weeks, we have seen federal, state, and local governments attempt to bridge the gap to address food insecurities, legislate moratoriums on evictions, and create stimulus packages to assist the millions left unemployed furloughed indefinitely by COVID-19. This modern-day advancement will play out in all aspects of our lives. Moving beyond 2020, I believe we will see educational programs, workforce programs, and medical services addressing shortfalls in our underserved communities. Whether it is providing stable, virtual connectivity or access to affordable, quality housing; or healthy, fresh food sources, we appear to be on the cusp of real change in our society. Now that COVID-19 has revealed the inequities, we are obligated to do more to close the gap. The new normal will dramatically impact society at large but, more specifically, these vulnerable and marginalized populations.

Moving forward, the energy of advocacy demonstrated after the George Floyd murder is being actively funneled through communities of marginalized people across the United States. While we are not certain when we will leave this pandemic experience behind us, we have seen an increased demand for justice for the vulnerable, the marginalized, and the underserved. There are many unknowns about our collective future and challenges beyond our control; therefore, I encourage everyone who reads this to take charge of the things you can control and to provide whatever support you can to help our most vulnerable populations overcome the stressors amplified by the pandemic.

We have seen painful evidence that the virus does not discriminate. The virus acts efficiently and cruelly by exploiting our weaknesses. First-hand, we have seen how it ravages through crowded urban areas just as we have seen it sweep through rural areas. The answer is the same across the board. We must protect ourselves and each other. That is the only way we can "slow the spread," stop this virus and return to some semblance of our lives pre-COVID-19. What is clear is now that we see the truth that the ingrained inequalities in our country diminish people's safety and must not return. We should consider equal health under the law as surely as we expect equal justice under the law. As we enter this nation's rebirth and rethink our "social justice movement," we must do our due diligence to be in the game no longer on the sidelines. It is my belief that, in the end, we will come out of this experience victorious.

DEDICATION

This chapter is dedicated to the woman who gave me life, my mother, Malois Everett. My only wish is that you could read this chapter and share your thoughts with me about my contribution. Mother has been living with dementia for over 20 years; she is my rock and the source from where I draw strength in times of weakness. As I witness challenges that vulnerable populations experience due to COVID-19, I draw from her strength to keep a positive outlook on what the future holds. Thank you, Mother, for all that you have done and continue to still do.

ACKNOWLEDGMENTS

Special thanks to Pamela Hall for inviting me to contribute a chapter on this most important topic. Indeed, this chapter was challenging to write while witnessing the impact of COVID-19. Additionally, I must thank my wonderfully brilliant wife, Kimberly Gray Roberts, for being my muse, research assistant, and major supporter during this endeavor. I immensely enjoyed the enriching exchanges we had about the various topics covered in this chapter. Thank you for embarking on this journey with me emotionally, physically, and intellectually.

REFERENCES

CDC. (2020, August 14). Mental health, substance use, and suicidal ideation during the COVID-19 pandemic--United States, June 24-30, 2020. https://www.cdc.gov/mmwr/volumes/69/wr/mm6932a1.htm#:~:text=Overall%2C%2040.9%25%20of%20respondents%20reported,increased%20substance%20use%20to%20cope

Czeisler, M., Lane, M., Petrosky, M., Wiley, E., Christensen, J., Nijal, A., Weaver, M. D., Robbins, R., Facer-Childs, E. R., Barger, L. K., Czeisler, C. A., Howard, M. E., & Rajaratnam, S. M.W. (2020). *Mental health, substance use, and suicidal ideation during the COVID-19 pandemic—United States, June 24–30, 2020.* Centers for Disease Control. https://www.cdc.gov/mmwr/volumes/69/wr/mm6932a1.htm?s_cid=mm6932a1_w#suggestedcitation

Evans, G., & Kantrowitz, E. (200). Socioeconomic status and health: The potential role of environmental risk exposure. *Annual Review of Public Health, 23*(1), 303–331.

Grief, S., & Miller, J. (2017). Infectious disease issues in underserved populations. *Primary Care: Clinics in Office Practice, 44*(1), 6785.

Kaiser Family Foundation. (2020, January 11). Communities of color at higher risk for health and economic challenges due to COVID-19. *National Academies Press*. https://www.kff.org/coronavirus-covid-19/issue-brief/communities-of-color-at-higher-risk-for-health-and-economic-challenges-due-to-covid-19/

King, J. S. (2020, June 25). Perspectives: Covid-19 and the need for health care reform. *The New England Journal of Medicine.* https://www.nejm.org/doi/full/10.1056/NEJMp2000821

Madrigal, A., & Meyer, R. (2020, March 12). Coronavirus: The Atlantic's most crucial coverage of COVID-19. *The Atlantic*. https://www.theatlantic.com/health/archive/2020/03/coronavirus-covid-19-the-atlantics-most-crucial-coverage/607906/

Stephenson, J. (2020, June 19). *COVID-19 outbreaks among food production workers may intensify pandemic's disproportionate effects on people of color.* https://jamanetwork.com/channels/health-forum/fullarticle/2767667

University of Utah Health Sciences. (2020, September 8). COVID-19 deaths among black essential workers linked to racial disparities. *Medical Express*. https://medicalxpress.com/news/2020-09-covid-deaths-black-essential-workers.html

U.S. Bureau of Labor Statistics. (2020). *Employment situation news release*. https://www.bls.gov/news.release/archives/empsit_08072020.htm

WhiteHouse.gov. (2020). *Remarks by President Trump after tour of the Centers for Disease Control and Prevention*. https://www.whitehouse.gov/briefings-statements/remarks-president-trump-tour-centers-disease-control-prevention-atlanta-ga/

CHAPTER 20

KEMETIC YOGA

Coping, Healing, Wellness

T. Conswello Davis

From an historical perspective, African Americans/Black people exude resiliency. We have had to endure horrendous atrocities and conditions in different environments to survive. Historically, these experiences are documented. It is fascinating to ascertain people's strength which continues to embody light and resistance. Many in the African American or Black community continue to move forward despite traumatic episodes, incidents, and experiences. As Meyer (2020) observes:

> Given this history, it should be clear that the capacity of non-immigrant Africans in America, those enslaved as chattel who built this country's wealth and their progeny, to survive and oft times thrive in the worst of human circumstances is beyond remarkable, and possibly the miracle of modern times.

Consequentially, African Americans/Blacks continue to cope with managing life during a pandemic and despite racial trauma.

The coronavirus pandemic exposed the depth of healthcare disparities and limited medical care access for many African Americans/Black

Coronavirus and Vulnerable People: Addressing the Divide in Harm and Responses and Exploring Implications for a More Peaceful World, pp. 327–331

Americans. African American/Black communities do not have ample access to health care or wealth and financial support to pay for health care. Therefore, many will continue to live without receiving the necessary medical services and support due to all American citizens. The pervasive lack of medical and health insurance for this particular racial group in America is historical and intergenerational. The coronavirus (COVID-19) is that it attacks the two most important systems of the body, respiratory, and immune systems. The population most affected by the virus: African Americans.

It has been determined that three major factors contributed to the higher COVID-19 rates of African Americans/Black. One is preexisting conditions such as diabetes, hypertension, and obesity that disproportionately impact the African American community. Many African Americans/Blacks have jobs that are categorized as essential but are not in the health professions, where protective equipment was often provided. People of color disproportionately hold these essential jobs, including bus drivers, train operators, and custodians. As we continue to uncover why there is an increase in mortality rates for African American/Black women giving birth, the most pervasive reason is structural inequities and social determinants of health that are influenced by implicit bias and racial discrimination (Zarefsky, 2020).

As a mental health professional, I began thinking about the various forms of coping mechanisms employed during crises like the pandemic. These coping mechanisms are integrated into our lives to alleviate stress, anxiety, depression, and trauma. It was apparent that many of the pre-existing conditions prevalent within the African American/Black community can be mitigated via implementing coping strategies and wellness practices. This may include applying coping mechanisms to counteract the effects of hypertension, diabetes, and obesity. Another question is, "How do we help and support the population by implementing coping and wellness that ultimately facilitates the healing of trauma for individuals? The additional questions I posited were, "What are some effective coping and wellness methods to promote within the community?" What are some of the evidence-based coping mechanisms to educate and teach the community? And "What are forms of coping and wellness that encourages healing?

A tool that provides a system of coping and wellness that can facilitate healing is yoga. It is an evidence-based form of coping that empowers and supports wellness. Yoga promotes mental and physical health, partly due to its impact on the hypothalamic-pituitary axis that moderates the release of cortisol and modifies its adverse effect on cardiovascular, neuroendocrine, and central nervous systems (Moscoso et al., 2019).

A deep breathing technique is perfect for relaxation and to alleviate anxiety, high blood pressure, and stress. The breath transcends an individual to develop a calm and peaceful state, which transitions an individual into meditation. The meditation helps reduce stress, control anxiety, empowers, enriches sleep, supports emotional health, develops self-awareness, increases focus and concentration, and relieves pain. The breath facilitates the flow of energy throughout the body. In Kemetic yoga, the movement, poses, and postures are facilitated via the breath. The benefits of yoga include but are not limited to improved stress-related autonomic measures, such as blood pressure and heart rate, diabetes risk reduction through weight loss, decreased waist circumference, lower perceived stress, lower body mass index, and reduced depression and stress for post-menopausal women (Moscoso et al., 2019, p. 202).

While the overall goal of yogic practices is to facilitate and awaken spiritual awareness, there are also many documented physical benefits. These include improved functioning of all bodily systems, and in particular, strengthening of the immune system. Other benefits include the slowing of the biological aging process and an overall reduction of stress indicators. Individuals experience clear thinking processes, improved intellectual skills, enhanced creativity, and an overall increased appreciation for living are also some of the many benefits of yoga practice (Glassey, 2012, p. 32). "Kemetic Yoga embodies coping, healing and wellness. Kemetic yoga can be utilized to support African American/Black communities with active coping, wellness, and empowerment. Kemetic Yoga refers to the entire spiritual system of self-development created by the sages of ancient Egypt. It is a worldview that recognizes the nature of reality and our place in the universe. Kemetic Yoga understands our connection to our ancestors' spirits and the true nature of Divine Universal Forces (deities properly called Neteru) (Hotep, 2020a).

In Kemetic yoga, the breath is the life force. The breath is the most powerful. We refer to the breath as the "shu." The shu is the force that helps us heal, connect with our senses, and facilitates energy movement throughout the body. When we apply the breathwork into our daily lives, it becomes the most incredible coping mechanism. We can take deep breaths to release the negative energy and tension and transition into relaxation. From relaxation and deep breathing, one can transcend oneself into mediation. Meditation and visualization are both utilized in Kemetic yoga. Meditation helps activate the body's natural ability to heal itself. The process of meditation puts individuals in touch with the life force that flows through the body. The life force is accessed through controlled breathing. Visualization and breath control are used to move the life force through the body and into areas where known ailments exist (Hotep, 2020b, p. 27).

As we move through Kemetic yoga poses, the breath helps us become in tune with the body. We notice where we feel the energy and resistance in the body. The breath is used to help alleviate the resistance and facilitate energy flow out of the body. Yoga postures are supposed to be done in a manner that is in harmony with the body's physical anatomy and physiology. The Yoga Skills Method (YSM) demands that they also are performed in such a manner as to be in harmony with the exact way that energy moves and operates in the bioenergetic body (Hotep, 2020a). The poses and postures transfer the energy through the body so individuals can ground themselves and feel, define emotions, and learn about the body's resistance.

This system is slower and more methodical than the traditional methods of yoga. By slowing everything down, we put more emphasis on developing the yoga skills of patience and concentration. The respiratory system receives a more profound development because you are challenged to use the breath to flow through the forms (Hotep, 2020a, p. 4). The yoga movements and postures place primary emphasis on controlling the breath to move and circulate life force. In the same way that we have a physical body with specific anatomy and physiology and operate in a particular manner, we also have a spiritual or energetic body with specific anatomy and physiology and operate on the circulation of life force. We are born with this life force, and it is replenished from a substance in the air, the sages of ancient Kemet (Egypt) called Ankh (Hotep, 2020b, p. 2).

Kemetic yoga posits the seven principles of MA'AT. MA'AT is the Kemetic symbol for universal justice, balance, and harmony. Ka is the ancient Kemetic symbol for spirit. The principles of MA'AT are empowering and may resonate with individuals. MA'AT is a goddess that represents divine order. The principles are truth, justice, balance, righteousness, harmony, reciprocity, and order. The posture MA'AT Ka in Kemetic yoga is very powerful. The benefits of MAAT Ka are healing. It opens the energy channels and allows for the flow of life force through the body, which corrects imbalances in the body. In the same way that MAAT brings balance and harmony to the universe, the body should also manifest balance and harmony to activate the self-healing ability that we all naturally possess. The open supply of oxygen to various organs like the kidneys, liver, lungs, heart, lymph nodes, optic nerves, and sex organs. This specific posture also helps muscles and joints in the back, spinal column, neck, and back muscles, strengthening knees and opening hip joints (Hotep, 2020b, p. 56).

The benefits of Kemetic yoga are numerous. There are many components to this form of yoga which can be taught to individuals in community centers, neighborhood parks, schools, studios, and offices. It will help individuals who cannot afford therapy to heal trauma and establish effective coping skills and healthy wellness practices. Kemetic yoga encourages self-reflection and empowerment. Even if mental health professionals teach the just the breathwork for deep relaxation breathing and meditation, they will experience results. Educating African Americans/Blacks about the advantages of yoga and the self-healing element may encourage individuals to establish it as a form of effective coping. As mental health professionals, we must meet our clients where they are. The African American/Black community is capable of living healthy and fulfilling lives. We must acknowledge how dominant society does not advocate and support our existence. We must adjust accordingly. The adjustments must be made so that we can continue to survive and thrive. The adjustment I foresee making an enormous impact within our community is improved mental health and wellness. We must embrace learning how to alleviate medical ailments and facilitate our healing. It is especially important as mental health professionals serving our communities to promote effective coping mechanisms for African Americans/Blacks considering the pandemic. We know the community may not have all the resources necessary. Hence, we can help them learn useful and valuable methods of coping, healing, and wellness.

REFERENCES

Glassey, D. (2012, August). *Why yoga works: Glands, biochemicals, and cerebral spinal fluids*. Kemetic Yoga skills teacher training supplement, Kinetic Yoga Skills course.

Hotep, Y. (2020a). *The complete teaching training manual*. Kemetic Yoga Skills course.

Hotep, Y. R. (2020b). *Understanding the yoga skills method and kemetic yoga*. Kemetic Yoga Skills Course.

Meyers, L. J. (2020, May 15). Culturally-grounded is conceptualizing and contending with COVID-19. *Association of Black Psychologists*. http://www.abpsi.org/COVID/Culturally%20Grounding%20Conceptualizing%20by%20Linda%20James%20Meyers.pdf

Moscoso, D. I., Goese, D., Van Hyfte, G. J., Mayer, Z., Cain, L., Kobiernicki, F., Cano-Garcia, A., Unzueta, C., Ormaza, L. T., & Jones, K. (2019). The impact of yoga in medically underserved populations: A mixed-methods study. *Complementary Therapies in Medicine, 43*, 201–207.

Zarefsky, M. (2020, May 13). *Why African American communities are being hit hard by COVID-19*. American Medical Association. https://www.ama-assn.org/delivering-care/population-care/why-african-american-communities-are-being-hit-hard-covid-19

CHAPTER 21

RADICAL POTENTIALS IN A TIME OF CRISIS

Whose Vulnerability Is It Anyway?

Mark Lance and Matt Meyer

We live in interesting times.

While crisis alone does not force people to think about or act deeply upon the root causes of the troubles around them, it does not hurt either. Thus, any crisis may be linked to the opportunity for more openly radical thinking about how we can, in deep and lasting ways, change the world, our community, or our own lives. Our question, then, is what the current series of crises enables?

The COVID-19 pandemic has transformed global society, already causing massive alterations in social interaction patterns, perhaps only temporarily but in unprecedented ways. The global economic shutdown in response to COVID has caused increased and unmasked crisis levels in capitalist "development," which had previously been unthinkable for many. Yet despite physical distancing, widespread health fears, and a sense of "all in the same boat" community-building, the racial and white supremacist divisions which have long fueled contemporary economics and given rise to tremendous health and social disparities globally also

Coronavirus and Vulnerable People: Addressing the Divide in Harm and Responses and Exploring Implications for a More Peaceful World, pp. 333–349

saw an unprecedented transformation in this period—with estimates of up to 26 million people in the streets protesting racialized police violence and militarism in the U.S. in June 2020 alone (Black Lives Matter Protests, 2020).

The effects of the pandemic in the United States., occurring as they did against these backdrops of structural classism (poverty, homelessness, lack of access to healthcare), racism, and ableism and exacerbated by breathtaking levels of incompetence among national leaders, have been devastating. The official death toll was well over 150,000 and steadily climbing as of August 2020, and estimates are that the number who died directly or indirectly from the disease is much higher and will continue to climb. We have no idea yet the number of people who will be permanently impaired as the result of organ damage (Miller et al., 2020)· Economically, the U.S. is facing perhaps the greatest depression in its history with obvious international consequences (Nicola et al., 2020). All of this, as noted, is inflected by the usual racist, classist, ageist, and ableist disparities.

In the midst of pandemic lockdown, the U.S. experienced an explosion of racist incidents, including police murder of innocent and unarmed African Americans. The subsequent anger at white supremacist violence seemed sudden, with a looting fury and consistently lasting many days and weeks. In recent U.S. history, a particular murder has often set aflame an underlying powder-keg of anger at daily harassment and structural oppression—from Emmett Till to Martin Luther King Jr, from Eleanor Bumpers to Michael Stewart, from Eric Garner and Mike Brown to George Floyd. The cry "Black Lives Matter" arose in 2015 in direct contrast to the apparent reality that, in U.S. society, the life of a person of African descent mattered little other than as free or cheap labor. In New York City (like many others), a curfew was issued to quell the rage; the last time such a closing took place in the international "city which never sleeps" was in 1943, when an economically challenged U.S. was experiencing "racial unrest" and a recently-returned African American World War II veteran was shot by a White police officer in Harlem when trying to intervene in what he saw as brutality against a Black woman who was being arrested.

Nonetheless, the current uprisings seem different, if only because of the breadth of recognition they appear to create. Not only have we seen large protests with radical demands—police abolition or defunding—in every major U.S. city, but solidarity, empathy, and unity in cities throughout the world. Beyond this, even if it is often superficial, we have seen antiracist statements by hundreds of corporations and by mainstream institutions such as the National Football League, NASCAR, and Republican politicians. The Southeast (college football) Conference finally joined with the Black community in demanding that Mississippi change its state flag away from its traditional Confederate proslavery insignia, and football gets results. Nearly every candidate for the Democratic Party candidate responded in some way with calls for police reform. And the millions in the streets have spanned generations and included sizable support from white folks. Of course, this is not to say that the demands of those in the streets have been accepted at the highest levels. But institutions of power that have denied or ignored the reality of white supremacy for centuries are suddenly feeling the need to respond in some way. And that matters.

Our fundamental point is that this extraordinary explosion of energy around one of the "original sin" cornerstones of U.S. society and empire is taking place, not so coincidentally, during a time of unprecedented social and economic challenge: a plague, a depression, and an uprising. Though many have already died needlessly and many more will follow, the existential question for those seeking lasting peace with justice, a "new normalcy" throughout society which will center less around greed, militarism, and anti-democratic systems, is what institutions are the truly vulnerable ones? How can we best understand this moment to build better movements out of it?

Interesting times indeed.

SECTION I: CONSCIOUSNESS (CHANGES IN PUBLIC AWARENESS AND THE VULNERABILITY OF SELF-CENTERED GREED)

While it is too early to have data on specific changes in public attitudes, much less to assign quantitative values to them, it is clear that a number of features of our current economic system that usually remain carefully concealed from the eyes of the nonprivileged are bursting into view as a result of the COVID pandemic and subsequent social restrictions. Of course, health care is a constant source of discussion, and with that is a growing awareness of the massive disparities in U.S. healthcare (see Editorial Board, 2020; Facher, 2020; Reynolds, 2020; Slavitt, 2020)· Mass unemployment highlights the injustice of tying health care to employment status. In a pandemic, anyone who decides not to seek medical care for economic reasons is a threat to everyone who comes in contact with them. This means that lack of healthcare is recognized by many not merely as a matter of justice but also as a self-interest. If you stay in public while sick because of a lack of healthcare, you can kill me.

Beyond this, we are seeing mainstream portrayals of nurses as heroes. In language usually reserved for soldiers, the elite's public elements laud their work, noting their extraordinary hours and low pay, and recognizing their sacrifice as many on the frontlines die. Nor are nurses alone in their newly found visibility. Under capitalism, we are systematically taught not to notice the legions of people who clean our workplaces, staff grocery stores, or make deliveries. And if we occasionally and superficially acknowledge these people's existence, rarely do we treat them as crucial parts of our lives, even less as heroes. And yet, in a recent letter denouncing the rising militarism of Donald Trump's response to the protests, Marine Corp General "Mad Dog" Mattis echoed a sentiment that has become commonplace in the time of COVID:

> The pandemic has shown us that it is not only our troops who are willing to offer the ultimate sacrifice for the safety of the community. Americans in hospitals, grocery stores, post offices, and elsewhere have put their lives on the line to serve their fellow citizens and their country. (Goldberg, 2020)

Vulnerable Americans quarantining across the country suddenly have been thrust into the realization that their ability to obtain food and medicine depends on others. And those others are generally the lowest paid, least secure people in the country. It is no exaggeration to say that COVID has made our economic interdependence visible.

A second dimension of social life coming into high focus as a result of COVID concerns the work structure. Perhaps most obviously, people are becoming acutely aware of the massive disparities in work conditions. For instance, many academics are privileged to retain their jobs, even if they have to reconfigure them and devote extra hours to converting to online systems. Others are deemed essential and must work under conditions that risk their lives, while still others are simply out of work. There has been a nearly instantaneous mass increase in unemployment but also an increase of awareness about schemes to provide support to people in shutdown industries proliferate around the country. And the fate of pre-kindergarten through high school public education, all but gutted by accelerating privatization and federal constraints since the turn of the century, is undergoing more rigorous debate, as parent groups are becoming empowered, growing in numbers as they advocate more intensely for the physical and emotional safety of their children. Teacher unions are beginning to sound more like worker-advocates again, threatening militant actions unless the entire school environment is deemed safe. Community members are crossing local lines to think and act strategically about how best to safeguard education as a whole for the long term (see Germanos, 2020; Jones, 2020; Will & Schwartz, 2020).

Because and beyond this, the very possibility of changing work environments is now clear. We see think pieces in the media asking whether various industries should not remain work-from-home even after the pandemic (Friedman, 2020). Mass transit being a major vector for transmission highlights disparities in commuting possibilities. Finally, governmental responses to COVID have transformed generations of common wisdom regarding the possibility of large-scale economic intervention. There is a familiar pattern whenever budgetary debates open up at national or state levels. Virtually no discussion arises concerning military or police budgets, but the immediate response is that we cannot afford the expense whenever new social programs are proposed. Nowhere was this more apparent than in debates around single-payer health programs. The idea that these would cost a trillion dollars over a decade, whether true or not, was supposed to imply that the idea was a wild flight of fancy (Brownstein, 2020). And yet, within a month, the government had dumped twice that amount into the economy. Just like that. Two trillion dollars, with more soon to follow. Suddenly, it is protestations about the disasters of public spending that sound absurd … as absurd as they have always been, from the average citizen's point of view.

SECTION II: THE GROWTH OF MUTUAL AID NETWORKS AND THE VULNERABILITY OF TRADITIONAL INDIVIDUALISM

It is not uncommon to see a growth in grassroots mutual aid in moments of crisis (Solnit, 2010). The combination of the crisis generated by COVID—sudden poverty and homelessness for many, the inability of at-risk people to safely access necessities, lack of basic medical services—and the utterly incompetent federal government response led quickly to the creation of local grassroots networks of community support. In many cities, these networks were first launched by experienced activists, but they quickly attracted Nongovernment organizations, churches, liberals connected by loose neighborhood networks, and even local government (Jun & Lance, 2020). Such efforts build capacity. They create connections across communities, generations, races, and so forth. When people work together for a common purpose, new levels of trust arise. And that means that there are new possibilities for more radical action in the future. Mutual aid responses to a crisis of this magnitude teach people not only that the government is unable to provide the conditions of a just and flourishing life but that we can do it ourselves.

There is a good deal of discussion of such networks rising during a crisis—often under the name "spontaneous organization"—but most case studies involve relatively short-term crises such as floods and earthquakes. The COVID crisis has already shown a "staying power" beyond what we have typically deemed social emergencies. As we wrote this in August 2020, the daily infection rate in the U.S. is higher than it has been at any point. Hospitals in many states are at capacity, and even the most optimistic predictions call for another six months before vaccines are readily available. Beyond this, there is no reason to think that this outbreak is unique. Conditions of mass factory farming, population density, and global warming suggest that we are likely in for cycles of such outbreaks for the foreseeable future.

And further, there is simply no reason to think that governments will be able to respond adequately to meet people's material and social needs under such conditions. All these points together suggest that we might be in for some more profound social changes than we have seen in disasters past. New networks, new grassroots habits, new forms of collective power may well emerge in the coming months and years.

In the U.S. colony of Puerto Rico, an increase in mutual aid networking has followed several years of both traditional and expressly colonial crises: hurricanes, earthquakes, and deepening economic incursions in the form of a congressionally controlled PROMESA debt plan. Though organizers have forthrightly proclaimed that "the crisis is colonialism," the mutual aid response to the COVID-19 pandemic went beyond pro-independence speeches. Not only did health care workers set up networks to reach widespread populations in rural areas, but an emphasis on alternative medicine also became a focus of crisis response. Thus, the practice of acupuncture, both to assist in building respiratory strength or viral immunity and to ease hypertension, anxiety, and depression (which were exacerbated the pandemic), became widely used. For a general discussion of Puerto Rican resistance in the context of the COVID-19, see interviews with Dr. Fernando Cabanillas, MD, Rachel of Colectivo Feminista, Luis Rosa and Oscar Lopez Rivera, in *Puerto Rico: Colonialism is the Virus*, People's Strike Broadcast (May 1, 2020) (available at https://youtu.be/G6LBJR9gbyg). For Puerto Rico COVIID-19 mutual aid work, especially focused on acupuncture and alternative health (see interviews with Jose Santini & Rita Cordoba, 2020).

An August 2020 assessment of why the U.S. was faring more poorly than any other affluent nation could not have been clearer in summary: With a "tradition of prioritizing individualism over government restrictions" and an "aversion to collective action," the so-called richest nation on earth suffered a "unique failure" based on putting partisanship ahead of public health (Leonhardt, 2020).

SECTION III: BLACK LIVES MATTER AND THE VULNERABILITY OF THE FUNDAMENTAL IDEA THAT THEY DO NOT

In late May 2020, the latest police murder of a Black man, George Floyd in Minneapolis, ignited the entire country and many parts of the world.

Building on both the movement's anger and organizational capacity for Black Lives (M4BL), Black Lives Matter's group structure, and many related but unaffiliated grassroots groups connected to the overall Black liberation movement, the response to Floyd's murder has been astonishing. Not only every major U.S. city, but many small towns and cities worldwide have seen massive protests, confrontations with police, and upsurged in awareness across all sectors of society from corporations, government at multiple levels, professional sports, and entertainment, to the grassroots. It almost seems that the U.S. suddenly woke up and noticed that it was a white supremacist society.

Of course, part of the importance of a responsible cross-generational dialogue between academics and activists is to put the appearance of "suddenness" into a proper context. For example, the *New York Times* announced on the eve of one of the most anticipated July 4, 2020, Independence Day celebrations in recent history that "Black Lives Matter May Be the Largest Movement in US History" (Buchanan et al., 2020). Most of us in analytic left circles, both academics and grassroots activists, understood the ironies of that headline. Indeed, while the current historic moment is generating sustained, multigenerational, interracial, youth-led, Black-led demonstrations and consciousness-raising, sadly, there is no "mass movement" in the U.S. as of yet.

This *Times* declared "movement" shares much with the "civil rights movement," a name bestowed on the uprisings in the 1960s by elite revisionists hoping to contain the radical development of King, SNCC, Black Power, and related forces from veering too close to the human rights affirmations of Malcolm, the Black Panthers, and others. Let us be clear: the great U.S. historian and organizer Vincent Harding, author of Dr. King's "Beyond Vietnam" speech delivered one year to the day before his inevitable assassination in 1968, corrected the characterization of what took place in the U.S. from the mid-1950s through the mid-1970s as a "Black-led, southern-based freedom movement" (Harding, 2010). The phrase "civil rights" was rarely, if ever, uttered by those we credit with shaping those times.

To be sure, movements require more than just a month or two of demonstrations, more than an organization or three with a national membership, and a series of popular webinars under their belt. And though the hashtag #BlackLivesMatter is surely more than simply a massively popular Twitter feed, it and all of the local elements of the distinct but related Movement for Black Lives still do not make up what historically can be defined as a movement. There is neither a coalition structure nor a clearly stated campaign strategy. More importantly, there are multitudes of organizations, and a good number of newly emerging coalitions as well, which rally heartily under the BLM banner but do not associate with what the group named Black Lives Matter (BLM) actually is or wishes to be.

In absolutely no way this is meant as a negative commentary on the many extraordinary local, regional, and national BLM and M4BL spokes-people, organizers, and activists. It is simply to state that BLM, as currently encompassed organizationally and also as experienced in national mobilizations over the past months, does not definitionally fall into the category of "movement." The Montgomery Bus Boycott was a glorious, months-long, ultimately successful campaign that eventually sparked a movement. Neither Dr. King's Southern Christian Leadership Conference nor the larger NAACP could or should be considered "movements"—though they were central to the coalitions which *made up* the movement. And Black Lives Matter, whatever the *New York Times*, mainstream foundations, or corporate entities vying for favor among their "customers of color" say, has provided the key slogan for a moment where more diverse groupings of people have flooded out in frustration and hope than at any previous junction. It IS the stuff out of which movements are made. But without a great deal more on-the-ground organizing, it is not yet a movement.

We might better understand this time as a "moment at war" (Meyer, 2020). When the young Black female mayor of Atlanta, Georgia is informed that the old White governor of her southern state is suing her over her order that city residents must wear life-saving face masks in public, there is something unusual even within the madness of the U.S. electoral arena. When BLM-related protests in Portland, Oregon (see Humphrey, 2020) devolve into scenes where federal U.S. troops emerge from unmarked cars with no signifying badge, name tag, or identifier, picking off targeted and unarmed protest leaders who are then taken away without charges, words, or legal justification of any kind, something unusual is going on even for a country grown used to militarized policing. The closest thing we have seen within the U.S. is what were called "disappearances" in Latin America in the 1980s. It is the mark of the petty dictator (Devereaux, 2020) which, of course, is what U.S. life was under Trump. And it goes well beyond anything directed by the White House (Lorber, 2020). It is America at war.

Most of the responses to recent protests remain purely symbolic: writing "Black Lives Matter" on a DC street, changing the flag of Mississippi, changing the racist names of a few sports teams, removing monuments to racist figures, and so forth. One never knows what level of staying power such moments will have. But for all that, the breadth of influence is enormous, and the demands of the core elements of this uprising are radical. Perhaps abolitionist sociologist Ruth Wilson Gilmore said it best when asked about the true meaning of the call to defund or abolish the police or prisons. "It only means changing one thing," Gilmore (2021) noted. What is that one thing, according to that activist-scholar? Simply put: "Everything."

The combination of broad social awareness, strong radical cores across nations, and new social networks are what have led to radical change at many points historically. Across the actions, events, webinars, and organizations, it may be that we do not yet have something fully approaching a campaign and do not yet have what has traditionally been understood as a full-fledged movement. But we have the building blocks of these things at a clearly historical juncture ... and more people talking and acting in ways which evidence an awareness of this.

SECTION IV: NEW BROAD INITIATIVES AND THE VULNERABILITY OF THE EMPIRE

For many of us who came of age politically in the 1970s, the 1980s, and earlier, the initials "BLM" still signify the "Black liberation movement"—and harken back to a time when people of African descent asserted leadership over many campaigns for radical social change and liberation. In the United States, this meant for some a move to "free the land" and look towards the southern base of territory, which remains majority Black under largely white business and political control. For others, this meant a deepening of worker and workplace organization building. For still others, a focus on internationalism, decolonization, and Pan-Africanism took the fore. Too little is still understood of the 1970s–1980s period of fight-back and backlash, of the scores of political prisoners still suffering under the repression of those times, and the solidarity provided by some intent on living up to the principles of self-determination and accountable work under the leadership of liberation forces.

Out of that period of new internationalism and cross-disciplinary creativity, the field of peace studies was born. Despite the Reagan era's reactionary core, a waning of traditional empire-building from Europe and North America was already underway. Therefore, it is not surprising that one of the first global analysts to predict the U.S. empire's imminent fall was peace researcher Johan Galtung. It is tempting to reflect upon a future end of empires, free of the conflicts that the most unequal form of development necessitates. However, the rise of regional superpowers appears more intricately linked to a reemergence of new forms and geographies of imperial control rather than their dissolution.

Galtung, the Scandinavian intellectual often cited for his accurate predictions two decades beforehand regarding the timing of the collapse of the Soviet Union, based his predictions on "synchronizing and mutually reinforcing contradictions" which suggest that deepening social crisis as economic, political, and military forces are no longer able to dictate the social order within a given empire. In the last years of its decline, Galtung (2009) wrote at the time, the U.S. is likely to experience a period of reactionary fascism. This would include, he asserted, a U.S. capacity for extreme global violence; a vision of U.S. exceptionalism as the "fittest nation" on the planet with a "manifest" destiny to rule over others; a belief in a coming final war between good and evil; a cult of the strong state leading the fight of good against evil; and a cult of the "strong leader." Reading these assertions in Trump's era, the COVID-19 pandemic and the Black liberation uprisings and subsequent repression suggest a preciseness beyond even what Galtung's admirers expected.

Fast forward to 2020: Within the U.S., a new coalition called People's Strike is emerging as a Black-led, southern-founded network bringing together a multigenerational grouping across geographic, racial/ethnic, gender binary, and ideological lines. With principles of "unity not uniformity," "mutual aid," and supporting frontline workers and one another through the multiple crises, it stands a more promising chance of building a united front building anything seen over the past century. But People's Strike would be unthinkable without the Occupy movement, without the environmental mobilizations of the 2000s, without Seattle and the Global Justice uprisings, and without the "our revolution" electoral momentum of Vermont's Bernie Sanders, whose utterance and continued use of the word "socialism" was almost cathartic for the U.S. political scene. U.S. fear of the "S" words (strike and socialism) has clearly diminished, as the Democratic Socialists of America (DSA) passed the 70,000-membership mark, making it one of the largest left groups in over 100 years of U.S. politics.

Beyond the U.S., this historic moment will require an understanding of the "movements of movements"—as defined, discussed, and brought together in Jai Sen's (2018) two-volume PM Press book subtitled "What Makes Us Move?" and "Rethinking Our Dance." More than ever, we must understand that future movements will be much more than a single united front or a simple political thread. We must act with an awareness, for example, that this moment at war is inextricably intertwined with the global war against mother earth, which has been waged across ideological lines by imperialists as well as the sub-imperialist corporate forces in Brazil, Russia, India, China, South Africa and beyond. We must be in tune with the evolving World Social Movement and People's Assemblies processes, much of which has been positively shaped by the "movements of movements" notions espoused by Sen and others. We must work in tandem with others countering these assaults, such as the First Ecosocialist International, founded in Venezuela; and such as a burgeoning decolonization movement led by still occupied and colonized peoples who are most profoundly connecting strategic, tactical, and conceptual issues of human and planetary liberation. The predominantly U.S. People's Strike group provides a promising set of possibilities across the lands, peoples, and histories of too-often divided mass campaigns in North America. But there must be more.

Within our virtual spaces, and as we emerge from a coronavirus cocoon, organizations and individuals have to take this opportunity to passionately dream together and to dispassionately yet lovingly critique our dreams so as to construct realities that can better withstand the crushing onslaught of a dying empire and the violent emergences of competing sub-empires.

SECTION V: STRATEGIC AND TACTICAL PRIORITIES

So, where are we? We are at a historical point where the existing public health and economic power structures are deeply stressed and potentially collapsing. Consequently, we witness a huge increase in grassroots, truly democratic efforts, including mutual aid. We see a huge rise in radical protest while broadening and deepening efforts at building people-based local alternatives. We are seeing political initiatives—from reformist demands for universal health care, free community-based education, and guaranteed jobs and income, to radical demands for labor solidarity across borders, police and prison abolition, and the rollback of militarism worldwide.

Neither capitalism, imperialism, nor U.S. superpower politics are new to crisis. But the crisis of this moment has caused these inter-related systems to enter a new phase—within the backdrop of the dying U.S. empire. The U.S. executive branch has deployed troops against state governments that are perceived as oppositional to the current regime and long-standing militarized policing practices. The troops are new; the practices of repressive policing are not. Federal policies relating to health care, especially in response to the pandemic, spotlight an extremely racialized, class-based schism whereby "herd immunity" and the question of "reopening" aspects of society equate to the mass murder of at least tens of thousands of predominately Black, Brown, Indigenous, and poor people. The speed and scale of COVID-related deaths are new. Genocidal policies based on white supremacy, patriarchy, and capitalism are not. The economic crisis spurred on by this perfect storm of factors has led to a global downturn from which the empire, as such, cannot fully recover. But an end of U.S. ability to fulfill its former imperial dreams does not mean an end to U.S. aggression, externally or internally. The weakening of the U.S. is new; the manner in which the brunt of this collapse will be borne on the backs of the most vulnerable is not.

What, therefore, should our priorities be at a time like this?

For one, thinking, talking, and acting more boldly should be a prerequisite to campaign building in this period. Even in New York City and New York State, where successes in "flattening the curve" of the COVID-19 virus has meant immediate relief in terms of hospital and health care, where a mildly liberal governor has become a national hero to many, even in this internationalist, liberal epicenter which has momentarily passed the curse of being the global coronavirus epicenter, the carrot, and stick, divide-and-conquer ruling class reform maneuvers seem to have a more limited effect than usual. Robert Cuffy, a young leader of the emerging People's Strike Movement (see https://peoplesstrike.org/) and a member of the Afro-Socialist Caucus of DSA who himself was a victim of a targeted violent right-wing attack, declared that "almost like an act of faith, the response has to be a revolution" (Solidarity National Committee, 2020).

Assassinated Black Panther leader Fred Hampton used to admonish, "It is time to settle our differences." The question now is 'Which Side Are You On?' and what form of militant resistance will you help organize for? If these questions keep being asked and concrete answers are sought to create constructive, alternative programs, positive things may emerge from the belly of the beast in this crisis-laden moment. We can be sure, at least, of two things: Nothing short of an ideologically diverse, non-sectarian, multigenerational, united front connecting a wholistic critique of racist, capitalist patriarchy will build into an effective movement for social change. And no such potentially emerging movement will be led by older males of Euro-American descent, whatever their charisma, skills, and access to money or media. This is a Black-led moment, within the U.S. and elsewhere, based not merely on past injustices but also on the contemporary realities of the working class and social conditions. The leadership of our movements must reflect the realities of our moment.

There are ironies to be faced, and we are moved to cite two icons of the "civil rights" era: one, a congressman who passed away just as these new realities were emerging, as if to pass the torch in definitive and irrevocable ways. John Lewis made his mark as a leader of young people as the Student Nonviolent Coordinating Committee spokesperson during celebrated August 1963 March on Washington for Jobs and Freedom. Lewis died on the same day as his fellow Atlanta Black leader: Reverend C.T. Vivian of the National Anti-Klan Network. Though spotlighted because of their roles in the church and the state, both of their ongoing decisions to build people's movements are significantly more important. Like many of his colleagues, C.T. could have rested on his 1960s laurels as a bona fide "friend of Dr. King" rather than choose to lead coalitions fighting against the Ku Klux Klan and the racist radical right. Once an elected Congressman, John could easily have decided to forget his past life and make his rags-to-riches story the focus of his last decades. Instead, ever the student organizer, Lewis worked to reach new generations about the importance of popular social mobilization; his comic book trilogy *The March* was more a legacy than any legislation (Lewis, 2016).

In one of his later interviews, Lewis (2016) reflected not on his days in Congress but on the movement, which enabled him to serve as an elected official. He characterized the Black-led justice campaigns in simple words but hard to replicate terms. They were all, he asserted, examples of "Love in Action." Eulogizing his old friend, Reverend James Lawson, Dr. King said he was the most strategic U.S. thinker of our time. He emphasized organizing over electoral work, movement-building above all else. Demanding that we understand Lewis not as a "Black leader" but as a true leader of "we, the people," he added that "we do not need bipartisan politics" to celebrate Lewis' life. He asked that we, freedom fighters, must determine to "not be quiet as long as any child dies in the first year of life in the United States, as long as the largest poverty group in our nation are women and children, as long as our nation continues to be the most violent culture in the history of humankind, and as long as our economy is shaped not by freedom but by plantation capitalism that continues to cause domination and control rather than access and liberty and equality for all" (O'Shea & Suggs, 2020).

Ironic also is the 2020 Presidential race, with the world watching in typical disbelief at what passes for democracy in "the land of the free." U.S. hypocrisy might be second only to India, loudly calling itself the world's largest democracy when a mere glance at occupied Kashmir reveals the opposite (Meyer & Nepram, 2019). Facing the realities of Trump and the loud and sharp outcries against his daily moves towards greater authoritarianism, militarism, nationalism, and the crushing of dissent, we are faced with an opponent in Biden, who has outwardly declared that "good, nonviolent" demonstrators should be left alone while those labeled as bad, anarchists, disrupters, antifascist, or whatever the "black mark" of the day might be, deserve whatever violence or repression they will surely get. The electorate was thus asked to choose between someone who would maim, kill, or imprison 9 out of 10 dissenters, attracting the ire of a sizeable percentage of an outraged population and, on the other hand, someone who would only maim, kill, or imprison 7 or 8 out of the above 10, but in such a way as to gain the acceptance or acquiescence—not scorn—of a similarly sizeable percentage. In either case, authoritarianism, militarism, and repression win.

The strategic priorities of the day mandate that we accept the leadership of our comrades of the South. The more successful 21st century revolutionaries—from the Zapatistas to those in Rojava and the camps of Western Sahara—have already learned that state power is less important than the need to build a new world in the shell of the old. The Latin American Peace Research Council insists that we do not even consider returning to a pre-COVID-19 normal, but that we build towards a "new normalcy" which will:

1. Guarantee the sustenance of life and attention to the material needs of the population: replacing the economic paradigm

of overproduction, speculation, capital accumulation, and exponential growth;

2. Restore value to life that takes into account future generations and puts an end to climate change, exploitation of living beings and natural assets, air and water pollution, and the destruction of forests and beaches, a paradigm that understands humans as part of the cosmos and just another species in the planet's biodiversity;
3. Replace the paradigm of what is "mine" with the paradigm of what is "ours," which recognizes that we are deeply interdependent, that there are no "others" but one common horizon;
4. Replace the logic of political representation with the logic of deliberative, direct participation;
5. Recognize different forms of knowledge, and promote their flourishing through the development of free and quality public education, based on dialogic, sentipensante (feeling-thinking), participatory and emancipatory educational strategies: an educational paradigm that promotes critical reflexivity, affection, and solidarity between peoples;
6. Conceive of health beyond illness; enhances diverse, ancestral, and emerging knowledge; and prioritize dignity, the sovereignty of bodies, and the healing of violence;
7. Recover the value of diverse memories, intersubjectivity, and singularity; which recognizes diversity as an inherent human characteristic and eliminates all forms of domination and discrimination;
8. Allow us to come together based upon our differences, in which our identities, eroticisms, and joys are not penalized: where no violence is exercised by reason of gender or sexual orientation; with no human trafficking, nor femicides; where subjects decide over their bodies and desires, care does not befall upon women, and parenthood is understood for its political and transformative potential;
9. Stimulates art and culture, understood as scenes of creation and experimentation which vindicate and renew our ways of knowing, inhabiting, and sharing the world;
10. Promote nonviolent action that assumes the construction of peace as a comprehensive and participatory process (Latin American Council for Peace Research, 2020).

There are many platforms, multiple manifestos, and countless coalitions, networks, and potential movements to follow. Radical transformation will require more than the application of tactical band-aids to piece together another few moments of familiar "good old days" feelings of "life during wartime" (Talking Heads, 1979). It will first require a transformation of our own thinking: that those we consider most vulnerable today might actually hold the keys to a new tomorrow. A vulnerable series of oppressive systems might cause much destruction in their downfall, but that destruction will still be better than a maintenance of old status quos. Our thinking must lead to unified action: as People's Strike has written, "unity not uniformity." But we must be prepared for continued dark times and the fight of our lives.

This ain't no fooling around.

REFERENCES

Black Lives Matter Protests 2020. (2020). https://www.creosotemaps.com/blm2020/

Brownstein, R. (2020). The eye-popping cost of Medicare. *The Atlantic.* https://www.theatlantic.com/politics/archive/2019/10/high-cost-warren-and-sanderss-single-payer-plan/600166/

Buchanan, L., Bui, Q., & Patel, J. (2020, July 3). Black Lives Matter may be the largest movement in U.S. history. *New York Times.* ttps://www.nytimes.com/interactive/2020/07/03/us/george-floyd-protests-crowd-size.html

Devereaux, R. (2020, June 6). Police attacks on protesters are rooted in a violent ideology of reactionary grievance. *The Intercept.* https://theintercept.com/2020/06/06/police-brutality-protests-blue-lives-matter/?utm_medium=email&utm_source=The%20Intercept%20Newsletter

Editorial Board. (2020, April 11). Opinion: Has the coronavirus pandemic provided urgency for universal health coverage? Yes and no. *Washington Post.* https://www.washingtonpost.com/opinions/has-the-coronavirus-provided-urgency-for-universal-health-coverage-yes-and-no/2020/04/10/de30bce6-7b40-11ea-9bee-c5bf9d2e3288_story.html

Facher, L. (2020, May 19). 9 ways COVID-19 may forever upend the U.S. health care industry. *Stat.* https://www.statnews.com/2020/05/19/9-ways-covid-19-forever-upend-health-care/

Friedman, Z. (2020, May 6). How COVID-19 will change the future of work. *Forbes.* https://www.forbes.com/sites/zackfriedman/2020/05/06/covid-19-future-of-work-coronavirus/?sh=724a55bc73b2

Galtung, J. (2009). *The fall of the US empire—and then what?* TRANSCEND University Press.

Germanos, A. (2020, August 4). Teacher protests erupt as #DemandSafeSchools takes off. *Common Dreams.* https://www.commondreams.org/news/2020/08/04/teacher-protests-erupt-demandsafeschools-takes

Gilmore, R. (2021). *Change everything: Racial capitalism and the case for abolition.* Haymarket Books.

Goldberg, J. (2020, June 3). James Mattis denounces President Trump, describes him as a threat to the constitution. *The Atlantic.* https://www.theatlantic.com/politics/archive/2020/06/james-mattis-denounces-trump-protests-militarization/612640/

Harding, V. (2010). *Hope and history: Why we must share the story of the movement.* Orbis Books.

Humphrey, W. (2020, July 17). Federal and local police team up in aggressive response to day 50 of Portland protests. *Portland Mercury.* https://www.portlandmercury.com/blogtown/2020/07/18/28652209/federal-and-local-police-team-up-in-aggressive-response-to-night-50-of-portland-protests

Jones, S. (2020, July 17). America's teachers face an impossible choice. *NY Magazine.* https://nymag.com/intelligencer/2020/07/teachers-back-to-school-protests.html

Jun, N., & Lance, M. (2020). Anarchist responses to a pandemic: The COVID-19 crisis as a case-study in mutual aid/ *Kennedy Institute of Ethics Journal.* https://kiej.georgetown.edu/anarchist-responses-covid-19-special-issue

Latin American Council for Peace Research. (2020, May 28). Latin Americans call for a more just and peaceful "new normal." *Waging Nonviolence.* https://wagingnonviolence.org/ipra/2020/05/manifesto-for-a-more-just-and-peaceful-new-normal/

Leonhardt, D. (2020, August 6). The unique U.S. failure to control the virus. *New York Times.* https://www.nytimes.com/2020/08/06/us/coronavirus-us.html

Lewis, J. (2016). *The march trilogy.* Top Shelf Productions.

Lorber, B. (2020, July 19). A constellation of threats: Far-Rightists respond to the Black-led uprising. *Three Way Fight.* http://threewayfight.blogspot.com/2020/07/a-constellation-of-threats-far.html

Meyer, M. (2020, July 20). Moments at war. In *Movements of Movements.* Open Source Website. https://movementsofmovements.net/openspace/moments-at-war

Meyer, M., & Nepram, B. (2019, December 1). 150 years after Gandhi's birth, authoritarianism in India must be met with resistance. *Waging Nonviolence.* https://wagingnonviolence.org/rs/2019/12/150-years-after-gandhis-birth-authoritarianism-in-india-must-be-met-with-resistance/

Miller, I., Becker, A., Grenfell, B., & Metcalf, J. (2020). Disease and healthcare burden of COVID-19 in the United States. *Nature Medicine, 26,* 1212–1217.

Nicola, M., Alsafi, Z., Sohrabi, C., Kerwan, A., Al-Jabir, A., Iosifidis, C., Agha, M., & Agha, A. (2020). The socioeconomic implications of the coronavirus pandemic (COVID-19): A review. *International Journal of Surgery, 78,* 185–193.

O'Shea, B., & Suggs, E. (2020, July 31). John Lewis' funeral: Remarks by Rev. James Lawson. *Atlanta Journal Constitution.* https://www.ajc.com/john-lewis/john-lewiss-funeral-remarks-by-rev-james-lawson/4HUU5KYIEBB4VBLQZPW54YIGIY/

Reynolds, K. (2020, May 14). Will COVID-19 bring us closer to universal healthcare? *Medical Economics.* https://www.medicaleconomics.com/view/will-covid-19-bring-us-closer-universal-healthcare

Santini, J., & Cordoba, R. (2020, June 1). *People's Strike Broadcast* [Facebook]. https://www.facebook.com/113492336999520/videos/3300196266691229

Sen J. (Ed.). (2018). *The movement of movements* (Parts 1 and 2). PM Press.

Slavitt, A. (2020, April 4). The coronavirus crisis will force us to reconsider universal health care. *Medium.* https://coronavirus.medium.com/the-coronavirus-crisis-will-force-us-to-reconsider-universal-health-care-d5e26380e744

Solidarity National Committee. (2020, July 3). On the attack on Robert Cuffy at the mass march to defund the NYPD. *Solidarity.* https://solidarity-us.org/on-the-attack-on-robert-cuffy-at-the-mass-march-to-defund-the-nypd/

Solnit, R. (2010). *A paradise built in hell: The extraordinary communities that arise in disaster*. Penguin Press.

Talking Heads. (1979). "Life During Wartime." from *Fear of Music*. Sire Records.

Will, M., & Schwartz, S. (2020, June 1). "Teachers cannot be silent": How educators are supporting Black students after protests. *Edweek*. https://www.edweek.org/teaching-learning/teachers-cannot-be-silent-how-educators-are-supporting-black-students-after-protests/2020/06

CONCLUDING THOUGHTS

The State of the Pandemic on Our Most Vulnerable

Pamela D. Hall

As this book concludes, America is still amid the COVID-19 pandemic. The U.S. count was as follows on December 19, 2021, a number still increasing: 50,636,126 confirmed cases and 802,969 deaths (CDC COVID tracker, 2021). Yet, what is noticeably missing from this data is an accurate portrayal of the social, economic, public health, and mental health impact that the pandemic has on vulnerable populations. The only data that the CDC releases regarding vulnerable populations are individuals in the prison industrial complex and individuals with preexisting conditions. The accurate count for race and ethnicity is not reported, and many states do not report those numbers either. The numbers are continuing to rise; people are still risking their lives and the lives of those close to them. This includes frontline workers, such as nurses and doctors who continue to treat patients. Other vulnerable groups such as warehouse workers, farmworkers, and grocery clerks are still leaving their homes, filled with angst and higher than normal stress levels. They go to work, often by way of public transportation. The reported cases of other vulnerable groups, such as those living in poverty, the multiple ethnic groups of the Black, Brown,

Preparing Quality Teachers:
Advances in Clinical Practice, pp. 351–355

and Indigenous People of Color, aka BIPOCs, are still disproportionately high. We have no accurate count of the number of cases amongst students or professors who returned to the classroom. Further, we do not know how many of our LGBTQ community members have been impacted.

These vulnerable groups are not privileged to stay at home and work. In fact, many of them may be sick or have lost their jobs, as millions of individuals file unemployment claims each week. The lack of health insurance also impacts testing and services, including possible hospitalization. Thus, many may try homemade remedies when symptoms arise. Schools are opening back up, yet those living in poverty, those considered "essential" workers, do not have the option to stay at home and continue educating their children from home. These "essential" works have to take the risk that their child will be exposed to the virus at school and bring it home to an elderly family member or a family member with a preexisting condition. Why? Because they do not have the privilege to work from home. They must work in order if they want to have the necessities of food, clothing, and shelter. Why? Because the era of neoliberalism has created a society of "I" and not "we," a society of greed and power over fairness and equity.

Higher education is taking a big hit, as professors alter their teaching styles to meet their students' needs via virtual learning. Some universities have had to close their doors permanently. Many adjunct faculty member's teaching loads have been reduced, creating financial strain and mental exhaustion. Faculty are asked to remain flexible and compassionate when they themselves also need compassion. Professors, many with children, are also having to navigate teaching and supporting their young children who are in school remotely. They are dealing with their teenagers suffering from great loneliness and sinking into anxiety and states of depression, if not suicidal ideation.

Many students report to their professors that they must work to pay tuition and help their families. They state that they are frightened every day when they go to their low paying yet demanding jobs—frightened because people will not wear their masks. When these consumers are confronted, they become threatening and belligerent. The students need a safe space to discuss such issues, and professors need to make that space available if they expect their students to succeed under such tenuous situations. Faculty members who have contributed to this book described how they, as well as their students, are navigating this "new normal."

Throughout the book, a common theme was that Black individuals from the diaspora who live in the U.S were disproportionately diagnosed and died from the coronavirus. Did these people have to die? Perhaps if they had not had so many preexisting conditions, those associated with current day systemic oppression and past historical trauma, the rates would not have been so high. If the large population of those vulnerable and so-called essential workers had health insurance they would not have endured such levels of heartache. Perhaps if many of them were not living in suboptimal conditions, they could have avoided the virus. Those that died may have been able to recover. Yet, as one of the coeditors points out, "healing is peace." Healing is necessary for peace. These individuals deserve healing and peace.

From the perspective of this book's contributors, healing has come in many forms. One is the training and workshops by the Association of Black Psychologists-South Florida Chapter that provided mental and spiritual support to these communities. The Haitian Mental Health Think Tank. Haitian contributors addressed *Soufras a Ayien* or Haitian suffering, and how the pandemic accentuated this suffering. Healing has also come through contributors who discussed Kemetic yoga and meditation practices as well as teletherapy. These professionals have seen an increase in need and responded to this need by these vulnerable populations. They also report the considerable need to support those suffering from continued trauma via sexual assault, domestic violence, systemic oppression, abuse, and neglect. They are reporting more men than ever asking for help. Black men from the diaspora rarely seek mental health support. However, the pandemic has changed this. That might be one silver lining. The stigma is being reduced for Black men because they realize they need support to make it through these very trying times. Calls and e-mails are flowing in from Blacks asking specifically for help from someone "who looks like me" and the LGBTQ community has been seeking therapists trained in working with their specific needs. Like the educators who contributed to this volume, mental and spiritual healers noted the need to do more self-care due to this increased work. For they too have lost family and friends during this pandemic.

Amid the pandemic, many of us have witnessed the mistreatment of BIPOC through police brutality and unfair criminal justice actions. Many people were on lockdown due to COVID, so they witnessed the 8 minutes and 46 seconds of a police officer with his knee on the neck of George Floyd as the victim cried out to his deceased mother. This sparked many protests and calls for police reform, but the killings did not and have not stopped. The trauma continues, no doubt contributing to more stress and possible cases of COVID-19. If many Americans had not been at home to witness the lynchings of George Floyd, Breonna Taylor, and many other BIPOC, they might have continued to turn a blind eye to this continued abuse. Fortunately, the stay-at-home order may have caused many allies to support these communities of color and to call for reform and healing. Contributors from South Florida People of Color (SFPoC), a racial healing organization, have also seen a surge in the need for diversity, equity, and inclusion training for schools, businesses, legal services, and universities.

SFPoC has held virtual anti-racism trainings to help people of all races and ethnicities have open dialogues and think about action steps to address this continued trauma.

This book discussed the impact of COVID-19 on vulnerable populations, but the contributors also provided voices and echoes of hope and stories of resiliency. Resiliency is in the DNA of many marginalized groups. That is how and why they have survived the systemic and institutional practices that have tried for centuries to wipe them out. That is how and why they have withstood the wave of neoliberalism that has come and gone as the government treated vulnerable communities as inhuman or as commodities. Many of the contributors suggest we must go back and fetch the past. Go back to past cultural practices, principles of spirituality such as communalism and respect for nature. Indigenous people and Blacks from the diaspora hold similar beliefs in this regard. They can attest to the fact that suffering brings strength and resiliency. As Blacks from the diaspora state, we must adopt the principle of Sankofa, which means "go back and fetch it." Go back to the past and incorporate ways of being and knowing that have sustained these people for generations. A common theme from the contributors was also the principle of Ubuntu--"I am because we are." As we practice the notion of collectivism and communalism, the echoes of hope will ring louder, and the vulnerable will prevail.

Some of the book's contributors introduced new concepts from their epistemology, such as ancestral liberation theology (alecia deon) or Melanated people from the Diaspora (Hall), BIPOC (Finley, Pate, & Roberts), Soufrans Ayisyen (Desir, Gentry, and Louis), and *Soufrans Ayisyen Syndrome (Jeanty)*. We hope that these concepts will be adopted and contribute to our understanding of vulnerable communities' strength, hope, resiliency, and spirituality.

Many of these chapters provide suggestions that can help the reader during these times. Reports are coming that a vaccine will not be ready for nearly a year, and with the winter months coming, the numbers may begin to surge again. Many BIPOC are mistrusting of the medical community. Many immigrants, such as those in detention centers, may now feel the American Dream is a continued nightmare for them. They fled their home countries where they were victimized and traumatized and risked their lives to make the voyage to America. Once they arrived, they only continued living in terror by being subjugated in unsafe facilities, abuse, neglect, and exposure to conditions that leave them vulnerable to contacting COVID-19. Yet, like so many other vulnerable communities, their cries for help fall on deaf ears.

Let us take a hint from the planet, Mother Maya. Some say that the stay-at-home order is allowing earth to replenish herself. There is less pollution in the air because of fewer planes in the sky and vehicles on the roads.

There is less eating out, so less waste. The animals in the sea are happy because fewer people are violating their home. There are reports that the bees are coming back. Some call this moment of stillness a form of peace that nature needed. And if we heed nature's call, we too should remain still and reset. Reset in ways that the busy lives we have been leading have not allowed us to. Though we may not control COVID-19, we can control how we react to this pandemic; we can control and manage ourselves and treat one another in a more just and peaceful manner.

What is peace? We often think of peace as a state of mind. I contend that peace is a verb; peace is about action. That action involves steps towards renewal—a renewal of our mind, body, and spirit. Peace means connecting with nature and seeing ourselves as living in harmony with nature, not conquering nature. Peace means being quiet, meditating, and reflecting. We must go beyond the pandemic to a place where we see one another as human beings, all striving for peace and a piece of the American Dream. In conclusion, let us all reflect on the fact that we stand on the land of indigenous people. And as we continue to navigate COVID-19, let us reflect on these words from Red Cloud:

> "I am poor and naked, but I am the chief of the nation. We do not want riches, but we do want to train our children right. Riches would do us no good. We could not take them with us to the other world. We do not want riches. We want peace and love."
>
> —Red Cloud, Makhpiya-luta (Gibby-Brown, 2020)

REFERENCES

CDC COVID Data Tracker. (2021, December 19). *CDC*. https://covid.cdc.gov/covid-data-tracker/?CDC_AA_refVal=https%3A%2F%2Fwww.cdc.gov%2Fcoronavirus%2F2019-ncov%2Fcases-updates%2Fcases-in-us.html#cases_casesinlast7days

Gibby-Brown, S. (2020, March 10). 50 wise Native American quotes on community, respect and more. *Everyday Power*. https://everydaypower.com/native-american-quotes/

EPILOGUE

Pamela D. Hall

The first COVID vaccine was administered on December 14, 2020. Since then, as of August 2021, over 60% of the United States has received at least one shot (Reuters, 2021). Yet, the hopes for herd immunity seem doubtful at present. This may be due in part to how vulnerable populations have been treated before and during this pandemic. As outlined in this book, vulnerable populations include BIPOC, the poor, LGTBQ+, the elderly, the homeless, victims of violence, those who are stigmatized because of mental health diagnoses, front-line workers such as nurses, immigrants, prisoners, and descendants of Africans enslaved in the America (DAEA). Vulnerable populations may be at risk for dangerous side effects, have illnesses that do not make them eligible for the vaccine, or are reluctant to take the vaccine. There have been media campaigns urging DAEA, BIPOC, and other vulnerable groups who have been historically and culturally infected by a system of oppression encouraging them to take the vaccine. In some cases, people are being incentivized to take the vaccine. Yet, there is a great deal of hesitancy that remains.

For descendants of DAEA, many people assume that the distrust and hesitancy are due to the Tuskegee experiment. However, as Harriet Washington points out in her book *Medical Apartheid*, DAEA have been the subjects of experiments without their consent from the days of slavery

Coronavirus and Vulnerable People: Addressing the Divide in Harm and Responses and Exploring Implications for a More Peaceful World, pp. 357–360

by medical practitioners such as J. Marion Sims. He did experiments on enslaved women without anesthesia and surgical procedures on infants diagnosed with neonatal tetanus. Using an awl, which is a tool used to pierces holes, this being forcibly pierced holes in infants' heads. All the infants died, as the procedure is fatal. Many studies have been done on prisoners and children as well without informed consent or with deception. What is called vaccine hesitancy to some may be a logical summation not to trust those who have inflicted pain on you and your loved ones for centuries. These individuals are also cautious because of past treatment by health care officials, without care and empathy.

Many students from colleges and universities are expected to attend classes in person this fall. Some have already colleges and universities have begun in-person classes. Students are anxious, and quite frankly, some students are afraid to return to campuses because they have not taken the vaccine. They are experiencing a great deal of anxiety around returning to in-person activities for fear that they may harm family members with autoimmune disorders or not eligible for the vaccine. Preexisting conditions, stress, poverty, and family history may be contributing factors that make these family members not eligible for the vaccine. There are also college professors and adjunct professors who have these preexisting conditions and cannot take the vaccine. They, too, are anxious, and some report panic attacks at the thought of returning the school. Some students and faculty members are anti-vaxers and will not be taking the vaccine. This pandemic and the consistent re-traumatization of vulnerable populations have indeed taken a toll.

In many cases, when we think about the vaccine, we think of it as though America is a monolithic society. If one were to believe the media campaigns, everyone is eligible to take the vaccine. Everyone does not include many of those described above, as America is not a monolith. Some individuals cannot take the current vaccine. So, the statement that everyone can take the vaccine is just as flawed as the clinical trials that were done to develop the vaccine. There were no clinical trials on special populations, such as individuals with preexisting conditions, autoimmune diseases, pregnant women, or children. This oversight suggests that these trials lacked reliability and are not useful for some vulnerable populations. It also makes one wonder about the mindset of the powerful and privileged individuals who decided not to do trials on vulnerable populations. Did they say this vaccine will be administered to the monolithic aspect of the population, with the notion that we will vaccinate the largest number of people eligible? Sounds sort of like survival of the fittest. It makes one wonder about philosopher Thomas Malthus writing entitled *Principle on the Population*. The notion behind Malthusian misery is that there will be too many people on the planet, and the resources, especially food, would not be available for everyone. Malthus events such as plagues would come along to reduce the size of the population, creating misery. Well, if it happens naturally, that is as it should occur. The results are still out with regards to whether COVID-19 was created in a lab or happened naturally. What is evident is that when the solution to the plague in the form of the vaccine does not consider all people when creating the vaccine, what results is an unequal distribution of resources and bias towards those less fortunate.

Whether individuals take the vaccine or not, whether those who have taken the vaccine will need a booster shot is yet to be seen. It is clear that vulnerable populations still are victims of this oppressive system which continues to discount them. As of February 2022, 75.3% of the population had received at least one dose of the vaccine. Of those that reported their race/ethnicity, 66% of the those not vaccinated are White. This is a narrowing of the gap from May 2021, when only 9% were Black, 14% were Hispanic, 6% were Asian, 1% were First Nation, less than 1% were Native Hawaiian or Pacific Islander (Nduga et al., 2022).

Further, as of June 2021, more than 33,093 238 cases were in the United States, and the daily average was over 15,000. This is a steady decline in cases since the vaccine started being administered from over 220,000 daily to 15,000. Yet, who are those 15,000? Are they the most vulnerable, those with preexisting conditions? So, the vaccine does not seem to be reaching the most vulnerable for myriad reasons. At the top of the list is continued systemic and institutional oppression.

Chapter 12 contributor Roni Bennett says racism is a preexisting condition. This perspective can be expanded to include systemic and institutional oppression as a preexisting condition. These preexisting conditions have compounded the trauma of the pandemic on the most vulnerable by rolling back time to days where there are more overt acts of oppression. State legislators around the country are passing bills that will make it extremely difficult for individuals that have been marginalized to vote. Other states are expanding abortion legislation to include heartbeat laws. This recently occurred in Texas, where it is illegal to have an abortion after six weeks, when most fetal heartbeats are detectable. In Florida, anti-trans and LGBTQ+ laws were passed on the first and second day of June, Pride Month.

America, how did we get so far gone? Perhaps we were always this way, for the country did start with the slaughtering of Indigenous people and captioning Africans, buying them, and enslaving them in this country for 246 years. Yes, the elderly were the first to receive the vaccine. However, that leaves out a large group of the who may have sickle cell, diabetes, sarcoidosis, and other autoimmune disorders such as lupus. We must ask ourselves why are the most vulnerable always an afterthought. There is much talk about herd immunity, yet it will not be achieved if vulnerable populations are continually left to fend for themselves without a living wage.

There is excitement in the air, and people are packing up their campers, dusting off their passports, having family reunions, and just enjoying social interaction or being hugged. Unfortunately, this may not be possible for many vulnerable populations. They do not have campers to pack up or the vacation days to take a trip, let alone the money to afford the trip. They are still waiting in food lines. Passports to leave the country are not likely for the thousands of individuals, children, and families who have crossed the borders and remain in detention camps. They are not trying to leave the country for respite; they are escaping trauma, sexual exploitation, gang violence, and poverty. The freedom we often take for granted is an escape from daily traumatic incidents for our immigrant and refugee communities.

In sum, one thing is for certain, those who are victims of oppression and those who care for them, such as all the contributors to this book, ***we are tired***. We are tired and weary. Yet, we contribute to march forward on the paths set forth by our ancestors. The Black male has been pushed so hard that he is seeking mental health support. That, in fact, is one of the silver linings of the pandemic. More people, such as Black males, are seeking mental health support, more vulnerable groups are starting to support one another in the activism and call for peace, equity, and justice. We recognize the strength in numbers. For we know, we must continue the work of our ancestors' hopes, dreams, visions, and prayers. We march forward towards equity, justice, and peace, making beauty from ashes. In the words of Maya Angelou (1978):

> You may write me down in history
> With your bitter, twisted lies,
> You may trod me in the very dirt
> But still, like dust, I'll rise.

Yes, vulnerable populations and those who support them continue to rise!

REFERENCES

Angelou, M. (1978). *And still I rise.* Random House.

Ndugga, N., Hill, L., Artiga, S., & Haldar, S. (2022, February 2). *Latest Data on COVID-19 vaccinations by race/ethnicity.* KFF. https://www.kff.org/coronavirus-covid-19/issue-brief/latest-data-on-covid-19-vaccinations-by-race-ethnicity/

Reuters. (2021, August 9). *Nearly 60% of Americans at least partially vaccinated against COVID-19—CDC.* https://www.usnews.com/news/us/articles/2021-08-09/nearly-60-of-americans-at-least-partially-vaccinated-against-covid-19-cdc

APPENDIX

Table A

Resources and Information

Name and Organization	Contact Information
Roni Bennet, Executive Director, South Florida People of Color	Website: https://southfloridapoc.org E: rbennett@southfloridapoc.org E: info@southfloridapoc.org
T. Conswello Davis, MA, MBA, CYT Goddess Health & Wellness, LLC	Website: www.ghw-llc.com E: goddesshwell@gmail.com
Alecia Deon	Website: aconjurewoman.com Website: roseandconcrete.com E: hello@roseandconcrete.com
Dr. Charlene Desir, The Empowerment Network (T.E.N), Global Haitian Mental Health Think Tank The Black Androgynous Genius Project	Website: https://tenglobal.org/ E: info@tenglobal.org P: 786-588-8855

(Appendix continued on next page)

Coronavirus and Vulnerable People: Addressing the Divide in Harm and Responses and Exploring Implications for a More Peaceful World, pp. 361–362

Table A (Continued)

Resources and Information

Name and Organization	Contact Information
Dr. Guy Jeanty, LMFT	Website: www.drjeanty.com
Jeanty Counseling & Consulting, LLC	E: DRJLMFT@gmail.com
Elizabeth Farrah Louis, PhD	Website:
Pamela D. Hall, PhD	https://www.linkedin.com/mwlite/in/dr-elizabeth-louis-53b76210
	E: eflouis2011@gmail.com
	Black Healer's Network
	Bhnetwork2020@gmail.com
Ruben Roberts,	Website: http://miamidadenaacp.com
President of the Miami Dade Branch of the NAACP	E: presidentofmiamidadenaacp@gmail.com
Mureen Shaw	E: r.roberts@rer-consulting.com
JoHanna "J" Thompson, MPA	Organization: The Jamaica Nurses'
	Association of Florida, Inc.
	Website: http://jamaicanursesoffl.org/
	E: jamaicanursesflorida@gmail.com
	Consultant with National Black Women's
	Justice Institute (NBWJI)
	Website: www.nbwji.org E:jthompson@nbwji.org

ABOUT THE EDITORS AND AUTHORS

EDITORS

Laura L. Finley, PhD, is Professor of Sociology and Criminology at Barry University in Miami Shores, Florida. She is the author, coauthor, or editor of more than 30 books, as well as numerous book chapters and journal articles. Additionally, Dr. Finley is a syndicated columnist with *Peace Voice* as well as an activist for peace, human rights, and gender equality. She serves as cochair of the Board of Directors for the Peace and Justice Studies Association and is a Board Member for The Humanity Project and Floridians for Alternatives to the Death Penalty. With Michael Minch, Dr. Finley coedits the *Peace Studies: Edges and Innovations* series.

Pamela D. Hall, PhD, is an Associate Professor of Psychology at Barry University in Miami Shores, Florida. Dr. Hall is actively involved in projects throughout South Florida involving the empowerment of children and families, particularly Haitian adolescents. From 2010–2015 Hall received a $296,000.00 grant from The Miami Children's Trust to implement a summer for Haitian middle and high school students called the Haitian Empowerment and Literacy Project (H.E.L.P). Dr. Hall also serves as a facilitator for South Florida People of Color, serves on the board for the Haitian Youth Community Center of Florida, is the President of the Board for the Alliance for GLBTQ Youth, and President-Elect for the South Florida Chapter of the Association of Black Psychologists. She has received numerous awards for her work and published scholarly articles on Haitian adolescents' and adults' spirituality and mental health.

AUTHORS

Roni Bennett is cofounder and executive director of the non-profit organization South Florida People of Color, which focuses on socialization and education to build empathy. It does that by offering programs that change hearts and minds. Factoring history's role in upholding racism, its efforts are aimed at increasing knowledge and communication between people who live racially segregated lives.

Karine Champagne is a Clinical Therapist with 14 years of experience. She graduated from Oakwood University with a BSW in 2003. She graduated from Alabama A&M University with an MSW in 2004. She is a proud product of two HBCUs. She is a passionate advocate for optimum mental health, especially among vulnerable populations such as women, children, and African Diaspora. She specializes in grief and loss, anxiety, depression, and trauma. Karine is the CEO of Geriwellness, which focuses on educating the public about mental health and healing from emotional wounds. She is a speaker, a psychotherapist by trade, but most importantly, a lover of people living out their best lives.

Conswello Davis is a Mental Health counselor/practitioner, doctoral student, author, public speaker, social justice advocate, spiritual and trauma specialist trained in Eye Movement Desensitization and Reprocessing (EMDR), establishing a unique professional identity in multicultural counseling. Ms. Davis is a world traveler who loves culture, practices yoga and meditation, and believes in promoting holistic health and wellness.

Pascale Denis received her medical degree in Psychiatry from Haïti and worked as a licensed psychiatrist for seven years before moving to the United States. She is a Licensed Mental Health Counselor in South Florida. Her approach expands on the disease or medical model of psychopathology by including contextual factors to understand and better treat patients. Specifically, she realized the value of addressing patients' culturally based beliefs about their illness, challenges, and interventions. In her private practice, she works with a diverse population, focusing on addressing challenges associated with acculturation for first- and second-generation immigrants, as well as issues around gender and affectional orientation. Sessions are conducted in English, French and/or Creole.

alecia deon is a queer, Caribbean immigrant living in the United States and surviving Sickle Cell Anemia. As a writer, visual artist, and independent scholar, she is committed to giving voice to her experience, empowering herself and others like her. In 2015, Alecia Deon graduated from the University of South Florida with a Bachelor of Arts degree in Africana Studies. While there, she was awarded a $20,000 David L. Boren Scholarship from the U.S. State Department to study Swahili culture and language in Zanzibar, Tanzania. She has spent over a decade working in various capacities within the education system, serving the needs of Black youth in South Florida. She has received scholarships and volunteered with the Sickle Cell Disease Association of Broward County. During Hurricane Irma, she launched a social media campaign and raised $3300 in 3 days to support vulnerable populations in South Florida and Houston, Texas. In fall 2019, her article "Between the Worlds of the Colonizer and the Conjure Woman" was published in *QED: A Journal in GLBTQ Worldmaking*. Through her work, she constructs a means for the disenfranchised to reclaim their truth, edify their best self, and fulfill their highest purpose.

Charlene Désir is a professor at Nova Southeastern University's Abraham S. Fischler College of Education. She received her doctorate from Harvard University. Dr. Désir's academic interest is in the social, psychological, and spiritual adjustment of immigrants, specifically psychosocial trauma, and how psychosocial issues affect social, cognitive, identity, and spiritual development. Dr. Désir has presented various papers on the topic of immigrants and their adjustment to the United States. She has also published on the topic of immigrant identity, spirituality, and becoming a reflective researcher. Dr. Désir founded The Empowerment Network (TEN). It is a global nonprofit organization that supports the personal, spiritual, and academic development of women and students in Haiti and the United States. She was the 2012 president and is presently the vice president of Kosanba-Vodou academic conference. Dr. Désir has worked as a school psychologist, a K–12 school counselor, an academic advisor, and a professor.

Luigi Esposito, PhD, is a Professor of Sociology and Criminology at Barry University, Miami Shores, FL (United States). He has coedited four books, presented academic papers in dozens of professional conferences in several countries, and published numerous articles and book chapters on neoliberalism, race and ethnic relations, social theory, mental health, gun politics, and globalization, and ethics. His research has appeared in various peer-reviewed professional journals, including *The Sociological Quarterly*, *The Western Journal of Black Studies*, *Humanity and Society*, *Journal of Aging and Identity*, *Studies in Symbolic Interaction*, *Theory in Action*, *Peace Studies Journal*, *State Crime Journal*, and *Perspectives on Global Development and Technology*.

Dr. Esposito has also served in various professional journals' editorial boards, including *Sociology of Race and Ethnicity*, *Humanity and Society*, and the *Western Journal of Black Studies*.

Laura L. Finley, PhD, is a Professor of Sociology and Criminology at Barry University in Miami Shores, Florida. She is the author, coauthor, or editor of more than thirty books, as well as numerous book chapters and journal articles. Additionally, Dr. Finley is a syndicated columnist with *Peace Voice* as well as an activist for peace, human rights, and gender equality. She serves as cochair of the Board of Directors for the Peace and Justice Studies Association. She is a Board Member for The Humanity Project and Floridians for Alternatives to the Death Penalty. With Michael Minch, Dr. Finley coedits the Peace Studies: Edges and Innovations series.

Pamela D. Hall is an Associate Professor of Psychology and Associate Dean of Graduate Studies for the College of Arts and Sciences at Barry University in Miami Shores, Florida. She received her PhD in Social Psychology from Ohio State University. Before arriving at Barry University, Dr. Hall taught at Hampton University. She holds the position of President-Elect of The Association of Black Psychologists, South Florida Chapter. Dr. Hall is an Afrikan-centered Psychologist who focuses on spirituality and well-being. Dr. Hall is actively involved in projects throughout South Florida involving the empowerment of children and families, particularly Haitian adolescents. From 2010–2015 Hall received a $296,000.00 grant from The Children's Trust to implement a summer for Haitian middle and high school students called the Haitian Empowerment and Literacy Project (H.E.L.P). Dr. Hall also serves as a facilitator for South Florida People of Color, serves on the board for the Haitian Youth Community Center of Florida, is the President of the Board for the Alliance for GLBTQ Youth, and President-Elect for the South Florida Chapter of the Association of Black Psychologists. She has received numerous awards for her work and published scholarly articles on Haitian adolescents' and adults' spirituality and mental health.

Jordana A. Hart is an associate of the law firm Hart & Associates. Previously, Jordana had a solo immigration law practice in Cambridge, Massachusetts, where she specialized in immigration and nationality law. She is a former associate of Ross, Silverman & Levy, LLP, an immigration law firm in Boston, MA. Jordana has a BA from Brandeis University and an MSc from Boston University. She graduated cum laude from Suffolk University Law School in Boston in 2004 with distinction in the International Law concentration. Jordana founded and chaired Suffolk Law School's Immigration Law Committee. Jordana has experience helping clients obtain

H-1B, L-1, E, and O visas and permanent residence through Labor Certification, National Interest Waiver, and other employment-based immigration options. She also has expertise in visas for victims of crime. Prior to law school, Jordana was a journalist with *The Boston Globe* for 12 years. Jordana is admitted to practice law in Massachusetts and is a member of the American Immigration Lawyers Association. She handles temporary protected status applications for Haitian national's pro-bono. Jordana was born in Montréal, Canada. She is a citizen of Canada and a lawful permanent resident of the United States. Jordana currently resides in Miami, FL. She speaks English, Spanish, and French.

Fanya Jabouin-Monnay, DMFT, LMFT—holds a doctorate in Marriage and Family Therapy with a Certificate in Medical Family Therapy and is a Licensed Marriage & Family Therapist in South Florida. She is the founder and clinical director of Family Matters Therapeutic Services, LLC, a private practice that provides mental health services to families, couples, individuals, and groups. Dr. Jabouin-Monnay also works as a family counselor for the Broward County School board, providing counseling and crisis services to middle and high school students. Her research focus is Brief Systemic Therapy with immigrant and refugee families. For the past 25 years, she has been instrumental and active in promoting refugee resettlement and acculturation issues for Haitian families. She is also trained as a Clinical Trauma Professional, and she is a state of Florida Qualified Supervisor for MFT and MHC registered interns. She is a nationally certified Youth Mental Health First Aid (YMHFA) Instructor, teaching adults who work with youth to learn strategies for helping someone in both crisis and noncrisis situations. Dr. Jabouin-Monnay works extensively with community groups, Haitian organizations, and churches to support efforts to meet Haitian individuals' mental health needs and the professionals who serve the community.

r. Guy Jeanty earned a doctorate in Marriage and Family Therapy from Nova Southeastern University. He has more than 20 years of experience in Family Systems Therapy, a treatment mode that he skillfully incorporates in working with clients. As a counselor, Dr. Jeanty has worked with the Department of Children and Families, providing court-mandated counseling to emotionally distressed children and families. He has conducted supervised therapeutic family visitations, mental health evaluations, and personality assessment. Dr. Jeanty has served as a board member of the American Association of Integrative Medicine, a board member of Broward County's Agency for Persons with Disabilities, a Faulk Professional Leadership Council member Faulk Center for Counseling in Boca Raton, FL. He is now a volunteer Family Mediator at the Broward County Court.

Alexandra Lavado is a Hispanic/LatinX immigrant who has been residing in South Florida for the last 23 years. She developed an interest in clinical child and adolescent psychology at a young age. As a high school student, she started a community service project that fundraised money, books, and toys for children with special needs and delivered them to the University of Miami's Debbie Institute. She also volunteered at the Debbie Institute for two years and helped children with developmental delays. In 2016 she graduated with a Bachelor of Arts in Psychology and Political Science and a Latin American Studies specialization from Syracuse University. Afterward, she has continued her studies in the clinical psychology program at Barry University. Her research has focused on examining the role of social support in the acculturative-stress-antisocial behavior relationship in Hispanic youth. As a clinical psychologist practicum student, she had the opportunity to work with Haitian children at the Lillie M. Williams Head Start Center and currently carries out her clinical internship with the North Miami Foundation for Senior Citizen's Services and works with the older adults' population. As her studies expand, she hopes her skills and knowledge of psychology can help address individual problems and serve as a medium to help bring social change to vulnerable populations.

Wim Laven, PhD, has two decades of experience working, researching, and teaching in the fields of peacebuilding, conflict resolution, and conflict management. His experiences range from maximum security prison and complex humanitarian disasters to reconciliation, small claims mediation, and the Special Olympics. He currently serves on the Peace and Justice Studies Association board and the International Peace Research Association board. He works as part of the editorial team for the *Peace Chronicle* magazine.

Elizabeth Louis is a Haitian American psychologist with clinical and research interests in global mental health, trauma, disaster mental health, and ethnic/racial minorities' well-being. Her experiences have led her to engage in community mental health work in Haiti and Rwanda to address mental health stigma and health disparities and incorporate culturally appropriate training for health/mental health professionals and laypersons in diverse settings. She is a recipient of local, state, and national awards, which attest to her commitment to mental health and service to marginalized and underserved populations.

Matt Meyer is an internationally noted author, historian, and organizer, elected in 2018 as Secretary-General of the International Peace Research Association (IPRA, the world's leading consortium of university-based professors, scholars, students, and community leaders). Meyer is the Senior

Research Scholar of the University of Massachusetts/Amherst's Resistance Studies Initiative, a position he has held since retiring from 30+ years as a tenured educator and teacher-trainer for the New York City Department of Education. He is also active with the International Fellowship of Reconciliation (IFOR) and the War Resisters' International (WRI), serving as Chair of IFOR's Financial Advisory Committee and Africa Support Network Coordinator for WRI. Meyer is author or editor of over a dozen books and one hundred chapters and articles, including CSP's *Connecting Contemporary African-Asian Peacemaking: From Satyagraha to Ujamma (2017)*, coedited with Vidya Jain; and PM Press' *White Lives Matter Most and other "little" white lies (2018)*. His first book, *Guns and Gandhi in Africa* (2000, coauthored with Bill Sutherland), included a Foreword by South African Nobel Peace laureate Archbishop Desmond Tutu, who wrote that Sutherland and Meyer "have looked beyond the short-term strategies and tactics which too often divide progressive peoples.... They have begun to develop a language which looks at the roots of our humanness."

Jordan M. Pate MS, MCAP, Registered Mental Health Counseling Intern (RMHCI), is the current Mental Health Therapist for Miami-Dade County Teen Court, a diversion program and second-chance initiative. She began her mental health inpatient field experience providing support to her clinical team for intervention strategies and advocating for client needs. While in pursuit of her master's degree, she transitioned into a career working closely with individuals living with substance abuse issues, later obtaining her Masters Certified Addiction Professional certification. Jordan's current focus is working with juveniles to provide restorative and rehabilitative therapeutic services from an Afrikan-centered paradigm and address disparities affecting Black individuals.

Ruban Roberts is CEO and founder of RER Consulting Enterprise LLC, a Training, Professional Development, Evaluation, Strategic Planning, and management services firm. Mr. Roberts enrolled at Barry University in Miami Shores, Florida, earning his Master's Degrees in Social Work and Business Administration. Mr. Roberts also generously contributes his time and resources to numerous governmental and non-profit organizations. He currently serves as the President of the Miami Dade Branch of the NAACP. He is an appointee to the following boards and workgroups: The Census 2020 Task Force appointed by Miami Dade County Board of County Commissioners (2019), Independent Review Board Work Group by Miami-Dade Board of County Commissioners (2016); the Juvenile Justice Statewide Advisory Group by Governor Rick Scott (2016). He also served as a Board member of the Miami Dade Economic Advisory Trust (MDEAT) appointed by the Miami Dade Board of County Commissioners

(2015); the Circuit Eleven Juvenile Justice Board Miami Florida (2003); and was an appointed workgroup member for Eliminating Mental Health Disparities (EMHD) (2005)—an initiative sponsored by the Center for Mental Health Services (CMHS) and the Substance Abuse and Mental Health Services Administration (SAMHSA).

LaTasha Russell received her doctorate in Clinical Psychology in Berkeley, California, 12 years after graduating from Spelman College in Atlanta, Georgia. Today, she is the President of The Association of Black Psychologists, South Florida Chapter. She has provided therapeutic sessions to individuals, groups, families, and couples in Los Angeles, Chicago, Virginia, Washington D.C., Singapore, Japan, and South Florida, where she now resides. She has worked in hospitals, drug, and alcohol rehabilitation facilities, battered women's shelters, lock-down detention centers, and community mental health agencies. At 39 years old, Dr. Tasha has helped to dispel the myths of going to therapy. As seen on *CBS4 Miami*, Dr. Tasha specializes in quickly getting to the core of an issue, which she calls "Drive-by Therapy."

Christian A. I. Schlaerth graduated from the University of Miami with his PhD in sociology in 2014. His dissertation was titled *Community-Based Philosophy and Service-Learning: A Case Study at Barry University*, where he investigated, with the use of qualitative methods, how service-learning is practiced at Barry University from both the perspectives of the faculty and the students. He has also published many articles and chapters about inequality, higher education, community-based philosophy, criminology, and contemporary theory. He served as an adjunct for many years at the University of Miami, Barry University, and Miami-Dade College. He has helped lead the movement to unionize adjuncts, which has colored his analysis of higher education. He often advocates for issues that impact adjunct instructors across the nation. He currently serves as an Assistant Professor of Criminal Justice and Sociology at Waldorf University in Forest City, IA.

Mureen Shaw is board-certified as a family nurse practitioner. She has worked in multiple area hospitals and in medical clinics in the South Florida region in family planning, occupational health, and urgent/walk-in care settings home healthcare. She is a member of the local nursing organization The Jamaican Nurses' Association of Florida, Inc. She has been an active Board member since 2001 and has held key positions as the Chair of the Education Committee (2013–2018). She partners with community humanitarian organizations such as the Kiwanis of Kendal to actively volunteer for international humanitarian mission trips. Dr. Shaw's passion is global population health and serving the needs of impoverished geographical areas. She participates in multiple yearly international medical and academic mission trips to Jamaica, Grenada, and Haiti's rural regions. She has been honored to have been a past recipient of The Greater Miami Chamber Health Care Heroes Finalists.

Michelle Collins-Sibley joined the faculty at the University of Mount Union—then Mount Union College—in 1994; she chairs the Department of Interdisciplinary & Liberal Studies (home to the Africana Studies, Gender Studies, and Peacebuilding and Social Justice Programs). For nearly a decade, she served as one of the lead faculty of the annual NEH Summer Seminar, ROOTS: African Dimensions of the Americas' History and Culture through the Atlantic Slave Trade at the Virginia Foundation for the Humanities in Charlottesville, Virginia. Publications include, " 'Becoming the Bear': A Meditation on Racial Battle Fatigue, Resistance & Grace in Academia," [Martin, ed. *Racial Battle Fatigue: Insights from the Front Lines of Social Justice Advocacy* (Praeger)], and, "If These are Our Values then What is Our Practice: #Black Lives Matter and an American Apocalypse" [Groarke & Welty, *Peace and Justice Studies: Critical Pedagogy* (Routledge)]. She currently serves on the boards of the Peace and Justice Studies Association and the Alliance Area Domestic Violence Shelter, and on the steering committee of the Ashland Center for Nonviolence.

JoHanna Thompson, MPA, is an Executive Management Consultant who earned a Master of Public Administration from New York University, Wagner School of Public Service, and an undergraduate degree in psychology from Columbia University. She prefers to be called J. J's career has been dedicated to creating collaborative spaces across an intersection of networks, fostering relationships, and maintaining a vision to increase the capacity of influencers, community organizations, programs, and campaigns working toward equitable social and transformational justice. J Thompson lends lived experience and expertise as a Social Impact Strategist, Public Administrator, Organizer, Guardian ad Litem, Therapeutic Foster Parent, Temporary Instructor, Interventionist, Restorative Justice Practitioner, facilitator, trainer, and Healer. A self-proclaimed agent of change and persuasion, J's personal commitment and approach to life aligns with community accountability, Structural Reformation, and the belief that *"one day change gonna come."*